INFORMATION SYSTEMS

FOR HEALTHCARE MANAGEMENT

Eighth Edition

INFORMATION SYSTEMS

FOR HEALTHCARE MANAGEMENT
Eighth Edition

GERALD L. GLANDON
DETLEV H. SMALTZ
DONNA J. SLOVENSKY

AUPHA

Health Administration Press, Chicago

Association of University Programs in Health Administration, Arlington, Virginia

Library of Congress Cataloging-in-Publication Data

Glandon, Gerald L.
  Information systems for healthcare management / Gerald L. Glandon, Detlev H. Smaltz, Donna J. Slovensky. — Eighth edition.
      pages cm
  Revision of: Austin and Boxerman's information systems for healthcare management.— 7th ed. / Gerald L. Glandon, Detlev H. Smaltz, Donna J. Slovensky. ©2008.
  Includes bibliographical references.
  ISBN 978-1-56793-599-8 (alk. paper)
1. Health services administration—Computer networks. 2. Health services administration—Data processing. 3. Information storage and retrieval systems—Hospitals. I. Smaltz, Detlev H. (Detlev Herb) II. Slovensky, Donna J. (Donna Jean) III. Title.
  RA971.23.A976 2014
  362.10285—dc23

                          2013014327

Acquisitions editor: Janet Davis; Project manager/editor: Jane Calayag;
Cover designer: Marisa Jackson; Layout: BookComp

Found an error or a typo? We want to know! Please e-mail it to hapbooks@ache.org, and put "Book Error" in the subject line.

For photocopying and copyright information, please contact Copyright Clearance Center at www.copyright.com or at (978) 750–8400.

Health Administration Press
A division of the Foundation of the American
   College of Healthcare Executives
One North Franklin Street, Suite 1700
Chicago, IL 60606–3529
(312) 424–2800

Association of University Programs
   in Health Administration
2000 North 14th Street
Suite 780
Arlington, VA 22201
(703) 894–0940

BRIEF CONTENTS

DETAILED CONTENTS

A TRIBUTE
to Dr. Charles J. Austin and Dr. Stuart B. Boxerman, Previous Authors of *Information Systems for Healthcare Management*

We express our sincere gratitude to distinguished scholars and emeritus professors Dr. Charles Austin and Dr. Stuart Boxerman. Their foundational work on this book established a new standard for training a generation of healthcare decision makers.

In the mid-1970s, when health administration programs started incorporating dedicated information systems courses into their curricula, Dr. Austin recognized the need to teach information system concepts in the context of managing clinical and business processes. At the time, no textbook existed to guide this novel approach, so Dr. Austin partnered with Health Administration Press (HAP) to create one.

Working closely with Daphne M. Grew and John R. Griffith (former director and co-founder, respectively, of HAP), Dr. Austin brought the book from concept to reality when the first edition, *Information Systems for Hospital Administration*, was published in 1979. Beginning with that early work and continuing through this eighth edition, Dr. Austin's vision of educating health administration students to become informed, key decision makers in technology adoption and implementation has been realized among the thousands of health administration graduates now employed by healthcare organizations.

Information Systems for Hospital Administration was a very important contribution to health administration education. However, the dramatic rate of change in the information technology (IT) industry and the proliferation of IT adoption models in healthcare organizations required the original edition to be updated every few years. Through subsequent editions and over the next 30 years, revisions were made to the book to address trends and advancements. Even the titles of each edition were changed slightly to reflect the evolution of IT in healthcare delivery.

The first two editions, titled *Information Systems for Hospital Administration*, were published during the era when hospitals were the primary driving force of the healthcare industry and administrators were the primary decision makers. As the industry grew to adopt a continuum-of-care orientation and encompass a range of other service settings, the title for the third, fourth, and fifth editions was changed to *Information Systems for Health Services Administration;* the content also was expanded for a broader administrative audience. The current title, *Information Systems for Healthcare Management*—one that has been in use since the sixth edition—represents another shift, emphasizing the application of IT in clinical areas and not just for operational or financial purposes.

Dr. Austin's dedication to maintaining the relevancy of this book, along with his partnership with Dr. Boxerman for the fifth and sixth editions as IT and its application in healthcare became more sophisticated and technical, resulted in an enduring educational resource for health administration students and healthcare managers alike. Since its inception, this book has been one of HAP's best sellers, another testament to its value to healthcare leaders. Most important, the book has influenced the increased use and improved understanding of information systems in healthcare organizations.

Although the eighth edition does not carry Dr. Austin's or Dr. Boxerman's name, it is the proud legacy of the commitment they each made in the prior editions. We believe, as they did, that health administrators must understand IT to exploit it as a managerial and clinical tool in a complex, rapidly changing healthcare environment. We appreciate this opportunity to continue their work, to keep this educational resource available to the next generation of healthcare leaders, and to teach how healthcare management can be improved by the intelligent use of information.

Gerald L. Glandon, PhD
Detlev H. (Herb) Smaltz, PhD
Donna J. Slovensky, PhD

PREFACE

The challenges of healthcare quality, cost, and access have been with us for more than half a century. Despite the rapid changes in information technology and its application to healthcare problems—and despite healthcare leaders' continuing struggle to come up with economic, political, and technological solutions—the problems persist even today.

With every "fix," we create additional challenges. Developments such as the electronic health record (EHR) as a repository for digital health information and the enhanced ability of providers, payers, and patients to share that information among themselves have appeared as solutions. Prior to the passage of the American Recovery and Reinvestment Act (ARRA) of 2009, which provides significant incentives for both hospitals and physicians to adopt EHRs, movement toward those solutions had been slow and challenges related to data privacy and security made some organizations reluctant to implement those solutions. In this era of the Patient Protection and Affordable Care Act (ACA), we are forced again to reexamine and update the use of information technology to support operational, management, and clinical decision making.

The study of healthcare information technology should no longer be delegated to a small subsection of the health administration curriculum. It has become central to all that a healthcare practitioner does and a healthcare management instructor teaches. The chief information officer (CIO) now is part of the executive staff of many healthcare delivery organizations. Fortunately for those in the field, new information technologies have raced far ahead of their utilization in healthcare. Such technologies present the CIO and the rest of the leadership team with challenges related to understanding their potential applications and implications, strategically planning their selection and implementation, ensuring that users receive sufficient training on their proper use, and finding a way to pay for them.

This eighth edition of *Information Systems for Healthcare Management* provides a comprehensive overview of healthcare information technology (HIT), including the effects of the external environment and government policies on its evolution; the expanded role of the CIO; the basics of hardware, software, and communication systems; the types of operational, management, and clinical applications; and the value HIT brings to the enterprise. The concepts included in the book reflect our broad vision of HIT management as a combination of technology, information, and manpower leadership.

The book is intended for current healthcare management students as well as practicing healthcare executives and managers. Although many of these readers may not fill a CIO role or be in charge of information systems, they will benefit from having a basic understanding of this expanding element of healthcare delivery. The book is suitable for a one-semester graduate or advanced undergraduate course in health information systems. It is also an extensive reference for healthcare managers and others involved in selecting and implementing HIT systems. Links to Internet sources are included to provide additional information on the major topics covered in each chapter.

All chapters have been updated to reflect mandates of the ACA and other new federal laws as well as to discuss the current (and potential future) challenges that HIT leadership and users face. Also new in this edition are current examples, an updated glossary, and a list of abbreviations. The three sections in this edition address those changes:

- Part I: HIT Strategic Alignment. The five chapters in this section reflect our view that successfully managing HIT today requires leaders who understand the influence of the external environment, including government interventions and policies. The same can be said about internal HIT activities and strategies. More than ever, achieving an alignment between the HIT strategic plan and the organizational strategic plan is critical. These chapters include a discussion of the implications of the ACA and ARRA, two laws that did not exist when the previous editions were published.
- Part II: Operational Effectiveness. The five chapters in this section center on the crucial elements that enable HIT to operate effectively and efficiently. New to this part is a chapter called "Systems Selection and Contract Management," a function of HIT management that is growing in importance.
- Part III: Strategic Competitive Advantage. To better organize the content, we moved the HIT project portfolio management chapter to this section.

Instructor resources—including a test bank, PowerPoints, answers or discussion points for the in-book Discussion Questions, and a case study—are available to professors who adopt this textbook. Please e-mail hapbooks@ache.org for more information.

ACKNOWLEDGMENTS

Developing a text of this scope requires the input and support of a host of individuals. This work, begun by Charles Austin many years ago, continues to be salient today. We owe Dr. Austin and his coauthor Dr. Stuart Boxerman, as well as the contributors to this book over the years, a substantial debt for starting the conversation about information systems in healthcare. We have a profound respect for the previous editions and the breadth of information included therein.

Dr. Glandon also thanks JaNean Whitlow, who spent endless hours gathering background information from the web and maintaining our massive list of references. Lorrinda Khan added great value to the design and structure of the text with her impressive editorial skills, and Angela Grace provided high-quality secretarial support.

Dr. Smaltz also extends his thanks to his entire team at the Ohio State University Wexner Medical Center (OSUWMC) for their dedication to continuously improving the practice of HIT management. In particular, Ben Walters and Ron Kibbe provided excellent counsel on information technology service management. Additionally, Phil Skinner, Benita Gilliard, Kevin Jones, and Jyoti Kamal of OSUWMC as well as Randy Carpenter of Health-South all provided sample exhibits and/or invaluable insight. Thank you to Paul Murphy of Encore Health Resources for his input into the section on the system selection process.

The responsibility for the remaining errors or oversights in this eighth edition lies entirely with us.

I

HIT STRATEGIC ALIGNMENT

CONNECTING THE STRATEGIC DOTS: DOES HIT MATTER?

Learning Objectives

1. List and define five major challenges facing healthcare delivery systems today.
2. Describe the complexity of these interrelated challenges for healthcare and healthcare information technology.
3. Illustrate the history, development, and current state of healthcare information systems.
4. Name and describe the four categories of healthcare information systems.
5. Analyze the key priorities of healthcare information systems today that will affect their future.

Healthcare Information Technology: The Future Is Now

Healthcare delivery continues to be an information-intensive set of processes. A series of Institute of Medicine (IOM 1999, 2001) studies suggests that high-quality patient care relies on careful documentation of each patient's medical history, health status, current medical conditions, and treatment plans. Financial information is essential for strategic planning and efficient operational support of the patient care process. Management of healthcare organizations requires reliable, accurate, current, secure, and relevant clinical and administrative information. A strong argument can be made that the healthcare field is one of the most information-intensive sectors of the US economy.

Information technology has advanced to a high level of sophistication. However, technology can only provide tools to aid in the accomplishment of a wider set of organizational goals. Analysis of information requirements in the broader organizational context should always take precedence over a rush to computerize. Information technology by itself is not the answer to management problems; technology must be part of a broader restructuring of the organization, including reengineering of business processes. Alignment of information technology strategy with management goals of the healthcare organization is essential. Despite these cautions, effective design, implementation, and management of healthcare information technology (HIT) show great promise (De Angelo 2000; Glaser and Garets 2005; Kaushal, Barker, and Bates 2001; Smaltz et al. 2005a).

An essential element in a successful information systems implementation is carefully planned teamwork by clinicians, managers, and technical systems specialists. Information systems developed in isolation by technicians may be technically pure and elegant in design, but rarely will they pass the test of reality in meeting organizational requirements. On the other hand, very few managers and clinicians possess the equally important technical knowledge and skills of systems analysis and design, and the amateur analyst cannot hope to avoid the havoc that can result from a poorly designed system. A balanced effort is required: Operational personnel contribute ideas on system requirements and organizational realities, and technical personnel employ their skills in analysis and design.

This chapter sets the stage for what is discussed throughout the rest of the book. It begins with a brief overview of the current healthcare environment as a driver of healthcare information technology (HIT) and then presents the future trends in healthcare related to HIT. Next is a brief history of healthcare information systems and the state of healthcare priorities today. The last part of the chapter presents a framework of information systems categories.

The Current Challenges in the Healthcare Environment

While nothing is more dangerous than predicting the future, Goldsmith (1980) looked into the future of healthcare in the late 1980s. He foresaw a vastly different landscape for the delivery of care than existed at the time. He documented a number of demographic, secular, and organizational changes that would shape that future. Such changes included the growing elderly population, the decline of the hospital as the center of the healthcare delivery universe, the oversupply of physicians, the expanded role of government in financing healthcare, the shift of financial risk from payers to providers, the expansion of health maintenance organizations (HMOs) in various forms, and problems related to the uninsured. He observed that to address issues such as continuity, linkage, coordination, and accountability, changes in the organization of the healthcare delivery system would be required. One can question the accuracy of specific predictions made in Goldsmith's forecast, but most cannot deny that he was correct in the change in focus. Looking back, it is clear that these issues require added emphasis on improving the management of both healthcare information and its technology.

The complexity and challenges in healthcare delivery are many. To give a sense of this, consider that delivery systems today must provide high quality, timely care that attains full transparency regarding costs and quality; be mindful of growing privacy and security concerns of patients; utilize idiosyncratic, personalized medicine as appropriate; adhere to best-practice evidence; and adopt care coordination across settings and time (Wanless and Ludwig 2011). On top of this, with the accountable care organization model becoming supported through healthcare reform, delivery organizations may have more financial incentive to effectively implement disease prevention and wellness (CMS 2012a).

Consequently, we define five factors driving the current changes in the healthcare system: (1) healthcare costs, (2) medical errors and poor quality of care, (3) access and health disparities, (4) evidence-based medicine, and (5) broad organizational change.

Healthcare Costs

Healthcare costs continue to spiral upward continuing a trend of the last 45 years; this is examined in more detail in Chapter 2 in our discussion of the healthcare triangle. The concern about persistent cost increases, and more important the value of dollars spent on healthcare services, appears to drive changes. A common belief is that high healthcare costs make the US economy less competitive and have different effects on different segments of the national economy. These contentions can be debated, and few have clear strategies to control costs, but we have seen and will likely continue to see cost control being implemented by government, by private payers, and even by consumers.

The evidence that we can control costs has been made more apparent by some recent popular analyses that examine differences in the utilization of services and costs across communities in the United States. Gawande (2009), for example, demonstrates a nearly twofold difference in healthcare expenditures for the Medicare population in communities that are otherwise similar in demographics and objective need for services. If these differences exist broadly, then some of the cost of healthcare may reflect practice patterns or other factors that we cannot justify. It is clear that better data—aggregated and compared across regions—will enable us to investigate the differences further. HIT at the organizational level, shared with regional and national entities, will be called on to address these issues.

Medical Errors and Poor Quality of Care

According to the IOM's 1999 landmark report, *To Err Is Human*, medical errors are a leading cause of adverse health consequences in hospitals. The report estimated that at least 44,000 and as many as 98,000 individuals die in hospitals per year as a result of preventable medical errors. Errors also resulted in greater direct and indirect costs borne by society as a whole. The report stated that "the total national cost associated with adverse effects [of medical errors] was approximately 4 percent of national health expenditures in 1996" (IOM 1999, 41). Further, in 2001 the IOM issued a blueprint, titled *Crossing the Quality Chasm,* designed to help organizations fix the delivery system.

More than ten years after the publications of the IOM reports, unnecessary deaths from medical errors (preventable and otherwise) and poor quality of care are still occurring at a high rate (Sternberg 2012). Estimation of the number of errors are difficult because no centralized reporting mechanism exists (Doheny 2009). We have seen the costs of poor quality and excessive medical errors, but the solutions to this complex problem are elusive.

Access and Health Disparities

The myriad problems arising from the failure of the US healthcare system to provide reasonable access to care have been well documented (Families USA 2012). While better information systems and exchange of information can address these challenges, they cannot directly solve all of them. Dealing with the uninsured will put a greater strain on the collection and reporting of clinical and administrative data at the organizational and system levels. The number of those uninsured is so large that the entire healthcare delivery system will be challenged as we implement policies to expand coverage. Data suggested that in 2010 just short of 50 million people were uninsured in the United States (DeNavas-Walt, Proctor, and Smith 2011). This estimate represented slightly more than 16 percent of the population and had been increasing since about 1980. However, according to recently released data, the number of uninsured dropped to 48.6 million (see Exhibit 1.1), representing 15.7 percent of the population, in 2011 (DeNavas-Walt, Proctor, and Smith 2012). This is a movement in the right direction, but the magnitude of the uninsured is still a current managerial challenge.

Evidence-Based Medicine

Evidence-based medicine grew in the late 1990s (Clancy and Eisenberg 1998) and has become mainstream, as indicated by the publication of at least one online evidence-based medicine journal (e.g., *Evidence-Based Medicine for Primary Care and Internal Medicine* launched in 1995). Landry and Sibbald (2001) define *evidence-based medicine* (EBM) as "an information management and learning strategy that seeks to integrate clinical expertise with the best evidence available to make effective clinical decisions that will ultimately improve patient care." It is a systematic approach to diagnosis

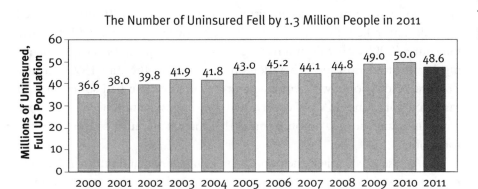

EXHIBIT 1.1
The Number of
Uninsured, 2011

The Number of Uninsured Fell by 1.3 Million People in 2011

SOURCE: Reprinted from US Census Bureau (2012).

and treatment that encourages the physician to formulate questions and seek answers from the best available published evidence. EBM has gained momentum as an important mechanism for improving healthcare delivery. Some even suggested that EBM could become the new paradigm for organizations to follow in providing care; in fact, Moskowitz and Bodenheimer (2011) recently proposed the concept of "evidence-based health," which requires the involvement of patients and their community, to expand the EBM model. To successfully incorporate EBM into healthcare, participants in healthcare organizations (i.e., physicians, patients, managers) must agree to follow the evidence wherever it applies (Ellwood 2003). For balance, widespread implementation of EBM may have bumps. Some have begun to caution that the transition to "evidence" given the proliferation of information on the Internet may apply pressure on providers (Diamond and Kaul 2008).

The focus of this book lies between two extreme views of the managerial world. The creation, storage, and retrieval of evidence for health management decision making necessarily involve HIT. The use of HIT, however, is associated with both costs and benefits. These costs and benefits need to be assessed, and healthcare managers need to develop their skills in using internal health information intelligently and entering into health information exchanges to support their organization's strategic and operational goals (Johnston, Pan, and Middleton 2002; Sidorov 2006; Williams et al. 2012).

Broad Organizational Change

Healthcare markets continue to change as they face ongoing efforts to manage costs, quality, and access. As these markets—and the major delivery organizations in the markets—adapt, HIT will be required to accommodate these changing needs accordingly. Market-driven healthcare reform and efforts to increase market competition, initiated in the 1990s, have evolved but still cannot be fully judged as to their effectiveness. Wilensky (2006) and Ginsburg (2005) provide interesting historical perspectives on the changing healthcare landscape. They demonstrate that in the mid-1990s, nearly 75 percent of people with employment-based insurance had some form of managed care, and HMOs constituted the largest component. Insurance companies and hospitals poured into this market because of the potential for profits.

As discussed earlier, the population of uninsured and underinsured US residents is still high, and disease prevention remains an elusive goal in most health plans today. This pressure will not subside in our opinion. Creating an organization and having the leadership in place to assist in meeting these and other challenges are essential. As we address in Chapter 4, the chief information officer (CIO) role will become even more essential in the future.

Future Challenges for Healthcare Information Systems

The factors that drive healthcare change today—costs, quality, access, evidence-based management, and organizational change—will not disappear in the foreseeable future because we have not solved the challenges associated with them. They also represent our future challenges. Look a little further out and see some other forces likely to alter the delivery of care. We have observed how technology has transformed banking, communications, retailing, and other industries. It seems, however, that healthcare and education are yet to fully absorb technology's ability to alter their respective landscape. We have identified five broad forces that will drive future change and potentially have profound impacts on information technology systems in and across organizations: (1) healthcare system change, (2) consumer empowerment, (3) connectivity, (4) transparency, and (5) tourism.

Healthcare System Change
The fundamental shift in thinking, partially expressed in the Patient Protection and Affordable Care Act of 2010 (discussed in Chapter 3), was largely overshadowed by the immediate emphasis on providing access to care for the uninsured population in the United States. Within that massive legislation were the seeds of experiments designed to identify other ways of operating the healthcare delivery system. Elements such as bundled payments, payment for outcomes, accountable care organizations, patient-centered medical

homes, and comparative effectiveness research all challenge the conventional fee-for-service payment and focus on the care of an individual patient. These changes will alter the sources of data that information management professionals will be required to identify, collect, store, analyze, and report. All of the challenges we face today will expand with the addition of sources of information and legitimate users of information outside of the normal organizational boundaries.

In the coming years, payment will be more oriented toward the outcomes generated and will cover the costs of a full range of services necessary to treat the patient. Already we are bundling Medicare payments for surgery and postsurgical care. Even broader ranges of clinical services—from presurgical assessments and testing to postsurgical clinical management and rehabilitation—are likely to be paid to a single provider. This expanded episode-of-illness system will fundamentally enlarge the sources of vital data that an organization must process. Because these data cross organizational lines, the episode-of-illness systems complicate how the data are linked and aggregated for reporting purposes. Starting in 2012, hospitals are penalized for excessive 30-day readmission rates, so leadership is demanding more information and intervention to make sure that patients are ready to be discharged and that essential follow-up care is provided.

Similarly, our responsibility for providing reasonable cost, high quality, and good access will shift from individual patients to populations. Monitoring and designing interventions to keep people healthy before they show up at the healthcare provider's door require a different type of thinking about data needs. For example, how do providers capture and assist the patient with uncontrolled diabetes living in the community but not yet showing up with out-of-control blood sugar?

Finally, as the government gets more directly involved in changing the system, it will fund research aimed at identification of positive changes. IOM (2009) identified the top 100 funding priorities as a means of guiding government research support. Brief descriptions of the ten priorities from the top quartile are as follows (IOM 2009, 107):

1. Compare the effectiveness of treatment strategies for atrial fibrillation, including surgery, catheter ablation, and pharmacologic treatment.
2. Compare the effectiveness of the different treatments (e.g., assistive listening devices, cochlear implants, electric-acoustic devices, habilitation and rehabilitation methods) for hearing loss in children and adults, especially individuals with diverse cultural, language, medical, and developmental backgrounds.

3. Compare the effectiveness of primary prevention methods, such as exercise and balance training, versus clinical treatments in preventing falls in older adults.

4. Compare the effectiveness of upper endoscopy utilization and frequency for patients with gastroesophageal reflux disease on morbidity, quality of life, and diagnosis of esophageal adenocarcinoma.

5. Compare the effectiveness of dissemination and translation techniques to facilitate the use of comparative effectiveness research by patients, clinicians, payers, and others.

6. Compare the effectiveness of comprehensive care coordination programs, such as the medical home, and usual care in managing children and adults with severe chronic disease.

7. Compare the effectiveness of different strategies of introducing biologics into the treatment algorithm for inflammatory diseases, including Crohn's disease, ulcerative colitis, rheumatoid arthritis, and psoriatic arthritis.

8. Compare the effectiveness of various screening, prophylaxis, and treatment interventions in eradicating methicillin resistant Staphylococcus aureus (MRSA) in communities, institutions, and hospitals.

9. Compare the effectiveness of strategies (e.g., bio-patches, reducing central line entry, chlorhexidine for all line entries, antibiotic impregnated catheters, treating all line entries via a sterile field) for reducing healthcare-associated infections (HAI), including catheter-associated bloodstream infection, ventilator-associated pneumonia, and surgical-site infections in children and adults.

10. Compare the effectiveness of management strategies for localized prostate cancer (e.g., active surveillance, radical prostatectomy [conventional, robotic, and laparoscopic], and radiotherapy [conformal, brachytherapy, proton-beam, and intensity-modulated radiotherapy]) on survival, recurrence, side effects, quality of life, and costs.

Clearly, these are comprehensive assessments that will strain even the best data collection, reporting, and analysis systems for healthcare.

Consumer Empowerment

Related in some ways to the reform of the delivery system is that consumers have become increasingly sophisticated in their selection and use of healthcare services. Empowered by the Internet, consumers are seeking medical information and joining together in support groups as they interact with physicians and other healthcare providers. Goldsmith stated that "the patient is in charge of the process. . . . The Internet has enabled patients to aggregate their collective experiences across disease entities" (Reece 2000).

Although providers express legitimate concerns about misusing and misunderstanding information obtained from the Internet, they realize that the trend of Internet use by healthcare consumers is clear and irreversible. Oravec (2001) suggested that the healthcare system should help develop approaches to empower consumers to use the Internet effectively as one part of a total healthcare strategy, rather than simply warn them about the potential hazards of using inaccurate or misunderstood medical or healthcare information. Further, Ellwood (2003) outlined a comprehensive set of recommendations that arose from a health reform meeting held in Jackson Hole, Wyoming, in 2002. The Jackson Hole Group looked to Congress to set up a "uniform, national information infrastructure and a process for its further development and implementation" (Ellwood 2003). The proposal called for four infrastructure-related developments, which include electronic health records; evidence-based clinical practices; public disclosure, analysis, and feedback of quality performance information; and genuine patient power and responsibility.

Evidence shows that the consumer empowerment/involvement movement is growing and is highly integrated with the need for information management in healthcare. For a comprehensive overview of the history of social networking and social media not applied to healthcare per se, see Boyd and Ellison (2007). PricewaterhouseCoopers Health Research Institute (2012) has published results of a consumer participation survey related to healthcare. The findings reveal that age matters in who trusts and shares information (younger patients are more likely to trust and share). However, young people in poor health are also more likely to engage in health-related social media. Consumers in general are likely to share through social media any (positive and negative) information on the care received, on experiences with medication/treatment, and on specific physician or provider. Interestingly, a posting on social media raises the expectations for responses to consumers' request for appointment, information, and complaint. Consumers appear willing to seek a second opinion and choose a hospital/facility, physician, or health plan on the basis of the information they found on social media. All of this suggests that consumer preferences and managing the information of consumers will be vital to provider survival and raise the demand on HIT professionals to help address these needs. The concerns of rising consumer populism as opposed to consumer empowerment have already been raised as systems struggle to meet rising consumer expectations (Simborg 2010).

Connectivity

Related to the rise of the consumers and their connectivity is how providers and payers will change the healthcare delivery system and HIT needs as a result. Social media needs a series of hosts for transmitting connected

information. Not long ago, people relied heavily on the phone to communicate, but that technology is being supplanted by e-mail, text, tweet, and
other mechanisms. This change is central for consumers, especially younger
consumers, and is certainly worthy of significant study. As a brief overview,
each year many bloggers post the top new technologies related to consumer
connectivity and technology. For example, Swayze (2011) indicated the following nine trends, many of which occurred by 2012: "(1) Android invasion,
(2) tablets galore, (3) Internet TV, (4) faster phones, (5) 3-D, (6) watching
TV on the go, (7) cameras you can afford, (8) faster laptops with better
graphics, and (9) techie cars."

The push toward connectivity has begun to permeate the health provider system as well. A good gauge of how this connectivity will proceed can
be seen in a report from the Federal Communications Commission (2012).
The Federal Communications Commission chair asked industry leaders to
evaluate the "opportunities and challenges" arising from the widespread
adoption of wireless health technologies. The result was the formation of the
mHealth Task Force, which examined how patient care can be improved and
made more efficient by the use of mobile health, wireless health, and e-Care
technologies. The task force aims to make these technologies best practices
by 2017; to this end, it identifies five broad goals (FCC 2012, 1):

Goal 1: FCC should continue to play a leadership role in advancing mobile health
adoption.

Goal 2: Federal agencies should increase collaboration to promote innovation, protect
patient safety, and avoid regulatory duplication.

Goal 3: The FCC should build on existing programs and link programs when possible in
order to expand broadband access for healthcare.

Goal 4: The FCC should continue efforts to increase capacity, reliability, interoperability,
and RF safety of mHealth technologies.

Goal 5: Industry should support continued investment, innovation, and job creation in
the growing mobile health sector.

The scope was broad in that the task force examined nine aspects of mobile
technology (mHealth), as seen in Exhibit 1.2.

The types of challenges in adopting this technology are the subject
of study for government and private specialists. For example, the National
Institute of Standards and Technology (2010) has been convening a number
of integrative forums to address such innovations as cloud computing. These
often have strong proponents but also focus on the challenges that new technology presents to cybersecurity.

EXHIBIT 1.2
Nine Aspects of
mHealth Activi-
ties Evaluated
by FCC mHealth
Task Force

- Medical devices that act as remote patient monitors used in clinical, home, mobile, and other environments
- Mobile medical and general health software applications that allow patients to upload or download health information at any time
- Medical body area network sensors that capture and wirelessly forward physiological data for further analysis
- Medical implant devices that allow neuromuscular microsimulation techniques to restore sensation, mobility, and other functions to paralyzed limbs and organs
- Medical device data systems that allow for the transfer, storage, conversion, or display of medical data through wired or wireless hubs, smart phones, or broadband-enabled products
- Mobile diagnostic imaging applications that allow doctors the flexibility to send or review medical images from virtually any place and at any time
- Patient care portals that can be accessed anywhere for self-reporting and self-management
- Accessible clinical decision support tools that allow doctors to help patients in real time with diagnosis, treatment options, and necessary medical calculations at the point of care
- Broadband-enabled HIT infrastructure that allows healthcare providers to share rich electronic health information with other providers, regardless of their provider organization and geographic area

SOURCE: Data from Federal Communications Commission (2012).

Transparency

The movement to greater transparency has been around for some time (Collins and Davis 2006), but it got a big national push with the federal government's Value-Driven Health Care initiative. An Executive Order signed by President George W. Bush (2006) established value-driven care consisting of four cornerstones: (1) interoperable HIT, (2) public reporting of provider quality information, (3) public reporting of cost information, and (4) incentives for value comparisons. This government support added to the growing evidence that the system could improve in a number of ways if consumers, providers, and payers had better information on which to base their decisions. Early efforts in this regard concentrated on price transparency (Deloitte Center for Health Solutions 2007), but a Commonwealth Fund report suggested that price transparency was not in itself an answer to cost problems but could enable the development of the following (Collins and Davis 2006):

- Valid benchmarks of provider performance
- Quality and efficiency reward programs by payers
- Informed choices by patients

The report pointed out, however, that without transparency in outcomes and information on the "total cost" of care, price transparency could not enable consumers to make better choices. As discussed earlier, some broader changes are coming in the future. In any case, increasing transparency puts added pressure on healthcare's data systems to report more data and ensure all information is accurate and timely.

Tourism

Medical tourism is an important element of the future that will affect HIT. The prospect of US healthcare organizations losing patients to providers in third-world countries on the basis of price for select procedures or therapies could pose a major challenge. In addition to system effects, the information technology world would be made more complicated because these patients would want information about their medical history, tests, and prior procedures to be sent overseas. In addition, when the patients come back home, their surgical case information would have to be returned and then integrated into existing records of any follow-up care. There are many reasons, however, that traditional international medical tourism may not make as big an impact as first thought. The inability of average patients to afford long-distance travel to seek care for most clinical problems puts a limit on medical tourism's scale and scope. Further, despite quality assertions and some review by Joint Commission International, the lingering hesitancy by many people to try this trend may keep this at bay for years to come.

However, if the notion of medical tourism were expanded to include regional or cross-border travel within the United States as opposed to seeking only international providers, the issue takes on a whole new level of importance. Reports are still incomplete and the evaluation scale is not clear, but in 2012 Wal-Mart joined a number of large US employers that are contracting with select national delivery systems (known as centers of excellence) to provide specialty services to employees and their dependents (Diamond 2012). Lowe's and Boeing are also mentioned in this context, contracting with healthcare organizations with a national name recognition, such as Cleveland Clinic, Geisinger Medical Center, Scott & White Memorial Hospital, Virginia Mason Medical Center, and Mercy Hospital Springfield. The services include spine care, transplants, and heart procedures (Elliott 2012; Zeltner 2012).

Historical Overview of Healthcare Information Systems

The evolution of HIT will fill a text by itself, but a brief overview will help you understand where the system began and where it is likely heading. Many fine, classic summaries (e.g., Collen 1995) can help in this process along with newly developed tutorials that effectively tell the history of healthcare information systems in the United States (e.g., National Training and Dissemination Center 2012). Exhibit 1.3 presents a list of the specific section of the Health IT Workforce Curriculum Components (a tutorial) that discusses the comprehensive history of HIT. It enables interested readers to absorb a broad perspective. Especially important to note in these historical presentations is how the medical education community and professional organizations grew and supported the infusion of HIT into the research and practice communities. For complete information on this and other courses, visit www.onc-ntdc.org.

The first computer systems in healthcare date back to the early 1960s, when a small number of hospitals began to automate selected administrative operations, usually beginning with payroll and patient accounting functions. These systems were developed by analysts and computer programmers hired by the hospitals, and they were run on large, expensive, and centralized computers referred to as "mainframes" (see Exhibit 1.4). Little attention was given to the development of clinical information systems to support patient care, and the paper medical record was the legal and clinical record of the treatment experience. The growth of medicine as a science that could benefit from systematic collection and analysis of information spurred analysts to expand computer applications to clinical medicine.

EXHIBIT 1.3
Detail of HIT Curriculum Component 5

Component 5: History of Health Information Technology in the U.S.

Unit 1.   Evolution of Health IT: The Early Years
Unit 2.   Evolution of Health IT: The Modern Era
Unit 3.   Evolution of Health IT: The HITECH Act
Unit 4.   Evolution of Public Health Informatics
Unit 5.   Evolution of Nursing Informatics and HIT Tools Used by Nursing
Unit 6.   History of Electronic Health Records (EHRs)
Unit 7.   History of Clinical Decision Support Systems
Unit 8.   History of CPOE and E-Prescribing
Unit 9.   History of Health Information Exchange
Unit 10.   History of Privacy and Security Legislation
Unit 11.   Software Certification and Regulation
Unit 12.   History of Mobile Computing
Unit 13.   History of Telemedicine
Unit 14.   History of Quality Improvement and Patient Safety
Unit 15.   Payment-Related Issues and the Role of HIT
Unit 16.   History of Health IT Organizations

SOURCE: Reprinted from National Training and Dissemination Center (2012).

EXHIBIT 1.4
Mainframe
Computer

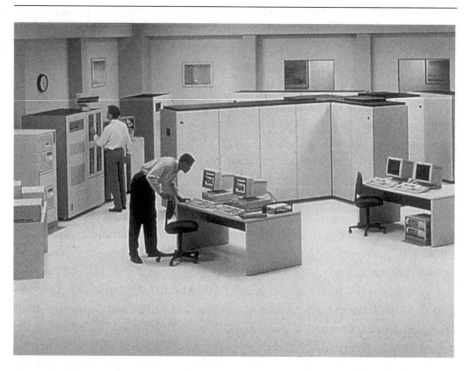

SOURCE: Courtesy of International Business Machines Corporation. Unauthorized use not permitted.

The medical record was still a relatively new concept, and standards for the paper version were established and widely adopted only in the 1960s. A few systems were developed for the electronic storage and retrieval of abstracts of inpatient medical records, but these systems contained limited information and were operated on a postdischarge, retrospective basis. The early "computer-based medical record" systems, such as COSTAR and RMRS, were attempts to capture the patients' experience in an easily retrievable manner.

Advances in technology during the 1970s expanded the use of information systems throughout all industries, and hospitals were no exception. These systems eventually became part of other healthcare settings such as clinics, physician office practices, and long-term-care facilities. Computers became smaller and less expensive, and some vendors began to develop "applications software packages"—generalized computer programs that could be used by any hospital, clinic, or physician's office that purchased the system. Most of these early software packages supported administrative operations, such as patient accounting, general accounting, materials management, scheduling, and practice management. Eventually, clinical systems were developed as well, particularly for hospital clinical laboratories, radiology departments, and pharmacies (for a description of current applications, see chapters 9 and 10).

As the scientific knowledge base of medicine expanded during this period with funding from the federal government, effectively diagnosing and developing treatment for patients began to tax the capacity of providers. Clinical decision support systems, such as MYCIN and HELP, were introduced to assist providers to apply the rules for diagnosis and treatment. While computers helped with retrieval of information, providers found that specialization became essential. Consequently, the collection, storage, analysis, and reporting of the expanding body of healthcare information required professional specialization of the HIT community as well. Organizations for medical records professionals (e.g., American Medical Records Association, which later became American Health Information Management Association), informaticists and researchers (e.g., American Medical Informatics Association), and HIT practitioners (e.g., Hospital Management Systems Society, which later became Healthcare Information Management Systems Society) supported the professionalization and specialization of the HIT workforce.

A virtual revolution in computing occurred in the 1980s with the development of powerful and inexpensive personal computers (PCs)—desktop devices with computing power and storage capacity that equaled or exceeded the large mainframe systems of the 1960s and 1970s. A second major advance in this period was the development of electronic data networks, whereby PCs and larger computing systems could be linked together to share information on a decentralized basis. An increasing number of vendors entered the healthcare software business, and a much larger array of products became available for both administrative and clinical support functions. The use of PCs in physicians' offices, particularly for practice management, became commonplace. This ad hoc proliferation of systems and applications to meet specific clinical and administrative needs contributed to the system-integration challenges providers face today.

The 1990s witnessed even more dramatic changes in the healthcare environment with the advent of market-driven healthcare reform and expansion of managed care. Much greater attention was given to the development of clinical information systems and strategic decision support systems to assist providers in achieving a critical balance between costs and quality in the delivery of care. These changes were supported by advances in technology, through the use of laptop computers and, today, notebook computers or the iPad. This portable hardware expanded the ability of clinicians and other caregivers to take the data-collection tool with them, access information from virtually anywhere, and communicate with others in the care team quickly.

At the same time, electronic data interchange and networking were used to link components of integrated healthcare delivery organizations and support enterprisewide information systems. As a result, healthcare organizations now employ Internet technology to support internal communications and external connections with patients and business partners. Similarly, telemedicine applications can link primary care providers at remote locations with clinical specialists at centralized medical centers. These technologies provide potentially better access to high-quality care at reasonable costs.

As an example, the Electronic Health Network (EHN), operated under the direction of Dr. Glenn Hammack at the University of Texas Medical Branch (UTMB) at Galveston, uses cutting-edge video, digital, audio, and telecommunications technology to deliver care (Blanchet 2005). While this major commitment to telemedicine has many components, the major activity is EHN's Correctional Managed Care Program, which has provided "prison health" to individuals incarcerated in Texas prisons since 1993. Today, the program is a full risk-capitated delivery system. In 2004, it had $330 million in revenue, covered 166,000 lives, and employed 3,700 workers. Texas is a large state geographically, and the technology enables UTMB to effectively connect clinical care in more than 100 locations for the Texas Department of Criminal Justice, Texas Youth Commission, Dallas County Jails, and Federal Board of Prisons in Beaumont.

The electronic medical record (EMR) used in the EHN is its key component. The EMR is a security encrypted, full-time web-enabled record that gives the physician access to medical records regardless of patient location. It contains a pharmacy system for identifying drug interactions, and clinical laboratory and radiology services can input data and images directly into the system. UTMB finds that the expanded capacity to reliably, remotely deliver quality care for less cost makes sense for the organization.

While hardware and software continued to emerge and to be implemented widely, many began to realize that information systems were being developed in partial isolation. The ability of products to seamlessly connect and transfer information was being impeded by the lack of rigorously defined standards. Consequently, many in the industry began to call for industry and, ultimately, government standards. Some of the standard-setting organizations today include the following:

- International Organization for Standardization (ISO) (www.iso.ch)
- American National Standards Institute (ANSI) (www.ansi.org)
- Health Level 7 or (HL7) (www.hl7.org)
- Healthcare Information Technology Standards Panel (HITSP) (www.hitsp.org)

- Current Procedural Terminology (specifically CPT-4) of the American Medical Association (www.ama-assn.org)
- Health IT Standards Committee (www.healthit.gov)

As addressed in Chapter 3, government got heavily involved in the setting of standards after 2000. For an outstanding review and history of HIT standards, see Amatayakul (2007).

Categories of Healthcare Information Systems

Computerized information systems in healthcare fall into four categories: (1) clinical information, (2) operational management, (3) strategic decision support, and (4) electronic networking and e-health applications.

Clinical information systems support patient care and provide information for use in strategic planning and management. Examples include computerized patient records systems; clinical department systems for pharmacy, laboratory, radiology, and other units; automated medical instrumentation; clinical decision support systems (computer-aided diagnosis and treatment planning); and information systems that support clinical research and education.

Operational management systems support non–patient-care activities in the healthcare organization. Examples include financial information systems, payroll, purchasing and inventory control, outpatient clinic scheduling, and office automation.

Strategic decision support systems assist the senior management team in strategic planning, managerial control, performance monitoring, and outcomes assessment. Strategic information systems must draw data from internal clinical and management systems as well as from external information on community health, market-area demography, and activities of competitors. Consequently, information system integration—the ability of organizational information systems to communicate electronically with one another—becomes very important.

Healthcare organizations also engage in *electronic networking*, which supports data interchange with external organizations and business partners for such activities as insurance billing and claims processing, accessing clinical information from regional and national databases, communicating among providers in an integrated delivery system, and communicating with patients and health plan members. Many of these applications are web-based, *e-health applications*. Computer applications in healthcare organizations are described in detail in chapters 9 and 10 of this book.

Healthcare Information System Priorities Today

Healthcare organizations and their leaders operating in this environment of change must understand the history and evolution of HIT. They also must keep an eye on how the future will likely unfold if they want long-term success. Most important, however, is that they must provide valid, reliable, and secure clinical and administrative information to assist healthcare leaders in making optimal clinical, operational, and strategic decisions today. To this end, organizations are developing sophisticated information systems to support clinical and administrative operations and strategic management.

This book is designed to meet the needs of a variety of healthcare information professionals as they strive to support their private and/or their organizational missions. As a result, the chapters that follow address both focused, detailed information needs and broader corporate information needs. We hope that this format is useful to those with clinical backgrounds, technical backgrounds, and business backgrounds. Because individuals with these three types of backgrounds must learn to work together to achieve common goals, it is vital for each not only to gain knowledge to support their own domain but also to gain a deeper understanding of other's perspectives.

The book addresses the priorities of today by embedding one priority in each chapter:

- *Chapter 2: External environment.* The strategic direction of any healthcare organization is influenced by the world outside its walls. Gaining a deep understanding of the fundamental forces of change and the ability to observe and anticipate that change is essential to the long-term success of the healthcare information professional. In this chapter, we explore the healthcare triangle of cost, quality, and access because these challenges prompt government and market changes that must be addressed by any organization. We also examine evidence-based medicine and management because this will likely be the mechanism of change in the delivery of healthcare services. Finally, the chapter compares domestic with international systems because the many aspects of the US healthcare world are and will continue to be influenced by developments in other countries.

- *Chapter 3: Government policy and healthcare reform.* The US delivery systems are being buffeted by government regulations and other interventions that affect cost, quality, and access. This chapter examines recent government interventions that change the HIT landscape. Our discussion starts with the appropriate role of government and quickly turns its focus on the healthcare reform legislation—the Patient Protection and Affordable Care Act of 2010. Related challenges and government programs are discussed as well, such as the HITECH Act, meaningful use of information technology, privacy and security, and healthcare information exchanges.

- *Chapter 4: Leadership.* Here, we examine the case of the healthcare chief information officer (CIO). To better manage the healthcare information enterprise, organizations need an appropriate structure. The roles of senior HIT managers are different today from those in the recent past, and thus their place within the organization must change as well. Senior-level HIT managers must become a part of the corporate strategy—both to understand organizational direction and to provide advice on the challenges that direction might impose from the information technology perspective. Similarly, HIT professionals must have a different set of skills to maneuver in the new organizational structure. CIOs must have leadership expertise and analytical/strategic thinking skills as well as be clinically savvy and technologically sound.

- *Chapter 5: HIT governance and decision rights.* To take advantage of the revised organizational structure and CIO leadership skills, HIT units must incorporate appropriate and effective governance structure. These are the necessary how-to components for ensuring that HIT infrastructure and operations reliably accomplish goals. The growing scale and scope of the information technology reach within the delivery system present major challenges to these assurances; thus, the importance of appropriate HIT governance expands accordingly.

- *Chapter 6: HIT architecture and infrastructure.* While leading successful HIT systems does not require an in-depth working knowledge of computer and communication technologies, a basic understanding of the physical and logical structure of information systems and their components is essential. This chapter offers an essential core lesson, clarifying the differences between hardware and software; providing examples of computer network structures; differentiating operating systems, utility programs, and application software; and exploring telecommunication concepts such as wireless technologies.

- *Chapter 7: HIT service management.* Operation of an HIT department has evolved and now consists of managing a complex set of interdependent elements. Unlike the other components of a healthcare delivery organization, all of HIT components must coordinate and communicate effectively, accurately, and securely. Consequently, service delivery and support services are vital to effective functioning. This chapter outlines the challenges of unplanned work and the necessity of implementing a process improvement framework for an organization. It also introduces the concept of an Information Technology Infrastructure Library and its components to assist HIT operations.

- *Chapter 8: Systems selection and contract management.* In the past, delivery organizations on the frontier of HIT development created their own information systems because integrated options from vendors were not available or adequate. Now, organizations purchase complex, integrated, and expensive HIT systems from a vast array of vendors. The selection of these systems constitutes a major financial, clinical, and administrative investment by an organization's leadership. The need to identify system requirements and ensure that vendors deliver those specifications in a timely manner requires a systematic approach to selection and contract management.

- *Chapter 9: Electronic health records.* In previous editions, the application chapter was small and primarily emphasized administrative/financial functions. This edition features two application chapters—Chapter 9 is devoted to the electronic health record (EHR) and Chapter 10 to management/administrative systems. Chapter 9 outlines the importance of EHR to the present and future of healthcare organizations. It discusses key capabilities, organizational benefits, costs of adoption, and methods of adoption/implementation. It follows up on meaningful use in the context of the EHR, the EMR, and the personal health record. In addition, it discusses related concepts such as the computerized physician order entry and constraints such as interoperability.

- *Chapter 10: Management/administrative and financial systems.* This chapter addresses the many conventional uses of HIT to support the overall goal of a delivery organization. The enterprise system applications include resource planning, financial management, scheduling, decision support, and research/medical education.

- *Chapter 11: HIT project portfolio management.* Successful HIT operations require conventional project management expertise. This chapter expands that necessary project management content to include HIT program and portfolio management techniques. The ultimate goal is to reach the synchronized stage of portfolio management. At this level, HIT leadership should regularly evaluate the portfolio with operational unit leaders. The evaluations should include both the risks and returns of the complete HIT portfolio.

- *Chapter 12: Knowledge-enabled organization.* Moving from operational effectiveness to achievement of strategic competitive advantage with HIT involves a transformation into a knowledge-enabled organization. The purpose of applying knowledge management is for it to become an integral part of the organization, thereby ensuring organizational success today and in the future. The chapter places a great emphasis on "baking in" the knowledge into workflows.

- *Chapter 13: HIT value analysis.* A formal, comprehensive valuation of a HIT system's direct and indirect costs will help organizations move to the next level of operational excellence. Too often, HIT decisions are based on partial assessments of both costs and benefits, a strategy that may spell doom in cost-competitive future scenarios. State-of-the-art valuation processes from other industries provide a full social benefit and cost assessment tool that will become part of our collective HIT future.

Summary

The management of healthcare organizations can be improved through the intelligent use of information. This requires systematic planning and management of information resources to develop information systems that support patient care, administrative operations, and strategic management. Change is occurring rapidly and persistently in the healthcare industry. Major forces of change that have a direct impact on the application of information technology include (1) continued pressure for healthcare cost containment, (2) concerns about medical errors and poor quality of care, (3) challenges from limited access to care and health disparities, (4) growth in the use of evidence-based medicine, and (5) need for broad organizational change. The US healthcare system is in the middle of fundamental change, and HIT plays a role in solving all the system's challenges.

As we look to the future, we see these five challenges remaining, so we need to consider the following: (1) healthcare system change, (2) consumer empowerment, (3) connectivity, (4) transparency, and (5) tourism. These, too, pose challenges and opportunities for HIT and healthcare leadership.

Healthcare information systems fall into four categories: (1) clinical information, (2) operational management, (3) strategic decision support, and (4) electronic networking and e-health applications. Clinical information systems support patient care and provide information for strategic planning and management. Operational management systems support non–patient-care activities, such as financial management, human resources management, materials management, scheduling, and office automation. Strategic decision support systems assist managers in planning, marketing, management control of operations, performance evaluation, and outcomes assessment. E-health network applications support electronic data interchange with external organizations and business partners, communication among providers in an integrated delivery system, and communication with patients and health plan members.

These environmental trends have resulted in a reordering of the information system priorities of healthcare organizations. To meet current and future challenges, HIT leadership needs a comprehensive view of healthcare information by considering external strategic alignment, internal strategic alignment, operational effectiveness, and achievement of strategic competitive advantage. The chapters that follow guide the reader through these four stages.

Web Resources

A number of organizations (through their websites) provide more information on the topics discussed in this chapter:

- Agency for Healthcare Research and Quality (www.ahrq.gov) is the health services research arm of the US Department of Health & Human Services that complements the biomedical research mission of its sister agency, the National Institutes of Health. It is home to research centers that specialize in major areas of healthcare and is a major source of funding and technical assistance for health services research and research training at leading US universities and other institutions.
- Bureau of Labor Statistics (www.bls.gov) has many components that report varied data regarding the US economy. Particularly, it presents detailed information on consumer prices at the national and state levels.
- Care Continuum Alliance (www.carecontinuumalliance.org/index.asp) is an organization dedicated to the improvement of population health.
- Centers for Medicare & Medicaid Services (www.cms.gov) offers access to a vast array of healthcare-related information regarding Medicare, Medicaid, research and statistics, and regulations.
- Institute for Healthcare Improvement (IHI) (www.ihi.org) is a not-for-profit organization leading the improvement of healthcare throughout the world. IHI's work is funded primarily through its fee-based program offerings and services as well as through support from foundations, companies, and individuals.
- National Association for Healthcare Quality (www.nahq.org) empowers healthcare quality professionals from every specialty by providing vital research, education, networking, certification, professional practice resources, and a strong voice for healthcare quality.
- National Committee for Quality Assurance (NCQA) (www.ncqa.org) is a private, 501(c)(3) not-for-profit organization dedicated to improving

healthcare quality. NCQA has been a central figure in driving improvement throughout the healthcare system, helping to elevate the issue of healthcare quality to the top of the US political agenda. Its mission is to improve the quality of healthcare with a vision to transform healthcare quality through measurement, transparency, and accountability.

- Office of the National Coordinator (ONC) for Health Information Technology (www.healthit.gov) is the primary federal agency responsible for coordinating efforts to promote and develop HIT infrastructure. The ONC was created in 2004 via an Executive Order and codified by the HITECH Act. Its aims are to improve quality of care while reducing cost, enhance coordination of care, encourage health information exchanges, and ensure a secure personal health record for the US population.

Discussion Questions

Because most developers are not clinicians and most clinicians are not developers, what measures are necessary to ensure the development of an effective healthcare information system?

1. What are the five most important challenges faced by HIT today, and why?
2. What are the five most important future challenges that will face HIT, and why?
3. In what ways may improved HIT assist in continuity, communication, coordination, and accountability of patient care? [Hint: Consider Goldsmith's discussion.]
4. How can HIT assist organizations in responding to the drivers of information technology changes?
5. Define and describe evidence-based medicine. Are there positive or negative aspects of this concept for the healthcare field?
6. Why is the improvement of clinical information systems a high priority to most healthcare organizations?
7. Order the following types of healthcare information systems from most important to least important to a healthcare organization, and discuss why you chose this order.
   a. Clinical information
   b. Operational management
   c. Strategic decision support
   d. Electronic networking and e-health applications

EXTERNAL ENVIRONMENT

Overview

As Chapter 1 indicates, the future of healthcare information technology (HIT) is now. While the bulk of this textbook addresses management challenges with HIT, some of the greatest challenges faced today are motivated by factors external to the healthcare organization in which most of you will work. This chapter looks at some key elements of the external environment and how that environment influences the healthcare delivery system overall and healthcare informatics in particular. Chapter 3 also addresses external factors but concentrates on government health policy—specifically healthcare reform. In this chapter, we discuss four aspects of the external environment in detail.

First, we examine what we call the *healthcare triangle*: cost, quality, and access. Efforts to address the interrelated challenges of this triangle occupy much of healthcare leadership's and researchers' time and energy. Much research has been done on each of these three elements, and we briefly introduce the challenges in Chapter 1. Despite these efforts, however, we are still far from identifying a solution to problems caused by any of the three sides of the triangle. Controlling costs, improving quality, and expanding access will continue to represent external challenges to healthcare delivery and HIT management in the years to come.

Second, we explore evidence-based medicine (EBM) and evidence-based management. While EBM was introduced in Chapter 1, the direct implication of this "innovation" was not fully developed. EBM might be considered a response to the challenges arising from the healthcare triangle. By using evidence for decision making in a more direct way, clinical and administrative healthcare leaders will need more intensive and more timely information from the HIT system.

Third, we address the broad issue of organizational change. Restructuring healthcare delivery organizations might be considered a response to the healthcare triangle as well, so we discuss the chief information officer (CIO) role in identifying and implementing broader organizational change.

Fourth, we examine international comparisons of healthcare delivery. The threat or opportunity posed by healthcare delivered outside of the organization or outside of the country must be identified and planned for. Although international threats were briefly addressed in the tourism section in Chapter 1, their implications were not fully analyzed.

Healthcare Triangle

By presenting the three main challenges—cost, quality, and access—facing the healthcare delivery system as an interrelated triangle (Exhibit 2.1), we are suggesting that efforts to achieve goals in any one of the areas will necessarily have an impact on the other two. For example, costs can be controlled easily but not without the resultant reductions in access to care or in quality of care. The challenge is to find ways to achieve goals in the three areas that are satisfactory to all participants. Who pays for care? Who might have limited or no access to care? Who might suffer from less-than-satisfactory quality of care? The answers are often different groups of people. The political considerations in finding a solution are substantial—as was evident in the debate surrounding the healthcare reform legislation passed by the Obama administration, a debate that continued to be a major focus during and long after the 2012 presidential election.

The study of how we measure healthcare systems' performance in these three areas keeps government agencies, foundations, and consultants busy. An effective way to organize the key elements of the triangle comes from work funded by the Commonwealth Fund (2006). The organization

EXHIBIT 2.1
The Healthcare
Triangle: Inter-
relations Among
Cost, Quality,
and Access

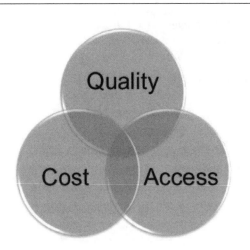

released *Why Not the Best?* to report the results from its assessment of the US healthcare system's performance. The analysis posed system questions, which do not directly reflect the performance of any individual organization or provider. However, it used measures that originate from elements of the delivery system. Organizations are going to be asked to provide some of these measures, which will put pressure on HIT. The five dimensions of overall performance and the 15 sub dimensions are presented in Exhibit 2.2.

Interestingly, *Why Not the Best?* reports a wide range of scores across the individual measures. Overall, the US system at that time scored an average of 66 in all measures when compared to a best-practice benchmark (Commonwealth Fund 2006). The implication is that the national healthcare system has achieved 66 percent of the target best-practice rating of 100 percent. Scores for the individual dimensions ranged from a high of 71 percent for both quality and equity to a low of 51 percent for efficiency. The US system scored highest for "adults with chronic conditions given self-management plan" at 89 percent and lowest for "physicians using electronic medical records" at 21 percent.

The point to notice here, however, is that for each of these indicators, the performance data are key, which means that completing a national report card (such as the *Why Not the Best?* publication) will require increased efforts by those responsible for HIT. The consideration of system performance measures will influence the HIT and organizational leadership to collect, analyze, and report a broader range of data than usual. They may have to identify that data for the patients they treat and for the potential patients in their service areas. While much of these data come from traditional sources (e.g., infant mortality rates, childhood immunization rates), other measures are relatively

EXHIBIT 2.2

Dimensions
of Health-
care System
Performance
Assessment

- Long, healthy, productive lives
  - Preventable mortality
  - Infant mortality
  - Life impacts of poor health
- Quality
  - Right care
  - Coordinated care
  - Safe care
  - Patient-centered and timely care
- Access
  - Participation
  - Affordability
- Efficiency
  - Overuse, inappropriate care, or waste
  - Access and efficiency
  - Variations in quality and costs
  - Insurance in administrative costs
  - Information systems to support efficient care
- Equity
  - Key roles of coverage, income, and race

SOURCE: Information from Commonwealth Fund (2006).

new to most hospital systems (e.g., chronic diseases under control, use of emergency department for conditions that can be treated by an ambulatory physician). Many of these indicators are based on population characteristics and are not usually items that individual organizations take the responsibility for collecting (e.g., health expenditures spent on administration).

Measuring performance is not the only approach to addressing the healthcare triangle. Other analysts have looked at combinations of factors as well. Baicker and Chandra (2004) examined the interrelationships among quality of Medicare beneficiaries' care, physician workforce, and spending. They found that states with greater spending actually had lower quality outcomes and that the composition of the physician workforce played a role in outcomes. Having more primary care physicians directed spending to more effective services and thus resulted in more desirable outcomes. Similarly, Yasaitis and colleagues (2009) reported on the link between quality of care and intensity of spending at the hospital level. They found that the relationship was mostly nonexistent and, if significant, was mostly negative.

HIT plays a central role in providing quality care, as explained in this book, and has the potential to improve efficiency and effectiveness. While it cannot solve efficiency and effectiveness problems, it serves as an important tool for government leaders and leaders of healthcare delivery systems in their efforts to find solutions.

Healthcare Costs

Healthcare costs continue to grow unabated. Government estimates state that the total national health spending reached nearly $2.6 trillion in 2010 and consumed about 18 percent of the US gross domestic product (GDP) (see Exhibit 2.3). This spending has been increasing steadily in the past 50 years (from $27.4 billion in 1960) and is expected to reach $3.3 trillion in 2015 (BLS 2012; CMS 2012b). To put the magnitude of this number into context, Exhibit 2.4 presents the data over time—from 1960 to 2010, including projections for 2015—on a per person (per capita) basis. In 2010, the United States spent $8,393 per person on healthcare, compared with the $147 spent per person in 1960; by 2015, we are expected to spend $10,272 per person. Exhibit 2.3 also shows health spending per capita and as a percentage of GDP for the same time frame (1960–2010). Healthcare expenditures are taking an ever-increasing portion of the goods and services produced in the United States, rising from only 5.2 percent of GDP in 1960 to 17.9 percent in 2010 and to an expected 18.2 percent by 2015.

Exhibit 2.5 analyzes the annual growth in healthcare spending by decade, from the 1970s through 2010 and projected data for 2015 (CMS 2012b). Healthcare spending increased faster than the GDP in all periods presented, although not always by the same amounts. These data suggest that regardless of good or bad economic times, Republican or Democratic presidents, and other factors, the result has been the same: The national health expenditure continues to grow faster than the GDP—the measure of the economy as a whole.

Exhibit 2.6 looks at the aggregate data in detail. It displays the spending by major healthcare delivery category for 2010. Hospital services represented the largest single category of spending at 31.4 percent, followed by physician services at 19.9 percent, prescription drugs at 10.0 percent, and nursing home care at 5.5 percent. It is interesting that research and construction constituted a substantial portion of spending at 5.7 percent. While these categories vary over time, they tend to remain stable for short periods. For example, Exhibit 2.7 presents the same national health expenditures breakdown by category—but for 1980. The big differences in this 30-year period (1980–2010) are a decline in the proportion of spending on hospital services (39.3 percent in 1980), an increase in the proportion spent on prescription drugs (4.7 percent in 1980), and a decrease in the proportion of research and construction expenditures (7.9 percent in 1980).

EXHIBIT 2.3

Select National Health Expenditures, GDP, Population, and Price Increases, 1960–2010

Component	Level						
	1960	1970	1980	1990	2000	2005	2010
National Health Expenditure (NHE)	$27.4	$74.9	$255.8	$724.3	$1,377.2	$2,029.1	$2,593.6
Research and construction	$2.6	$7.8	$20.1	$48.7	$87.5	$126.5	$149.0
Health services and supplies	$24.8	$67.1	$235.7	$675.6	$1,260.9	$1,860.9	$2,444.6
Gov. adm. and net private insurance	$1.1	$2.6	$12.1	$38.8	$83.0	$149.2	$176.1
Gov. Public Health Act	$0.4	$1.4	$6.4	$20.0	$43.0	$56.2	$82.5
Personal healthcare	$23.4	$63.1	$217.2	$616.8	$1,165.4	$1,697.2	$2,186.0
Hospital	$9.0	$27.2	$100.5	$250.4	$415.5	$609.4	$814.0
Professional services							
Physician services	$5.6	$13.0	$47.7	$158.9	$290.9	$416.9	$515.5
Dental services	$2.0	$4.7	$13.4	$31.7	$62.3	$87.0	$104.8
Other professional services	$0.5	$0.7	$3.5	$17.4	$37.0	$53.0	$68.4
						$1,165.4	
Home health care	$0.1	$0.2	$2.4	$12.8	$32.4	$48.7	$70.2
Nursing homes	$0.8	$4.0	$15.3	$44.9	$85.1	$112.5	$143.1
Retail outlet sales							
Prescription drugs	$2.7	$5.5	$12.0	$40.3	$120.9	$204.8	$259.1
Durable medical equipment	$0.7	$1.7	$4.1	$13.8	$25.1	$31.2	$37.7
Other nondurable	$1.6	$3.3	$9.8	$22.4	$31.6	$37.2	$44.8
Population (in millions)	186	210	230	254	282	295	309
GDP (billion $)	$526.0	$1,038.0	$2,788.0	$5,801.0	$9,952.0	$12,623.0	$14,526.5
General inflation (index)	29.8	39.8	86.3	130.7	172.2	195.3	218.1
Healthcare inflation (index)	22.6	36.7	77.6	162.8	260.8	323.2	388.5
NHE percent of GDP	5.2%	7.2%	9.2%	12.5%	13.8%	16.1%	17.9%

SOURCES: BLS (2012); CMS (2012b).

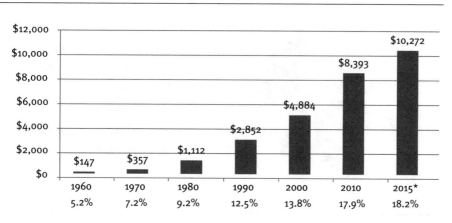

EXHIBIT 2.4

Per Capita National Health Expenditure (NHE) and NHE's Share of GDP, 1960–2015

Year and Percent of GDP

*2015 projection

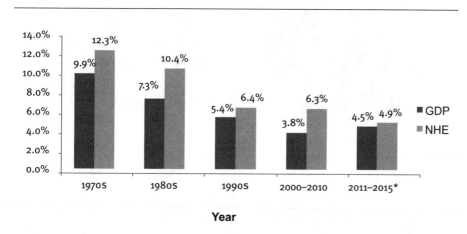

EXHIBIT 2.5

Annualized Growth Rates for NHE and GDP, 1970–2015

Year

*2015 projection

Another way to look at this is in terms of spending per year. Exhibit 2.8 presents the annual spending changes for select major categories, for total national health expenditures, and for GDP from 2000 to 2010. For the overall period, national health expenditures increased at an annual rate of 6.3 percent per year. Hospital services spending rose to slightly higher than the aggregate at 6.7 percent and as did prescription drugs expenditures at 7.6 percent, while physician services spending increased by less than the aggregate at 5.7 percent. National health expenditures and the major categories all increased faster than GDP, which was at 3.8 percent during this ten-year period.

EXHIBIT 2.6
National Health
Expenditure by
Major Service
Category, 2010

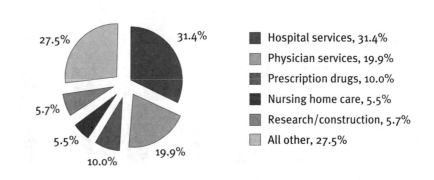

27.5%   31.4%

5.7%

5.5%

10.0%   19.9%

- ■ Hospital services, 31.4%
- ■ Physician services, 19.9%
- ■ Prescription drugs, 10.0%
- ■ Nursing home care, 5.5%
- ■ Research/construction, 5.7%
- ☐ All other, 27.5%

EXHIBIT 2.7
National Health
Expenditure by
Major Service
Category, 1980

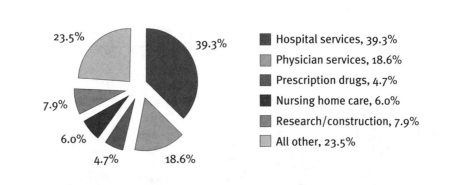

23.5%   39.3%

7.9%

6.0%

4.7%   18.6%

- ■ Hospital services, 39.3%
- ☐ Physician services, 18.6%
- ■ Prescription drugs, 4.7%
- ■ Nursing home care, 6.0%
- ■ Research/construction, 7.9%
- ☐ All other, 23.5%

To put all of this in perspective and get a better understanding of the factors that contributed to these overall changes in national health expenditures, you can decompose these overall changes into key component parts. Decomposition helps to determine the true magnitude of this overall change in healthcare spending and to aid in seeking solutions. The data in Exhibit 2.3 can be used to decompose the overall health expenditure changes; Exhibit 2.9 is a summary of the decomposition results for the 2000–2010 period. Again, overall national health expenditures increased 6.3 percent per year during this decade. Many factors contribute to this overall result, including the following:

- *Population growth.* During the 2000–2010 period, the US population grew by about 0.9 percent per year. Therefore, health spending per capita increased only 5.4 percent (6.3 percent – 0.9 percent) per year

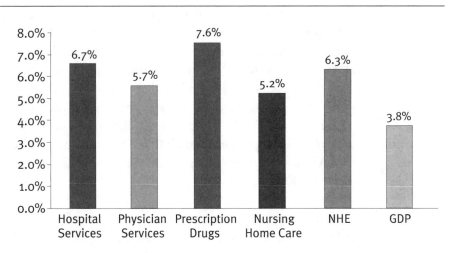

EXHIBIT 2.8
Annual Changes in Major Categories, NHE, and GDP, 2000–2010

during the decade. Population growth accounted for 14.4 percent of overall national health expenditure increases.

- *Inflation for the economy as a whole (measured by the Consumer Price Index).* Inflation was 2.4 percent per year during the 2000–2010 period. Therefore, real or inflation-adjusted health spending per capita went up 3.0 percent per year (6.3 percent [NHE] – 0.9 percent [population] – 2.4 percent [inflation]). Overall inflation increases accounted for 37.3 percent of health spending increases during this period. Of this remaining 3.0 percent per year, a substantial portion can be attributed to price increases for healthcare goods and services relative to general inflation.

- *Higher prices.* The medical care component of consumer prices climbed 4.0 percent during the 2000–2010 period. This increase was 1.6 percent (4.0 percent [medical care prices] – 2.4 percent [inflation]) more rapid than the overall inflation. Higher medical care prices accounted for 1.6 percent per year of the remaining real per capita increase of 3.0 percent per year, leaving a 1.4 percent annual increase unaccounted for. Relative medical care price increases accounted for 25.6 percent of overall health spending increases. The remaining 1.4 percent per year may be the result of two potential categories. One part represents greater spending due to increases in income, and the other part is residual.

- *Real income increases.* If you assume that health spending goes up at least as rapidly as income does, then real income increases should account for some of the 1.4 percent remaining. Real income (GDP adjusted for inflation) rose 1.4 percent per year during the decade

(3.8 percent [GDP] – 2.4 percent [inflation]). Real GDP accounted for at least 22.4 percent of the total increase. The other part of the 1.4 percent remaining can only be called a residual, but it represents quantity and quality of services. After controlling for population, inflation, relative prices of medical care goods and services, and real income increases, health spending increased by 0.0 percent per year (6.3 percent – 0.9 percent [population] – 2.4 percent [inflation] – 1.6 percent [medical care prices] – 1.4 percent [real GDP]). Quantity and quality increases accounted for essentially 0.0 percent of overall national health expenditures from 2000 to 2010.

This complex decomposition represents more than just an interesting exercise. As underlying causes of expenditure increase change, different solutions will arise. These solutions will affect how HIT leadership must collect and report key data. Decomposition also indicates that in aggregate, greater healthcare spending does not appear to be due to the expansion of services but rather a result of a complex mix of price increases and greater income. Cutting services further will not control expenditure increases; we must look at prices and perhaps the mix of services being delivered for solutions. This is further evidence that the external environment has a major impact on the healthcare system.

As our cost analysis suggests, healthcare expenditure growth will likely continue into the future; this trend is supported by federal government reports (see Exhibit 2.3). This analysis also indicates that not all of the healthcare cost problem can be attributed to healthcare prices or utilization, but both contribute substantially to it. However, cost analyses look backward and do not address the underlying socioeconomic factors that drive increases in spending in a more fundamental manner (Thorpe 2005). Among these

EXHIBIT 2.9
Decomposition of Annual National Health Expenditure, 2000–2010

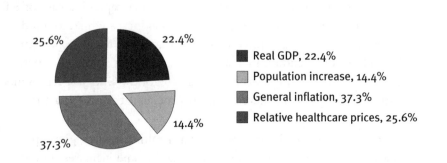

Real GDP, 22.4%
Population increase, 14.4%
General inflation, 37.3%
Relative healthcare prices, 25.6%

factors are modifiable "population risk factors such as obesity and stress," although Thorpe (2005, 1436) points out that rising disease prevalence and new medical treatments account for much of the increase as well.

Quality of Care

According to the Institute of Medicine's (IOM) 1999 landmark report, *To Err Is Human*, medical errors are a leading cause of adverse health consequences in hospitals (see Chapter 1). IOM followed up this study with a 2001 blueprint, *Crossing the Quality Chasm*, designed to help healthcare organizations fix the delivery system. The notion that quality in healthcare matters did not begin with these IOM studies, however. Most quality considerations for healthcare trace their origins to Avedis Donabedian.

He and his vast body of work conceptualized quality as a function of structure, process, and outcome—first in an article titled "Evaluating the Quality of Medical Care" (Donabedian 1966) and later and more formally in the classic book *The Definition of Quality and Approaches to Its Assessment* (Donabedian 1980). His work has become the foundation in that it continues to influence how we think about measurement and improvement of quality. He addressed many of the practical concerns regarding access to and use of patient clinical record data to measure and improve quality. In one of his more recent books, *An Introduction to Quality Assurance in Health Care*, Donabedian (2002) provided a guide to the many complex processes necessary for quality improvement. In his early work, he questioned access to and completeness of information in the traditional medical records (before the electronic medical record) and noted the challenges posed by physician record keeping. He even raised the notion of using direct observation, as opposed to paper records, as a means of collecting reliable, valid, and unbiased data. This innovative thinking occurred before the advent of most of the electronic record technologies that occupy our time today, and it continues to be an important consideration as a recent review of the evidence on the reliability and validity of quality measures suggests that more HIT work will be forthcoming in this regard (Chan, Fowles, and Weiner 2010). We urge you to read Donabedian's literature, including his 1988 article "The Quality of Care: How Can It Be Assessed?"

Davis and colleagues (2004) reported on the measurement of six domains of quality just from the perspective of the patient:

1. *Patient safety*—patient-reported medical error with serious health consequences
2. *Patient-centeredness*—patient assessment of quality of physician care, especially regarding involvement of the patient in care decisions

3. *Timeliness*—patient-reported waiting time for hospitalizations, elective surgery, and physician appointment
4. *Efficiency*—patient-reported coordination of care
5. *Effectiveness*—patient-reported ability to follow up on care ordered by the physician
6. *Equity*—patient-reported influence of income on ability to receive care

Combining the foundation of quality from Donabedian, the challenges regarding medical errors from the IOM, and the concept of patient-perceived domains from Davis and colleagues led to the conceptualization of quality of care in terms of a more comprehensive set of measures. The Agency for Healthcare Research and Quality currently assists providers and researchers in navigating the complex and expanding quality measurement space by creating and hosting the National Quality Measures Clearinghouse (www.quality measures.ahrq.gov/index.aspx). This comprehensive source of information on quality metrics even includes a tutorial that addresses the desirable attributes of a quality measure; selection of a measure for a particular purpose; use of measures for improvement, accountability, and research; validity of clinical measures; and paradigm for classifying measures (delivery or population based). The source collects and provides documentation for thousands of potential metrics and contains helpful classification schemes. For example, it presents measures by disease/condition, treatment/intervention, and health services administration. Of the 2,105 measures, 212 are listed by the National Committee for Quality Assurance. As an example of the types of information available, Exhibit 2.10 lists the nine items related to childhood immunization status (notice the subtle differences between the nine measures). This set of measurements gives an idea of the complexity of assessing quality.

Further, Davis and colleagues (2004) reported some of the problems with quality and the variability in the level of quality. Doing something about quality requires identifying a methodology and training people to monitor, assess, and improve quality of care. This has led to the formation of a host of associations, programs, and sources that have the common goal of organizing healthcare professionals around the task of improving quality or some aspects of service delivery in the US healthcare system (see Exhibit 2.11). All of these initiatives rely on the HIT function to provide data.

To demonstrate how vital information management is to the future, Senator Max Baucus (D-Montana) proposed in an article that two basic reforms be implemented to improve the system (Baucus 2005). First, the way that providers are paid must be changed to a system that encourages value and efficient, effective, patient-centered care. Second, more spending on (i.e., investment in) information technology is needed. Baucus asserted that these changes would result in a more transparent and value-based healthcare

1. Childhood immunization status: Percentage of children 2 years of age who had four diphtheria, tetanus, and acellular pertussis (DTaP); three polio (IPV); one measles, mumps, and rubella (MMR); three H influenza type B (HiB); three hepatitis B (HepB); and one chicken pox (VZV) vaccines by their second birthday (combination #2)

2. Childhood immunization status: Percentage of children 2 years of age who had four diphtheria, tetanus, and acellular pertussis (DTaP); three polio (IPV); one measles, mumps, and rubella (MMR); three H influenza type B (HiB); three hepatitis B (HepB); one chicken pox (VZV); and four pneumococcal conjugate (PCV) vaccines by their second birthday (combination #3)

3. Childhood immunization status: Percentage of children 2 years of age who had four diphtheria, tetanus, and acellular pertussis (DTaP); three polio (IPV); one measles, mumps, and rubella (MMR); three H influenza type B (HiB); three hepatitis B (HepB); one chicken pox (VZV); four pneumococcal conjugate (PCV); and two hepatitis A (HepA) vaccines by their second birthday (combination #4)

4. Childhood immunization status: Percentage of children 2 years of age who had four diphtheria, tetanus, and acellular pertussis (DTaP); three polio (IPV); one measles, mumps, and rubella (MMR); three H influenza type B (HiB); three hepatitis B (HepB); one chicken pox (VZV); four pneumococcal conjugate (PCV); and two influenza (flu) vaccines by their second birthday (combination #6)

5. Childhood immunization status: Percentage of children 2 years of age who had four diphtheria, tetanus, and acellular pertussis (DTaP); three polio (IPV); one measles, mumps, and rubella (MMR); three H influenza type B (HiB); three hepatitis B (HepB); one chicken pox (VZV); four pneumococcal conjugate (PCV); and two or three rotavirus (RV) vaccines by their second birthday (combination #5)

6. Childhood immunization status: Percentage of children 2 years of age who had four diphtheria, tetanus, and acellular pertussis (DTaP); three polio (IPV); one measles, mumps, and rubella (MMR); three H influenza type B (HiB); three hepatitis B (HepB); one chicken pox (VZV); four pneumococcal conjugate (PCV); two hepatitis A (HepA); and two influenza (flu) vaccines by their second birthday (combination #8)

7. Childhood immunization status: Percentage of children 2 years of age who had four diphtheria, tetanus, and acellular pertussis (DTaP); three polio (IPV); one measles, mumps, and rubella (MMR); three H influenza type B (HiB); three hepatitis B (HepB); one chicken pox (VZV); four pneumococcal conjugate (PCV); two hepatitis A (HepA); and two or three rotavirus (RV) vaccines by their second birthday (combination #7)

8. Childhood immunization status: Percentage of children 2 years of age who had four diphtheria, tetanus, and acellular pertussis (DTaP); three polio (IPV); one measles, mumps, and rubella (MMR); three H influenza type B (HiB); three hepatitis B (HepB); one chicken pox (VZV); four pneumococcal conjugate (PCV); two hepatitis A (HepA); two or three rotavirus (RV); and two influenza (flu) vaccines by their second birthday (combination #10)

9. Childhood immunization status: Percentage of children 2 years of age who had four diphtheria, tetanus, and acellular pertussis (DTaP); three polio (IPV); one measles, mumps, and rubella (MMR); three H influenza type B (HiB); three hepatitis B (HepB); one chicken pox (VZV); four pneumococcal conjugate (PCV); two or three rotavirus (RV); and two influenza (flu) vaccines by their second birthday (combination #9)

EXHIBIT 2.10
Sample Measures from the National Quality Measures Clearinghouse

SOURCE: Reprinted from Childhood Immunization, National Quality Measures Clearinghouse, www.qualitymeasures.ahrq.gov/browse/by-topic.aspx.

- Agency for Healthcare Research and Quality (AHRQ): www.ahrq.gov
- Ambulatory Care Quality Alliance (AQA): www.aqaalliance.org
- American Medical Association Physician Consortium for Performance Improvement (AMA-PCPI): www.ama-assn.org/ama/pub/category/2946.html
- American Society for Quality (ASQ): www.asq.org
- Institute for Healthcare Improvement (IHI): www.ihi.org
- Institute of Medicine (IOM): www.iom.edu
- The Joint Commission: www.jointcommission.org
- Leapfrog Group: www.leapfroggroup.org
- National Association for Healthcare Quality (NAHQ): www.nahq.org
- National Committee for Quality Assurance (NCQA): www.ncqa.org
- National Initiative for Children's Healthcare Quality (NICHQ): www.nichq.org
- National Quality Forum (NQF): www.qualityforum.org
- Nursing Quality Network: www.nursingqualitynetwork.org

system. He even wrote in the conclusion that "I hope that my colleagues in Congress will see the wisdom of that approach" (Baucus 2005). Today, the message in this article reflects the thinking of a politician considering fundamental reform of the healthcare system. In fact, some of its features appeared in the Patient Protection and Affordable Care Act of 2010.

Since the early days of HIT, the literature has presented evidence of HIT's positive impact on quality. Buntin and colleagues (2011) in a systematic review found that 92 percent of the literature found HIT provided positive or mixed benefits. Among Buntin and colleagues' many findings is that research that examined specific information technology tools was less likely to demonstrate positive results than research that explored comprehensive information technology systems. The evaluation methodology suggests that this should not have been the case. More research on this topic is needed to fully understand the role of HIT on quality of care. Appari and colleagues (2012) conducted a large-scale study of US hospitals and found that institutions that adopted HIT had patients who displayed significantly greater likelihood of adherence to recommended medications (for acute myocardial infarction, heart failure, pneumonia, and surgical care) than patients of non-HIT adopters. Appari and colleagues looked separately at all computerized physician order entry (CPOE) and electronic medication administration record (eMAR) systems. This study suggests HIT's positive impact on quality because adherence to recommended medications is a necessary element in overall quality-of-care improvement.

The complexity of systematically measuring and evaluating HIT impacts makes the studies that do exist somewhat unsatisfying, however.

HIT's effect on outcomes is difficult to identify immediately because several steps occur between the implementation and use of an HIT system and the final clinical outcome; the best system in the world will not work if the operators (physicians) do not use the system correctly. Thus, many studies instead examine the intermediate outcomes, such as adherence to practice guidelines, rather than the patient outcome. For example, Jamal, McKenzie, and Clark (2009) found that most studies (14 out of 17 they reviewed) demonstrated evidence of improved compliance with guidelines but essentially no positive impact on patient outcomes. Similarly, Black and colleagues (2011) found little evidence of HIT's positive impact on quality when they examined a host of systems, including clinical decision support and distant technologies.

Despite substantial progress in measurement and improvement of care, serious caveats exist. Baron (2007) suggests that information technology may not be an easy answer to improvement despite its substantial promise. For example, an electronic health record's failure to adequately structure information means that retrieving and using vital patient data will be difficult for users. In addition, in many ambulatory care settings, neither teams nor resources exist to implement improvement initiatives despite the availability of good data.

Access to Care

In addition to the quality of care challenges, the US healthcare system suffers from myriad problems related to individuals with poor access to care. As with quality, the concept of access can be addressed in many ways, making full understanding and finding viable solutions difficult (ACHE 2008; Feinson 2004). One type of access problem, for example, may arise from people living in remote, rural parts of the country that do not have healthcare facilities and personnel close by. "Close by" can apply to distance or travel time. Crowding also can present an access barrier. If available facilities are underdeveloped to meet the needs of the local population, crowding can result. Other access barriers stem from the interrelated issues of lack of insurance, fear of public programs, literacy and cultural competency, and transportation (Feinson 2004). For this discussion, we primarily consider the financial aspects of access challenges.

Many residents in the United States have no health insurance, making obtaining care a cost-prohibitive undertaking. As described in Chapter 1, although the number of uninsured decreased in 2011, it remains a large population—comprising about 48.6 million people (Exhibit 1.1). One thing is certain, US residents consistently rank access at or near the top of "the most urgent" healthcare-related concerns, as reported by the Gallup organization (Saad 2009).

People without access to care are, generally, those without insurance. Because they do not have a usual source of care, the uninsured consistently exhibit behaviors that contribute to poor health outcomes, which ironically often cost more. Specifically, those without insurance (Families USA 2012)

- use the emergency department as the regular source of care
- obtain few (if any) health screenings and preventive care,
- often delay or completely forgo medical services,
- are typically sicker and may die earlier than those with insurance, and
- pay more for medical care.

Problems of the uninsured are systems challenges, but they manifest in clinical care, and thus HIT, directly. A number of studies have demonstrated that lack of insurance and variations in the type of insurance have a negative impact on the stage of diagnosis and care for patients with cancer (Bradley et al. 2008; Farkas et al. 2012; Halpern et al. 2007). Other views exist, however, in that the uninsured are not uniform; in fact, many of them could pay for insurance, pay for care, and receive substantial healthcare (O'Neill and O'Neill 2009). The challenges of insurance, access to care, and cost/quality outcomes are at the center of the Patient Protection and Affordable Care Act, which is discussed in more detail in Chapter 3.

The bottom line is that as solutions to access-to-care barriers for uninsured individuals emerge, the US healthcare system will face a capacity problem. With improved access, more people (perhaps 25 to 30 percent of the population) will gain meaningful access to basic care and insurance. This will strain the public health and emergency systems, on which many Americans rely, to provide adequate care (Book 2005, 579).

Impact of the Healthcare Triangle on HIT

A host of external factors related to cost, quality, and access will influence healthcare delivery organizations. Importantly, each factor has direct implications for HIT. The real issue, however, is whether the growth of cost per se genuinely constitutes a problem. Are we getting value for this investment in healthcare goods and services? Many studies explore this problem and propose solutions, including a 2010 Institute of Medicine report titled *The Healthcare Imperative: Lowering Costs and Improving Outcomes.* Any review of the literature will demonstrate that identification of and solutions to cost increases dominate the published articles, and these studies (e.g., Cutler, Rosen, and Vijan 2006) suggest that investments in healthcare have been relatively cost-effective overall.

Improving quality requires greater accuracy, reliability, and timeliness of clinical information at the individual patient level (Metzger, Ame, and

Rhoads 2010). As quality improvement efforts take hold, organizations will need to be able to collect and share information across components of their systems. Identification of best practices involves sharing of information across units and institutions. Further, delivery organizations will increasingly be required to provide access to high-quality care to meet the needs of patients in their communities. These may not be patients in the traditional sense; thus, reliably obtaining information about them is essential. Sources, validation, and security of this information will pose future challenges to HIT. Organizations must adopt greater standards of transparency in reporting quality and cost information (Aron and Pogach 2009). However, if the challenges of improving quality from HIT investments prove too great a barrier as we have observed, the likelihood of sharing information across systems is in doubt.

Similarly, access involves a number of challenges that HIT must address. First, expanded access to 30 to 50 million more people strains delivery systems and HIT's ability to collect, monitor, and report across a host of environments. Second, by nature, many of the currently uninsured are challenging to serve. Often, they have different, more complex acute and chronic medical problems than those with insurance. On average, they are less likely to have higher education, positive home environment, and nutritional history or prior medical records at a healthcare facility. These make the newly insured less likely to comply with forms/paperwork or general medical treatment. Gathering data and validating data are, thus, more difficult.

From a cost perspective, access and quality further increase cost pressures. Efforts at reducing duplicate tests and procedures, eliminating fraud and abuse, reducing excess administrative costs, and redesigning processes all entail HIT involvement.

Evidence-Based Management

As defined in Chapter 1, EBM is a systematic approach to diagnosis and treatment that encourages the physician to formulate questions and seek answers from the best available published evidence. Relatedly, the past decade witnessed a corresponding increase in the emphasis on *evidence-based management* (Kovner, Fine, and D'Aquila 2009; Pfeffer and Sutton 2006; Walshe and Rundall 2001). In fact, Kovner, Fine, and D'Aquila's book *Evidence-Based Management in Healthcare* suggests that this topic has become mainstream in the training of future healthcare leaders. While experience, judgment, intuition, and a good sense of the political environment are still critical skills, administrative decision making increasingly relies on information. While some may discount the value of information in the management process—stating that management is still more an art than a science—the other end of the spectrum are the technocrats who argue that management and information are inseparable and that all management decisions need to be completely rational and based entirely on an analysis of comprehensive information. The resulting revision in the method of managerial decision making that relies more on data has now become part of the culture of healthcare organizations (Center for Organization, Leadership, and Management Research 2006). This new culture relies heavily on organizational information systematically gathered, stored, analyzed, and reported by a wide array of health informatics professionals. Many of the challenges emerging for EBM will also arise for evidence-based management—the management application of the EBM concept.

The most obvious example of the potential value of evidence-based management is in reducing the high levels of variation in management (and clinical) practices observed across healthcare delivery organizations. Over the last 40 years, a growing body of evidence regarding variation in care points to the problems that variations generate (Wennberg and Gittelsohn 1973). The investigations and evidence mounted, and Gawande (2009) wrote an accessible article that clarifies the evidence and importance of these variations. If we manage patients and organizations without valid, reliable information, then healthcare costs rise and quality falls (Fisher, Bynum, and Skinner 2009; Fisher et al. 2003).

Organizational Change

The stress of the evolving environment has been a major driver of organizational change along a number of dimensions (Bigalke, Copeland, and Keckley 2011). These changes fall into a number of categories but include some key elements:

- Securing information from physicians, hospitals, and post-acute providers regarding safety, quality, and healthcare outcomes
- Employing scientific evidence for recommended treatment protocols
- Facilitating coordination of care across entities with greater investment in information technologies
- Actualizing consumer decision making by providing choices in type of care and location of care delivery

Each of these strategies involves the use of information technology in new ways; they currently strain HIT operations and will continue to generate strain in the future. The first bullet in particular poses technical and political challenges for HIT as it entails gathering information from multiple sites. These data are collected from entities that are separate geographically, culturally, and by ownership. Interoperability is a necessary step in enabling that to happen, and even the government recognizes that true interoperability is a work in progress (see www.healthit.gov/providers-professionals /ehr-interoperability for a discussion of this topic and revisit it from time to time for updates).

Much of what is envisioned in today's healthcare reform appears similar to the managed care initiatives pushed as a solution to cost issues in the early 1970s. Back then, organizations responded to the growth of managed care by consolidating (Cuellar and Gertler 2003), purchasing medical practices (Morrisey et al. 1996), and improving efficiency and effectiveness (Enthoven and Singer 1996). Managed care, which flourished in the 1990s, was designed to help contain costs by providing financial incentives to squeeze out inefficiency in the delivery system. However, another way to contain costs is not just to provide care but to truly make the system more efficient. Much of the growth of managed care was not due to consumers choosing it as the preferred method of service. People selected managed care options to avoid paying higher premiums in alternative insurance plans (Gilmer and Kronick 2005). Consumer backlash to managed care arose because of fear of restrictions on access to care. This sentiment was fueled by physicians who did not support managed care because its plans placed limitations on the delivery of care and reduced physician reimbursement (Ginsburg 2005). Health maintenance organizations, in particular, came under heavy criticism from consumers and physicians. The political battle over the Patient's Bill of Rights, which was developed in response to the managed care restrictions, is a reflection of these consumer and physician concerns. Whether the current responses to health reform can avoid the problems of the managed care era is open to speculation.

The managed care movement did not end with the criticisms we mentioned. Accountable care organizations, bundled payments, and other elements of the healthcare reform legislation suggest that basic tenets of managed care survived—but under different terminology. Some form of assigning responsibility to providers for the full continuum of care, rather than for individual units of service, will be part of the healthcare future. For HIT, the implications are staggering. Collecting, storing, retrieving, and analyzing patient data across this continuum require increases in the amount of data and changes in the types of data needed (e.g., inpatient, outpatient, rehabilitation, prescription drug). Furthermore, as stated, these data will come from separate entities. Leaders of HIT must become more strategic in assessing many data-related options and meeting the changing needs of their organization (Chapter 4 addresses this in depth).

A potential fundamental change in the healthcare landscape might come from an international comparison of outcomes, costs, and efficiency.

Again, a growing body of evidence suggests that the US healthcare system does not measure up to international comparisons across a host of dimensions:

- *Overall.* Patient perspectives suggest that the US system does not compare well or favorably with the systems of a select set of English-speaking countries (Davis et al. 2004), such as Australia, New Zealand, Canada, and the United Kingdom, all of which outperform the United States from the patients' perspective; some might argue, however, that even in English-speaking countries, responses to common questions may not have exactly the same meaning.
- *Outcomes.* Most of the comparisons of outcomes point to problems in the US system. The Commonwealth Fund's "National Scorecard on the U.S. Health System Performance" presents a broadly consistent set of comparisons. For example, the percentage of "sicker" adults reporting a medical, medication, or lab error in 2008 for select developed countries reveals that the US rate (at 32 percent) was double the rate of the best-performing country—the Netherlands (at 16 percent)—and was substantially above the second "worst" performer—Australia (at 28) (Schoen and How 2011).
- *Access.* As most of the American populace expect, access is poorer in the United States. For example, the percentage of adults reporting at least one of three access problems was 40 percent in the United States versus 34 percent in New Zealand and 9 percent in the United Kingdom (Schoen and How 2011). The three access problems indicated in the report were not getting care because of cost, did not fill prescriptions because of cost, or skipped prescription doses because of cost.
- *Efficiency.* In terms of efficiency, the United States scored worse compared with other countries across a number of measures. For example, the percentage of adults who went to the emergency department (in the previous two years) for a condition that could have been treated by a primary physician was 26 percent for the United States versus 21 percent for Canada (the next highest) and 6 percent for Germany (the lowest among the reported countries) (Schoen and How 2011).
- *Expenditures.* Health spending was highest in the United States. Data are not available (as of this writing) for 2013 but have been reported for 2009. In 2009, adjusting for cost of living, spending per capita was $7,960 in the United States versus $5,352 in Norway, $5,144 in Switzerland, $4,363 in Canada, and $3,487 in the United Kingdom (Squires 2012).

International comparisons may present a competition challenge for US healthcare delivery. If medical tourism—defined as "overseas travel for medical, cosmetic and dental health care" (Medical Tourism Corporation 2012)—increased, it might directly address the challenges of the healthcare triangle. According to the marketing materials of Medical Tourism Corporation, the value of medical tourism is that it enables people to

a. save on medical costs;
b. avoid the long wait for medical services in their home country;
c. get better quality medical care or diagnostic services;
d. protect their privacy.

These benefits are not totally documented at this point, but the threat of medical tourism and its potential advantages exists. Much is still being considered, and the data reported on volume and growth are too unreliable for now. (For an interesting overview of these issues, see India Knowledge@ Wharton [2011].) What we do know is that at least some of the results from the United States's adverse performance in international comparisons may be due to less-than-adequate use of HIT in its healthcare system (Anderson et al. 2006). Anderson and colleagues document that while delivery organizations in the United States employ fewer resources (e.g., beds, nurses, physicians) per capita, they spend more than twice as much as other OECD (Organisation for Economic Co-operation and Development 2007) countries. The authors argue that a major portion of that performance difference can be explained by the following factors (Anderson et al. 2006):

- The United States is at least a decade late in making HIT a national initiative. Germany started at a national level in 1993.
- The United States has not relied on a centralized government role in motivating HIT adoption.
- The United States invests significantly less per capita on HIT. Data suggest that in 2005 the United States had invested $.43 per capita, Norway had invested $11.31 per capita, Germany had invested $21.03 per capita, and Canada had invested $31.85 per capita.

These estimates point to the potential reasons the United States lag the rest of the developed world in cost, quality, and access measures. However, they also point to a great potential for improvement with the assistance of a concerted HIT leadership and management.

Summary

Change is occurring rapidly in healthcare. While much of that change will be internal to the technologies and processes in healthcare delivery organizations, much will be derived from forces external to the organization and even external to the United States. Major forces of change that have a direct impact on the application of HIT include (1) the healthcare triangle, (2) growth of evidence-based management for decision making, (3) the need for healthcare organizational change, and (4) greater emphasis on international comparisons for performance assessment.

These environmental trends present challenges to healthcare leaders overall but to HIT leadership particularly. Addressing the healthcare triangle must involve improved access to and use of health information and HIT. These challenges involve not only internal operational responses but also the need to interface with organizations and agencies outside of the host institution. Hospitals, physician practices, and other elements of the provider network must learn to gather, store, retrieve, and analyze information more efficiently. Organizational leaders are learning to use data as evidence in making decisions; thus, they will demand more reliable and valid data, presented in understandable formats and in a timely manner. Further, information from external organizations (regionally and nationally) will need to be integrated and made available to those clinical and administrative decision makers as the decision frameworks expand. Finally, comparisons and competition from international providers may enlarge the scope of the information required.

Web Resources

A number of organizations (through their websites) provide more information on the topics discussed in this chapter:

- American Health Quality Association (www.ahqa.org) is a national membership organization that promotes and facilitates fundamental changes designed to improve the quality of healthcare.
- American Society for Quality (http://asq.org/index.aspx) is a global organization that focuses on using tools and ideas to make the world better.
- The Commonwealth Fund (www.commonwealthfund.org/About-Us .aspx) has the broad charge to "enhance the common good." Its mission is to improve access, quality, and efficiency in the healthcare system with special emphasis on low-income, the uninsured, minority Americans, young children, and the elderly.
- Henry J. Kaiser Family Foundation (www.kff.org) is a leader in health policy analysis and communication dedicated to providing a trusted, independent analysis of key policy issues. While it has many key agenda items, cost and coverage are central to its work and are a great source of data and analysis.

- Institute of Medicine (www.iom.edu/About-IOM.aspx) is an independent, nonprofit organization that provides authoritative advice to decision makers and the public on healthcare issues. With a strong clinical focus, IOM has specific initiatives in coverage and access to care as well as quality and patient safety.
- National Quality Measures Clearinghouse (www.qualitymeasures.ahrq .gov/index.aspx) is the source of comprehensive information on quality measures for healthcare.
- Robert Wood Johnson Foundation (www.rwjf.org/en/about-rwjf.html) is a large philanthropy devoted to the public's health. Among its many topics are cost of care, quality of care, and access/barriers to care.

Discussion Questions

1. Why do national concerns over cost of care affect those responsible for managing information systems within healthcare institutions?
2. Why do national concerns over quality of care affect those responsible for managing information systems within healthcare institutions?
3. Why do national concerns over access to care affect those responsible for managing information systems within healthcare institutions?
4. What information would you assemble for healthcare leadership in your organization to monitor healthcare cost? Would that differ if you work in a hospital versus a physician practice or other organization?
5. What information would you assemble for healthcare leadership in your organization to monitor healthcare quality? Would that differ if you work in a hospital versus a physician practice or other organization?
6. What information would you assemble for healthcare leadership in your organization to monitor healthcare access? Would that differ if you work in a hospital versus a physician practice or other organization?
7. What organizational challenges do you anticipate with changes necessary to control cost, improve quality, and expand access in your organization?
8. How much synthesis of external information will be necessary for effective evidence-based management? Who is best able to provide that synthesis?

GOVERNMENT POLICY AND HEALTHCARE REFORM

Learning Objectives

1. Describe a justification for government intervention in business processes.
2. List five major types of government intervention into the healthcare business, and explain the need for government to invest in healthcare information management and healthcare information technology (HIT).
3. Describe the eight components of the administrative simplification portion of the Health Insurance Portability and Accountability Act.
4. Assess your organization's readiness for transactions and code set development.
5. Analyze why privacy and security are important and why HIT has a key role in protecting privacy and security.
6. Assess four key questions to answer in developing privacy policies.
7. Describe HIT leadership's role in responding to legislation.

Overview

Much has been written regarding the details of the federal, state, and local government policies that have direct and indirect influences on healthcare information technology (HIT) and its leadership in healthcare organizations (Blumenthal 2006; Feldstein 2001; Goldsmith, Blumenthal, and Rishel 2003; Kleinke 2005; Poon et al. 2006; Taylor et al. 2005). This chapter does not present an exhaustive list of those impacts. Its goal is to provide HIT leadership with the awareness of the potential effects of healthcare legislation on HIT business practices; the tools to identify and respond to current healthcare legislation; and the strategic vision to plan for future challenges that may arise from government interventions. The chapter has three sections:

1. *Government's role in HIT*. This section provides the justification for government intervention in business processes. Understanding why government gets involved will assist you in responding to legislation and anticipating future actions.
2. *Specific healthcare legislations.*
    a. Health Insurance Portability and Accountability Act (HIPAA) of 1996. This major set of legislative and administrative interventions has fundamentally changed HIT for the last decade and will likely change it in the future. It is a complex array of interventions that have been implemented in ways not fully anticipated when the legislation was passed in 1996. This section presents some basic policies and procedures designed to respond to select HIPAA requirements.
    b. American Recovery and Reinvestment Act's Health Information Technology for Economic and Clinical Health Act. This legislation arose from the economic crisis of 2007–2009 but became an enabler, nonetheless, of electronic health record adoption in the United States.
    c. Patient Protection and Affordable Care Act of 2010. This controversial health reform legislation is designed to expand coverage to the uninsured and to improve quality of care and provider accountability.
3. *HIT leadership roles*. The external environment and government have direct, indirect, and substantial roles in healthcare operations. Leaders must understand those roles today and anticipate roles in the future. This section presents an action plan for HIT leadership.

Government's Role in HIT

Three questions must be asked in assessing the role of government in HIT:

1. Why does the government (at any level) get involved in healthcare or any business practice? Is there justification for government intervention?
2. If yes, how much and what types of intervention are justified?
3. What triggers those interventions?

The easy answer to these questions is that the government recognizes the challenges that the healthcare field faces regarding cost, quality, and access to care (see Chapter 2 or Gauthier and Serber [2005]). Further, the government has an obligation to intervene to provide access to high-quality, affordable care to all residents.

Justification for Government Intervention

The generic argument for government intervention is that the marketplace does not perform its normal function of optimizing resource-production efficiency and resource-allocation decision making as classical economics theory suggests (Santerre and Neun 2004). As a result of the market's failure, government can—and some say should—intervene to fix the problem. Key reasons for intervention include problems with public goods, externalities, imperfect consumer information, and monopoly. Public goods are those that producers cannot easily exclude people from consuming, and consumption by one person does not reduce the availability for others to consume. A classic example is national defense, but medical research that leads to cures for disease is another. Externalities are costs or benefits related to a market action that parties not related to the transaction incur. For example, cigarette smoking may impose costs on those not involved in the decision to smoke. Imperfect information may give rise to government involvement in markets because people are concerned that profit-seeking businesses may take advantage of people's inability to make informed choices. In each of these cases, the market does not reliably provide the optimal quantity. (See Santerre and Neun [2004] for an extensive discussion of these issues.)

If the market fails to produce a good or service for any of these reasons, government is empowered to intervene in the public interest. Generally, the "fix" is to develop and implement policies that approximate what the market solution would generate, if possible. For healthcare, that intervention is justified because of asymmetric information between purchasers and providers and significant uncertainty about future need for services (Arrow 1963; Poterba 1996). However, some have argued that government interventions are designed to benefit those special interests that influence politicians rather that society as a whole (Blumenthal 2006; Feldstein 2001; Goldsmith, Blumenthal, and Rishel 2003; Kleinke 2005; Taylor et al. 2005).

Examples of the range of government intervention are included in Exhibit 3.1. Correcting externalities has been one of the major reasons for government intervention. HIPAA, described later in this chapter, can be considered an intervention to force a market solution that would not occur without direct government support. Funding for medical research is a more traditional example of this type of intervention and is briefly described as it relates to funding for HIT. The other categories in the exhibit are not directly relevant to this book but are still worthy of note.

A significant amount of research in HIT has been funded by the federal government. A primary source of this funding for research and demonstration projects comes from the National Library of Medicine (NLM, www.nlm.nih.gov). The importance of the NLM to current initiatives and emerging features of HIT make it a major change agent. HIT leadership should be

EXHIBIT 3.1
Types of Gov-
ernment Market
Intervention

Purpose	Government Initiative
Provide public goods	Funding of medical research
Correct for externalities	Tax on alcohol and cigarettes
Impose regulations	Federal Drug Administration
Enforce antitrust laws	Limit hospital mergers
Sponsor redistribution programs	Medicare and Medicaid
Operate public enterprises	Veterans Administration hospitals

SOURCE: Reprinted from Feldstein (2001). Used with permission from Health Administration Press, Chicago.

familiar with NLM funding priorities. Exhibit 3.2 presents the eight primary functions of the NLM. Assisting healthcare organizations with developing the data systems to support both their clinical operations and health services research is a major portion of NLM's charge. Using the justification for government intervention argument, the government funds these (and other) crucial activities because it believes that private organizations will not spend

EXHIBIT 3.2
Primary Func-
tions of the
National Library
of Medicine

The National Library of Medicine

1. assists the advancement of medical and related sciences through the collection, dissemination, and exchange of information important to the progress of medicine and health;
2. serves as a national information resource for medical education, research, and service activities of Federal and private agencies, organizations, and institutions;
3. serves as a national information resource for the public, patients, and families by providing electronic access to reliable health information issued by the National Institutes of Health and other trusted sources;
4. publishes in print and electronically guides to health sciences information in the form of catalogs, bibliographies, indexes, and online databases;
5. provides support for medical library development and for training of biomedical librarians and other health information specialists;
6. conducts and supports research in methods for recording, storing, retrieving, preserving, and communicating health information;
7. creates information resources and access tools for molecular biology, biotechnology, toxicology, environmental health, and health services research; and
8. provides technical consultation services and research assistance.

SOURCE: Reprinted from the National Library of Medicine (2004).

sufficiently on them. Further, the findings from these efforts will benefit the entire US healthcare system by enabling the development and testing of new technologies and infrastructure support.

Government Intervention in the Healthcare Field

For most industries, the government largely allows the market to determine costs, efficiency, quality, availability, and firm survival. With the exception of enforcing property rights and legal contracts, the government's role is minor.

Healthcare is different from other industries, however. The government gets involved in healthcare—and, by extension, HIT—because the government has a broad obligation to protect the health and welfare of the population. That obligation extends beyond ensuring that markets function and property rights are enforced (Feldstein 2001). Finding that the health of the population is at risk makes intervention to improve patient safety vital. Evidence that this risk is real comes from a series of prestigious studies, such as the Institute of Medicine's 1999 and 2001 reports. Further, published estimates that nearly 50 million people are uninsured and many more are underinsured (DeNavas-Walt, Proctor, and Smith 2012; Gauthier and Serber 2005) bring another call for government intervention. Lack of insurance has an effect on the health of the population because lack of insurance may actually lead to preventable morbidity and mortality (a negative health outcome), which in turn cost the US healthcare system more than $65 billion per year (Ayanian et al. 2000; IOM 2003).

As discussed in earlier chapters, healthcare costs have been rising rapidly both in absolute terms and relative to the gross domestic product. These increases in cost are largely paid by governments; thus, budget considerations drive government interest as well. In 2010, 39.2 percent of personal health expenditures were paid by Medicare and Medicaid alone. All levels of government have a major stake in payment rates (CMS 2012b). The conclusion is that quality, access, and cost provide a justification of the government's role in healthcare and thus in HIT. (See Chapter 2 for more details on the expenditures for healthcare services.)

Government and Business Practice

Given that government intervention can be justified, how much and what types of intervention are justified? With respect to HIT, patient information privacy and security are the major foci of government intervention. The argument is that social interest in having patient healthcare information protected cannot be left to individual providers. Good business practice dictates that much of what comes under the guise of government intervention should be followed irrespective of the regulations. As addressed in detail in the next section, HIPAA has, among other features, enhanced privacy regulation.

Because healthcare delivery organizations are responsible for the health and welfare of their patients, it only makes sense to adopt strict privacy standards even in the absence of government regulation. Therefore, information system managers in healthcare facilities must develop policies and procedures to protect the security of information contained in automated systems throughout the organization.

Government can extend into healthcare business practices in a number of potential ways. Goldsmith, Blumenthal, and Rishel (2003) argue for the need for government-sanctioned and government-supported standardization of at least communication protocols and nomenclature. Without a direct government role, healthcare organizations will adopt technology slowly and in a haphazard fashion. Blumenthal (2006) provides three business arguments justifying government intervention. First, no compelling business case exists for investment in HIT. Better performance is not routinely rewarded in healthcare, and, in fact, poor performance and providing more services generate greater revenue. The savings from implementing HIT do not go to providers but rather benefit insurers and others. Second, for real system benefits to be seen, all components of the fragmented US healthcare delivery system must participate. Without this participation, benefits are incomplete. Interoperability among providers is a necessary step for true sharing to occur, and government needs to impose common communication standards. Third, fraud-and-abuse regulations do not allow physicians to receive subsidies from hospitals. Blumenthal (2006) makes a strong case for the failure of the market to achieve the desired results, and thus government must become more actively involved. HIT leadership must be aware of specific government interventions to effectively manage their organization.

The bottom line is that government has intervened in healthcare markets in significant ways, such as through the Health Insurance Portability and Accountability Act (HIPAA), Health Information Technology for Economic and Clinical Health (HITECH) Act, and the Patient Protection and Affordable Care Act (ACA). The issue with regard to HIT intervention, however, is still somewhat open, but a growing body of evidence suggests that HIT investment will have positive results (Buntin et al. 2011). Economic recovery funding through the HITECH Act implicitly assumes that this investment is good for quality and potentially for cost savings.

Specific Healthcare Legislations

Health Insurance Portability and Accountability Act

As an example of legislation that has had far-reaching effects on HIT, HIPAA has no equal. Begun as a mechanism to ensure that individuals could retain access to health insurance when they changed jobs (portability) (Flores and Dodier 2005; Schmeida 2005), HIPAA also contains a second provision called *administrative simplification* that has far greater impact (CMS 2005a):

> The Administrative Simplification provisions of the Health Insurance Portability and Accountability Act of 1996 (HIPAA, Title II) required the Department of Health and Human Services (HHS) to establish national standards for electronic healthcare transactions and national identifiers for providers, health plans, and employers. It also addressed the security and privacy of health data. As the industry adopts these standards for the efficiency and effectiveness of the nation's healthcare system will improve the use of electronic data interchange.

As this general provision indicates, HIPAA anticipated the development of electronic record keeping in healthcare. The healthcare field was not able internally to develop the standards and rules governing these new technologies for collecting, storing, and transmitting health information (another example of potential market failure mentioned earlier). Many realized that strict government controls would have to be put in place to enable healthcare providers to develop systems that met internal needs and facilitated the transfer of information across institutions (Blumenthal 2006; Goldsmith, Blumenthal, and Rishel 2003; Kleinke 2005). The electronic medium also raised concerns with security and privacy that the government felt it should address. In simple terms, administrative simplification involved setting standards, mandating health plan and provider compliance, and establishing privacy elements (CMS 2005b).

The complete text of HIPAA's Summary of Administrative Simplification Provisions is provided in Exhibit 3.3. Each of the five provisions presented in the exhibit is important because of what it implies. While the translation of these broad provisions to policy details has evolved incrementally since the passage of HIPAA in 1996, the details are now emerging as a result of a series of negotiations among all of the interested parties. Exhibit 3.4 shows the eight components of the administrative simplification provisions that were promulgated to meet the five provisions listed in Exhibit 3.3.

The HIPAA overview reveals specific details of these standards and the timing of their implementation (CMS 2005a). Steps to achieving the goals of improving patient quality and enhancing efficiency through the use of electronic records were developed in stages. The first step was to make employers obtain a national identification number for healthcare transactions. Next, providers were required to have a commonly determined standard identifier—the National Provider Identifier (NPI). These rules set the stage for creating a regional or national data set of electronic information transmission by uniquely identifying the payer source and the provider. This seems

EXHIBIT 3.3
HIPAA's
Summary of
Administrative
Simplification
Provisions

Standards for electronic health information transactions. Within 18 months of enactment, the Secretary of HHS is required to adopt standards from among those already approved by private standards developing organizations for certain electronic health transactions, including claims, enrollment, eligibility, payment, and coordination of benefits. These standards also must address the security of electronic health information systems.

Mandate on providers and health plans, and timetable. Providers and health plans are required to use the standards for the specified electronic transactions 24 months after they are adopted. Plans and providers may comply directly, or may use a health care clearinghouse. Certain health plans, in particular workers compensation, are not covered.

Privacy. The Secretary is required to recommend privacy standards for health information to Congress 12 months after enactment. If Congress does not enact privacy legislation within 3 years of enactment, the Secretary shall promulgate privacy regulations for individually identifiable electronic health information.

Pre-emption of state law. The bill supersedes state laws, except where the Secretary determines that the State law is necessary to prevent fraud and abuse, to ensure appropriate state regulation of insurance or health plans, addresses controlled substances, or for other purposes. If the Secretary promulgates privacy regulations, those regulations do not pre-empt state laws that impose more stringent requirements. These provisions do not limit a State's ability to require health plan reporting or audits.

Penalties. The bill imposes civil money penalties and prison for certain violations.

NOTE: Provisions in the original legislation have been modified by subsequent legislation, including the ACA.
SOURCE: Reprinted from CMS (2005b).

EXHIBIT 3.4
Eight Major
Components
of HIPAA
Administrative
Simplification
Provisions

1. Employer-identifier standard
2. Enforcement
3. National provider-identifier standard
4. Security standard
5. Transaction and code sets standard
6. Place-of-service codes for HIPAA transactions
7. Health insurance reform for consumers (HIPAA Title I)
8. Medicaid HIPAA administrative simplification

SOURCE: Information from CMS (2005a).

insignificant when viewed from within a healthcare organization because they have always used unique numbers to identify patients and to keep patient records distinct. The NPI was novel when applied across organizations, however. The timing of the NPI mandate is current in relation to this discussion in that after May 23, 2007, "healthcare providers may only use their NPIs to identify themselves in standard transactions" (CMS 2005c).

Transactions and *code set standards* warrant additional commentary because they are so vital to the effective implementation and use of the electronic record. The precise definition of these standards is also still in flux. According to the Centers for Medicare & Medicaid Services (CMS 2005d),

> Transactions are activities involving the transfer of healthcare information for specific purposes. Under the Health Insurance Portability & Accountability Act of 1996 (HIPAA), if a healthcare provider engages in one of the identified transactions, they must comply with the standard for that transaction. HIPAA requires every provider who does business electronically to use the same healthcare transactions, code sets, and identifiers. HIPAA has identified ten standard transactions for Electronic Data Interchange (EDI) for the transmission of healthcare data. Claims and encounter information, payment and remittance advice, and claims status and inquiry are several of the standard transactions. Code sets are the codes used to identify specific diagnosis and clinical procedures on claims and encounter forms. The HCPCS, CPT-4 and ICD-9 codes with which providers are familiar, are examples of code sets for procedures and diagnose.

This generic statement gives rise to an array of specific rules designed to enable organizations to collect data in a consistent manner. Unless everyone uses a common nomenclature for defining all clinical and administrative terms, there will be no capacity to communicate. *Interoperability* is the term that describes the goal to its fullest extent. To assist providers and others in this pursuit, CMS has provided information on the web that can be easily accessed and applied. The posted information is a series of checklists to be used by healthcare organizations to determine their readiness; download the information from www.cms.gov/Regulations-and-Guidance/HIPAA -Administrative-Simplification/EducationMaterials/Educational-Materials .html. In addition, CMS makes available a series of ten documents, listed in Exhibit 3.5, to assist organizations in dealing with issues appropriate to their particular need. (Discussing these documents is beyond the scope of this book; however, HIT leadership must be aware of their existence and importance.)

The Need for Information Privacy and Security

HIT "systems contain sensitive information. Clinical systems process medical information about individual patients; human resources information systems

EXHIBIT 3.5
Checklist Aids
for Transactions
and Code Set
Development

The HIPAA Information Series for Providers consists of ten papers that can aid healthcare organizations in transactions and code-sets development as well as other HIPAA issues:

• HIPAA 101
• Are You a Covered Entity?
• Key HIPAA Dates and Tips
• What Electronic Transactions and Code Sets Are Standardized Under HIPAA?
• Is Your Software Vendor or Billing Service Ready for HIPAA?
• What to Expect from Your Health Plans
• What You Need to Know About Testing
• Trading Partner
• Final Steps for Compliance with Electronic Transactions and Code Sets
• Enforcement

These documents can be downloaded from www.cms.gov/Regulations-and-Guidance/HIPAA-Administrative-Simplification/EducationMaterials/Educational-Materials.html.

contain personal information about employees; and financial and decision-support systems include proprietary data used for planning, marketing, and management of the enterprise" (Stahl 2003). HIPAA has placed special emphasis on privacy, and the implications of safeguarding privacy to HIT leadership are expansive.

To give some idea of the nature and extent of privacy and security issues even after HIPAA's enactment, the Health Privacy Project (www.healthprivacy.org) has compiled anecdotes reported in the national press. The sheer number of events suggests their importance. In 2012 *Healthcare Finance News* reported the top ten security breaches for that year (McNickle 2012). These breaches affected many institutions, including the Utah Department of Health, Emory Healthcare, and the University of Arkansas for Medical Sciences. Following are examples from the Health Privacy Project's (2007) web publication, *Health Privacy Stories*:

• "The California state Department of Health Services inadvertently revealed the names and addresses of up to 53 people enrolled in an AIDS drug assistance program to other enrollees by putting benefit notification letters in the wrong envelopes. . . . The department learned about the mix-up after 12 people in the drug assistance program phoned to say they had received letters addressed to someone else. . . . The department is looking into ways to make the system more foolproof, such as using envelopes with window addresses, said health services Director Sandra Shewry. HIV/AIDS services and advocacy groups said this was the first known breach of that database. 'I would hope this is an anomaly,' said Jeff Bailey, director of client services for AIDS Project Los Angeles" (Engel 2007).

- "A desktop computer containing personal information for up to 38,000 patients treated at Veterans Affairs Department medical centers in Pittsburgh and Philadelphia over the past four years was reported missing from the Reston, VA offices of VA contractor Unisys Corp. The VA and Unisys [say] the computer contained names, addresses, Social Security numbers and dates of birth. It may also have included insurance carrier and billing information, claims data and medical information" (Robeznieks 2006a).

Needless to say, ensuring the security of clinical information systems must be a top priority for healthcare leaders and HIT managers alike. Clinical information systems refer to the following types of health and healthcare records:

1. *Patient care systems* include information technology used in the course of providing care, services, or treatments, such as order entry and results reporting; electronic medical records; and lab, pharmacy, and radiology systems. Data contained in these systems—including medical histories, medication lists, physician orders, diagnoses, treatment plans, and test results—are extremely private and thus should be accessible only to those involved in care delivery. Breach of security in this instance has legal and ethical ramifications for the healthcare delivery organization.

2. *Public health information systems*, according to Stahl (2003), "support disease prevention and surveillance programs. Protecting public health requires the acquisition and storage of health-related information about individuals. Public health benefits sometimes conflict with threats to individual privacy. Individuals concerned about privacy who avoid clinical tests and treatments may endanger the health of others in the community." For example, a person with a sexually transmitted infection may opt to not test and/or report the presence of the infection, which could then lead to the spread of the disease (Gostin, Hodge, and Valdiserri 2001). A security breach of public health information systems could lead to a person or groups facing discrimination in employment or insurance eligibility.

3. *Medical research information systems* are repositories of medical diagnoses, health conditions, disease data, risk factors, and other health-related details culled from patient records. The purpose of such a

system is to enable clinical researchers and other investigators to understand disease risks, patterns, and contributing factors observed in a patient population. Lau and Catchpole (2001) emphasized the importance of respecting the patients' privacy rights as well as protecting the information contained in these systems by restricting access and use to authorized personnel.

Following are some of the ways healthcare delivery organizations have addressed privacy concerns to comply with HIPAA standards:

- Form HIPAA task forces.
- Install a new compliance office or function dedicated to managing HIPAA-related challenges, or designate an existing office or function (e.g., chief information officer, medical records, risk management) to address or prevent issues (Marietti 2002).
- Use information system software designed by a vendor to meet the specific purpose, needs, and concerns identified by the organization. In this way, HIPAA patches to existing programs, and some in-house work is required to ensure the applications interface with one another (Wilson and McPherson 2002).
- Implement changes to some business processes and procedures. Marietti (2002, 55) projected that "80 percent to 85 percent of HIPAA compliance issues will depend on adjusting human behavior."

Findings from studies of the HIPAA regulations have emerged. First, the immediate impact has been on the research community. Evidence suggests that HIPAA compliance makes recruitment and retention of subjects into research projects more difficult (Wipke-Tevis and Pickett 2008). Second, some specific examples now exist regarding how process improvements (automated access verification) can assist organizations to demonstrate compliance (Hill 2006). Third, the change process is still incomplete because privacy and security rules are being revised/updated frequently, such as a new rule announced in January 2013 (HHS 2013). Checklists are still being published to help organizations meet HIPAA requirements (HIPAA Survival Guide 2013).

A number of studies have examined the impact of privacy rules on healthcare organizations, giving rise to a set of inappropriate responses (as observed by consultants) related to privacy (Upham and Dorsey 2007). Some concerns center on the application of privacy rules to other activities or innovations in healthcare. For example, in 2007 Paul Tang, then the chair of the board of the American Medical Informatics Association, indicated that electronic health record vendors often included contract provisions that may require providers to violate patient privacy standards (Conn 2007). Similarly, in the wake of mass tragedies, access to the perpetrator's health record often is cited as a reason to relax privacy constraints. Peel (2007) discussed this issue in the context of the Virginia Tech massacre in April 2007, in which a student killed 32 people on that campus. Peel concluded that privacy constraints would not likely prevent these events. More recently, there is the case of James Holmes—the gunman who opened fire at an Aurora, Colorado, movie theater, killing 12 and injuring about 50 people. Prior to the shooting, Holmes was reportedly being seen by a mental health specialist at the University of Colorado, where Holmes was a student (Meyer and Ingold 2012). The specialist contacted a university threat-assessment team but did not invoke a "72-hour psychiatric hold" because Holmes was leaving the university. Under pressure from news sources that are trying to piece together the events that led up to the tragedy, the University of Colorado released thousands of e-mails related to Holmes. However, the university did not make available any records or documents related to the crime or Holmes's mental health status (Meyer and Ingold 2012). As consumers continue to provide information over the Internet, the collection, availability, and security of their data will remain a major concern (Nelson 2006).

At the level of information sharing across organizations was a study commissioned by the California Healthcare Foundation to look at privacy from the perspective of developing regional health information organizations (RHIOs). The study was trying to determine what needed to be done at the systems level to facilitate RHIO development. It resulted in a number of findings and substantial recommendations on developing and implementing security policies for RHIOs. The analyses identified the following four key questions that must be addressed to develop privacy policies (Rosenfeld, Koss, and Siler 2007):

1. Who will have access to patient information?
2. Which information will be accessible?
3. What are acceptable purposes of patient information exchange?
4. What circumstances justify patient information exchange?

In addition, the study reported a number of common elements that are important to consider in developing privacy policies across organizational entities, including the following:

- Privacy policies are local.
- Organizations participating in the RHIO influence the privacy policies.
- Privacy policies need to be developed early and revisited often.
- Work on privacy policies is ongoing.

- Privacy policies are unique to the environment; thus, best practices have yet to follow.
- Building consensus on privacy policies takes time.
- The consumer role in privacy policy development is limited.

HIPAA was not the first effort by government to assure the public that the privacy of an individual's medical information would be secure. The Privacy Act of 1974 established key provisions to protect the privacy of patients (CMS 2005e). Enacted before the conception of electronic health records prevalent today, the legislation protected all patient records with "personal identifiers" (social security number or other). Under the Privacy Act, every patient can access and, if necessary, correct his or her individual records, and it generally prohibits disclosure of these records—but that applied only to federal agencies.

The individual's right to genetic privacy was also addressed in Oregon's Genetic Privacy Act of 1995, which provides legal protection for medical information, tissue samples, and DNA samples. Harris and Keywood (2001, 415) pointed out that individuals "have a powerful interest in genetic privacy and its associated claim to ignorance"; however, "any claims to be shielded from information about the self must compete on equal terms with claims based in the rights and interests of others." Further, Cummings and Magnusson (2001, 1089) stated that "As genetic privacy legislation is developed and enacted at state and federal levels, the needs of individuals must be balanced with the needs of institutions and of research in the larger context of societal needs."

Now, the Patient Protection and Affordable Care Act of 2010 has increased the rigor of the HIPAA rules further by requiring a unique Health Plan Identifier and both standards and rules for financial transactions.

Health Information Technology for Economic and Clinical Health Act

President Obama signed the American Recovery and Reinvestment Act (ARRA) in February 2009. This comprehensive stimulus package is designed to address the 2007–2009 economic crisis. ARRA contains many provisions, including tax relief (federal); unemployment benefit expansion; social welfare spending; and spending for specific sectors such as energy, education, and healthcare. The healthcare spending is diverse, allocating funds or subsidies for Medicaid, health research and construction, benefits for the newly uninsured, prevention and wellness, and research on the effectiveness of healthcare treatments, among many other provisions.

A major part of ARRA is called the Health Information Technology for Economic and Clinical Health (HITECH) Act. It is designed to promote the expansion of the electronic health record (EHR) because of its perceived social benefits. A total of about $22 billion was allocated to the HITECH Act, with the bulk ($19.2 billion) devoted directly to EHR adoption. An additional $2 billion went to the Office of the National Coordinator for Health Information Technology (ONCHIT 2011) to support the agency's varied activities for promoting information exchange, training health professionals for information technology, and enhancing interoperability. ONCHIT is the body responsible for implementing the incentives for EHR use and establishing an HIT Policy Committee and an HIT Standards Committee. These committees are charged with developing recommendations for adopting health information infrastructure and standards for information exchange, respectively (Recovery.gov n.d.).

Adoption of EHR

From a broad social perspective and consistent with our earlier justification for government intervention, the benefits of the meaningful use of EHRs include the following, as identified by HealthIT.gov (n.d.):

- Complete and accurate information
- Better access to information
- Patient empowerment

One can argue whether the government or private sector is better at realizing these goals, but some opine that the benefits of sharable electronic information accrue to society at large and thus cannot be fully captured by any private provider or organization. Consequently, investing in this public good can be justified.

Meaningful Use

The HITECH Act provides the authority to make changes that can improve healthcare quality, safety, and efficiency through the use of EHR and the exchange of electronic health information. ONCHIT has released regulations to define appropriate standards for the certification of EHR technologies and the means by which providers can receive financial incentives to adopt and use those systems (see www.healthit.gov/policy-researchers-implementers /about-certification). An example of one of the many features of the HITECH Act is the meaningful use provision, which offers incentives to organizations that adopt and implement EHRs. The underlying assumption is that EHRs can provide benefits to providers and patients. The benefits may not be realized, however, without sufficient intensity of use. Consequently, CMS developed a set of standards called *meaningful use*. These standards allow hospitals and individual providers deemed eligible to obtain incentive payments by meeting specific criteria; the incentives for adoption by clinical professionals are substantial, as seen in Exhibit 3.6.

For professionals applying in 2011, the maximum payment was $44,000 over the period. Notice the built-in incentives to begin the process early: The initial payment was lower for eligible professionals who delayed EHR. Eligible professionals for Medicare's incentive program include doctors of medicine, osteopathy, dentistry, podiatry, optometry, and chiropractic medicine. For Medicaid, the professionals who may participate include nurse practitioners, certified nurse midwifes, and select physician assistants. Hospitals eligible for participation in Medicare incentives include those receiving inpatient prospective payment, critical access hospitals, and Medicare

EXHIBIT 3.6
CMS Meaningful Use Incentive Payment Schedule for Medicare-Eligible Professionals

Payment Amounts	If a Medicare-Eligible Professional Qualifies to Receive First Payment in 2011	If a Medicare-Eligible Professional Qualifies to Receive First Payment in 2012	If a Medicare-Eligible Professional Qualifies to Receive First Payment in 2013	If a Medicare-Eligible Professional Qualifies to Receive First Payment in 2014	If a Medicare-Eligible Professional Qualifies to Receive First Payment in 2015
Payment amount for 2011	$18,000				
Payment amount for 2012	$12,000	$18,000			
Payment amount for 2013	$8,000	$12,000	$15,000		
Payment amount for 2014	$4,000	$8,000	$12,000	$12,000	
Payment amount for 2015	$2,000	$4,000	$8,000	$8,000	
Payment amount for 2016		$2,000	$4,000	$4,000	
Total Payment Amount	$44,000	$44,000	$39,000	$24,000	

SOURCE: CMS (n.d.[a], 2010b).

Advantage hospitals. Medicaid qualifications include inpatient hospitals with 10 percent Medicaid patient volume or any children's hospital.

The catch in EHR incentive participation is that the level of use must be deemed "meaningful." Incentive payments come in three stages. Stage 1 (implemented in the 2011–2012 period) involves installing certified information systems that capture structured patient data and give the ability to share that data with the patient or other healthcare professionals. Stage 2 (scheduled for 2014) requires more collection and reporting to advance clinical processes. Stage 3 (scheduled for 2016) requires actual improved outcomes. The HIT requirement for meaningful use is clearly detailed in Stage 1. Eligible providers must report providing all 15 Core Measures, a choice of 5 out of 10 menu objectives, and 6 clinical quality measures. The 15 Core Measures are listed in Exhibit 3.7. Each of the core measures has detailed definitions and reporting requirements. Consult this government publication for the specifications: www.cms.gov/EHRIncentivePrograms/Downloads/EP-MU-TOC.pdf. As an example, the following is the specification for the measure computerized physician order entry (CPOE):

> Requirement: More than 30 percent of unique patients with at least one medication in the medication list and seen by the eligible professional must have at least one medication entered using CPOE. You can be excluded from this core measure if you write fewer than 100 prescriptions during the reporting period.

EXHIBIT 3.7
15 Core Measures for CMS Meaningful Use Standards for Eligible Professionals

1. Implement computerized physician order entry
2. Perform drug–drug and drug–allergy checks
3. Maintain up-to-date problem list of current and active diagnoses
4. Use e-prescribing (eRx)
5. Maintain active medication list
6. Maintain active medication allergy list
7. Record demographics
8. Record and chart changes in vital signs
9. Record smoking status for patients aged 13 or older
10. Report ambulatory clinical quality measures to CMS/states
11. Implement clinical decision support
12. Provide patients with an electronic copy of their health information, upon request
13. Provide clinical summaries for patients for each office visit
14. Establish capability to exchange key clinical information
15. Protect electronic health information

SOURCE: CMS (2010a).

The ten menu objectives (see Exhibit 3.8) are also required, and their specifications are found on the website mentioned earlier. While this list of objectives gives you some choice, the first two are public health–oriented and thus one of the two must be selected. Basically, meaningful use demands that providers demonstrate that they can effectively communicate population-based information from their practice.

Eligible professionals also must report six clinical quality measures. Three of the six are core, and the three others can be selected from a large list of measures (see Exhibit 3.9). The three primary and three alternate core measures (which are available should the primary measures not apply to the provider's patient population) include the following:

- Primary measures
  - Hypertension: Blood pressure measurement
  - Preventive care and screening: Tobacco use assessment and tobacco cessation intervention
  - Adult weight screening and follow-up
- Alternate measures
  - Weight assessment and counseling for children and adolescents
  - Preventive care and screening: Influenza immunization for patients aged 50 or older
  - Childhood immunization status

The remaining three quality measures must be selected from the 38 measures listed in Exhibit 3.9.

EXHIBIT 3.8
10 Menu Objectives for CMS Meaningful Use Standards

1. Submit electronic data to immunization registries
2. Submit electronic syndromic surveillance data to public health agencies
3. Perform drug formulary checks
4. Incorporate clinical lab-test results
5. Generate lists of patients by specific conditions
6. Send reminders to patients for preventive/follow-up care
7. Provide patient-specific education resources
8. Provide electronic access to health information for patients
9. Perform medication reconciliation
10. Maintain summary-of-care record for transitions of care

SOURCE: CMS (2010a).

The set of reporting requirements that apply to eligible hospitals includes 14 core measures, 5 of 10 menu objectives, and 15 quality measures. Details on these items are found in the following documents posted on the CMS website (www.cms.gov/Regulations-and-Guidance/Legislation/EHR IncentivePrograms/Meaningful_Use.html):

- ALL Stage 1 EHR Meaningful Use Specification Sheets for Eligible Hospitals
- Hospital Attestation Worksheet
- Critical Access Hospital Payment Tip Sheet
- EHR Incentive Program for Medicare Hospitals
- EHR Incentive Program for Critical Access Hospitals—Spanish Version
- Medicaid Hospital Incentive Payments Calculations

We have only discussed Stage 1 of meaningful use. Stages 2 and 3 are on the books but are not yet fully developed, and Stage 2 meaningful use core and menu measures were not released until October 2012 and are not scheduled to be implemented until fiscal year 2014. Those working with HIT *must* know where to go for the latest information, as these requirements are updated and revised occasionally. This website offers relevant information: www.cms.gov/Regulations-and-Guidance/Legislation/EHRIncentivePro grams/Stage_2.html.

The evidence of the impact of EHR adoption for hospitals and physicians is disappointing, despite the financial incentives and emphasis. Davis (2009) reports, using detailed HIMSS Analytics databases, that by 2008 few hospitals had attained any of the top four levels of adoption. Only 5.8 percent of respondents reported implementing CPOE and clinical decision support

---

1. Diabetes: Hemoglobin A1c poor control
2. Diabetes: Low-density lipoprotein (LDL) management and control
3. Diabetes: Blood pressure management
4. Heart failure (HF): Angiotensin-converting enzyme (ACE) inhibitor or angiotensin receptor blocker (ARB) therapy for left ventricular systolic dysfunction (LVSD)
5. Coronary artery disease (CAD): Beta-blocker therapy for CAD patients with prior myocardial infarction (MI)
6. Pneumonia vaccination status for older adults
7. Breast cancer screening
8. Colorectal cancer screening

EXHIBIT 3.9
Clinical Quality Measures for CMS Meaningful Use Standards

(continued)

EXHIBIT 3.9
Clinical Quality
Measures for
CMS Meaningful
Use Standards
(*continued*)

9. Coronary artery disease (CAD): Oral antiplatelet therapy prescribed for patients with CAD

10. Heart failure (HF): Beta-blocker therapy for LVSD

11. Antidepressant medication management: (a) effective acute phase treatment, (b) effective continuation phase treatment

12. Primary open angle glaucoma (POAG): Optic nerve evaluation

13. Diabetic retinopathy: Documentation of presence or absence of macular edema and level of severity of retinopathy

14. Diabetic retinopathy: Communication with the physician managing ongoing diabetes care

15. Asthma pharmacologic therapy

16. Asthma assessment

17. Appropriate testing for children with pharyngitis

18. Oncology breast cancer: Hormonal therapy for stage IC-IIIC estrogen receptor/progesterone receptor (ER/PR) positive breast cancer

19. Oncology colon cancer: Chemotherapy for stage III colon cancer patients

20. Prostate cancer: Avoidance of overuse of bone scan for staging low-risk prostate cancer patients

21. Smoking and tobacco use cessation, medical assistance:
    (a) Advising smokers and tobacco users to quit
    (b) Discussing smoking and tobacco use cessation medications
    (c) Discussing smoking and tobacco use cessation strategies

22. Diabetes: Eye exam

23. Diabetes: Urine screening

24. Diabetes: Foot exam

25. Coronary artery disease (CAD): Drug therapy for lowering LDL cholesterol

26. Heart failure (HF): Warfarin therapy patients with atrial fibrillation

27. Ischemic vascular disease (IVD): Blood pressure management

28. Ischemic vascular disease (IVD): Use of aspirin or another antithrombotic

29. Initiation and engagement of alcohol and other drug-dependence treatment:
    (a) initiation, (b) engagement

30. Prenatal care: Screening for human immunodeficiency virus (HIV)

31. Prenatal care: Anti-D immune globulin

32. Controlling high blood pressure

33. Cervical cancer screening

34. Chlamydia screening for women

35. Use of appropriate medications for asthma

36. Low back pain: Use of imaging studies

37. Ischemic vascular disease (IVD): Complete lipid panel and LDL control

38. Diabetes: Hemoglobin A1c control (<8.0%)

SOURCE: CMS (2010a).

systems, which are level 4 or higher. Nearly 16 percent of respondents had not yet installed laboratory information systems, pharmacy information systems, or radiology information systems, which are the minimum necessary to advance from the bottom level of EHR adoption. Davis concluded that for hospitals to meet meaningful use criteria by 2013, they had to have reached at least level 4. The numbers for physicians were equally discouraging. EHR adoption in US hospitals and physician practices lags in comparison with adoption rates in other industrialized countries (Jha et al. 2008).

Patient Protection and Affordable Care Act

No single legislation in the past several years represents the government's attempt to address a host of social problems in healthcare more than the Patient Protection and Affordable Care Act. Signed on March 23, 2010, HR 3590 and the accompanying HR 4872 (Health Care and Education Reconciliation Act of 2010) proposed historic changes to the US healthcare delivery and financing system. Designed to expand coverage, the ACA contains a host of provisions with short-term and far-reaching implications. Due to its size, however, most individuals tend to focus on issues of importance to them only. For example, the American Hospital Association (2010) released a summary highlighting eight key features of the legislation important to AHA's constituents:

1. Coverage: expansion of insurance to more than 30 million Americans
2. Delivery system reforms: changes in incentives facing providers to enhance quality, reduce costs, and improve care coordination; this section has the accountable care organization authorization
3. Medicare and Medicaid payment: efforts to reduce the rate of increased spending on these programs, with hospitals being the major target; provisions for a drug discount program, payments to rural hospitals, and enhancements to primary care physicians are also included here
4. Workforce and graduate medical education: expansion and alteration of workforce training to alleviate the shortages in select portions of the healthcare workforce
5. Wellness and prevention: allocation of resources to the Prevention and Public Health Fund and insurer requirement to cover immunizations and screenings with zero cost sharing
6. Quality, disparities, and comparative effectiveness: begins the movement to pay for quality and penalties for hospital-acquired conditions
7. Regulatory oversight: provisions to identify and reduce fraud and abuse, including the continuation of the RAC audits
8. Revenue: to pay for much of these features, the law taxes high cost health insurance plans and imposes fees on select industries

Many of the ACA features cause stress for HIT, but the following deserve special mention. First, accountable care organizations (ACOs) assign responsibility (accountability) to the organization for patients who may not obtain all or even most of their care from the host organization (Kaiser 2012; Miller 2009). Finding the patient, effectively exchanging information with other providers, and ensuring the privacy and confidentiality of that information outside of organizational boundaries are a challenge. That information is exchanged both ways, so even if the institution is not sponsoring an ACO, it may be asked to provide clinical information on select patients.

Second, pay-for-performance initiatives demand greater linkages between provider cost and clinical performance than is customary (Rosenthal and Dudley 2007; Rosenthal and Camillus 2007). The discussion in Chapter 4, regarding management across organizational boundaries, is put to the test as clinical (chief medical officers and chief nursing officers) and financial (chief financial officers) leaders demand accurate and timely data for evaluation, improvement, and contracting purposes.

Third, expansion of covered lives is taxing to HIT in a number of ways. Having more patients can be a minor stressor, but (depending on current capacity) sufficient volume growth might require added facilities. In addition, at least some new patients are likely to be unfamiliar with the delivery system and thus less compliant with completing forms and documentations necessary to manage the care process. Further, some added patients may be "sicker" and may present new problems to the clinicians, testing the provider's documentation, coding quality, and select systems in unforeseen ways.

Fourth, as Gawande (2010) pointed out, there is a host of pushback efforts to the ACA as there was to Medicare and Medicaid decades before, which emphasizes Gawande's argument that "the battle for health-care reform has only begun." More than any individual ACA feature causing concern for HIT leadership is that the timing of implementation is highly uncertain. Planning for an unknown future makes life difficult for HIT management, but that may justify the salary that HIT leadership receives.

HIT Leadership Roles

While government involvement through HIPAA, the HITECH Act, and the ACA may seem difficult for information technology specialists to fully understand, it is particularly baffling for those outside of HIT. The consequence of this difficulty is that it requires HIT leadership (chief information officer [CIO] and others) to understand, anticipate, and explain the impact of these legislations. They must be prepared for new and/or changes in government regulations and policies by developing and then implementing a number of activities and programs, including comprehensive environmental scanning and organizational education, information security policies and procedures, disaster preparedness and recovery planning, and information privacy and confidentiality protection.

Environmental Scanning and Organizational Education

The first responsibility of HIT leadership is to fully understand the operational and resource implications of all legislations. Internally, the team must understand what it has to do differently as a result and determine what extra staffing, expertise (consultants), hardware and software, and time are needed. The steps for this activity are as follows:

1. Determine breadth and scope of impending or current legislation.
2. Assess current organizational readiness for the impact.
3. Perform a gap analysis within the organization.
4. Recommend strategies to meet legal/regulatory changes.
    a. Develop staffing and critical expertise needed to address changes:
    b. Specify hardware and software needs.
    c. Estimate total financial implications of the recommendations.
5. Identify clinical and other resources within the organization that are necessary in meeting the standards.
6. Outline a timeline for implementation with key dates and milestones.

Naturally, difficulty may be encountered in effectively accomplishing these tasks once the legislation is in place and the deadlines are looming. Consequently, HIT leadership should be constantly monitoring the horizon for proposed legislation to get a head start on planning for its passage. To do this, HIT leadership should be engaged with those responsible for legislative affairs within the organization (if such a role exists). Getting a "heads up" from this source is vital. State and national associations—such as the Healthcare Information and Management Systems Society, American College of Healthcare Executives, Healthcare Financial Management Association, and American Hospital Association, among many others—are good sources of this "pre" data. A body of literature is available as well that documents the many and varied impacts of HIPAA, the HITECH Act, and the ACA. It is important for HIT leadership, either directly or through surrogates, to monitor and stay up-to-date on this literature. For example, Houser, Houser, and Shewchuk (2007) use the nominal group technique (NGT) for gathering information regarding the impact of HIPAA privacy rules on the release of patient information. "The NGT approach is a consumer-oriented formal brainstorming or idea-generating technique that is assumed to foster creativity and to be particularly effective in helping group members articulate meaningful disclosures in response to specific questions" (Houser, Houser, and Shewchuk 2007, 2).

Because the nature of government legislation, such as HIPAA, can be highly complex, HIT leadership should be prepared to educate senior leadership on the implications of these regulatory interventions. Senior leadership includes the chief executive officer as well as the chief operating officer (if the organization has that position), chief medical officer, chief nursing officer, and chief financial officer. Generally, the person responsible for strategic planning, the head of the legal department, the head of human resources, and the head of development should be educated also in HIT-related legislative matters.

Information Security Policies and Procedures

Healthcare organizations must establish enterprisewide standards to maintain data security and protect the privacy and confidentiality of information, particularly patient records. Data security involves two essential elements: (1) protecting against system failures or external catastrophic events, such as fires, storms, deliberate sabotage, and other destructive acts of man and nature that could result in critical information being lost, and (2) controlling access to computer files by unauthorized personnel.

Disaster Preparedness and Recovery Planning

The HIT steering committee must ensure that effective data backup and recovery procedures are implemented at all processing sites throughout the organization. Critical data files should be copied to removable disk packs or tapes and stored in a secure location away from the processing sites, preferably in a different building. The CIO should develop a data backup plan for approval by the steering committee. The plan should specify which files require duplication and how often backup procedures should be conducted. Recovery procedures to be used if catastrophic events occur should also be included.

The need for disaster planning was underscored by the terrorist attacks in New York City on September 11, 2001. If that event was not convincing, Hurricane Katrina and the resulting challenges surely were. Disaster plans must be implemented, tested periodically, and refined. Testing of the plan provides training for employees and helps identify shortcomings in technology and procedures before they need to be used. A disaster-plan notebook should be developed and stored at the healthcare facility, at an off-site storage location, and at the homes of key employees who are involved in recovery procedures (Vecchio 2000).

Consultants can be used to assist in disaster planning and recovery. For example, IRM International offers a disaster recovery program that includes four phases: assessment, documentation consolidation, disaster plan development, and testing and refinement. See www.irminternational.com/rptcard .html for a disaster recovery report card that rates disaster-planning readiness.

In addition, data can be lost through computer viruses, which are increasingly prevalent and destructive. Each computer program should be inspected by virus-protection software every time the program is run. Acquisition of software should be subject to central review and approval, and particular care must be exercised to ensure that software downloaded from the Internet or obtained over networks is scanned and proven to be virus free. All incoming e-mail messages should be scanned for viruses, and employees should be trained not to open suspicious files attached to an e-mail, text, or any other electronic communication.

Information Privacy and Confidentiality Protection

As suggested in the earlier discussion related to HIPAA, the HITECH Act, and the ACA, protecting information privacy and confidentiality should be a major concern of the HIT leadership. A comprehensive information security policy should include three elements: (1) physical security, (2) technical controls over access, and (3) management policies that are well known and enforced in all organizational units (Stahl 2003) (see Exhibit 3.10).

Understanding the processes of information privacy and confidentiality is not a necessary step to successful implementation at the systems level. While the past decade offers many examples of how individual systems have accomplished these goals, evidence indicates that many organizations are still not compliant with basic security standards (Davis and Having 2006). Some in the healthcare field have called for systematic incentives from industry or insurers to induce organizations to adopt privacy and security technology (e.g., Lang 2006). Despite substantial improvements, however, violations of basic privacy rights by hospitals and other providers are still a challenge (Hiltzik 2012). For an up-to-date list of privacy rule violations and settlements, see www.hhs.gov/ocr/office/news/index.html.

Physical Security	Technical Safeguards	Management Policies
Hardware	Passwords	Written security policy
Data files	Encryption	Employee training
	Audit logs	Disciplinary actions for violations

EXHIBIT 3.10
Components of Information Security

Prior to implementation of HIPAA standards, the Mayo Clinic, based in Rochester, Minnesota, developed a comprehensive set of plans to keep electronic medical records secure. A multidisciplinary team formulated the policy and provided management oversight of the security program. Leaders of the Mayo Clinic effort suggested that a confidentiality policy should include the following elements (Olson, Peters, and Stewart 1998, 29):

- Access rights—who has access and for what reasons
- Release of information to the patient, other healthcare providers, and third parties
- Special handling, if any, for specific information (e.g., HIV results, psychiatric notes)
- Special handling, if any, for particular patients (e.g., employees or VIPs)
- Availability of medical information, including retention policies
- Integrity of medical information, including authentication, completeness, and handling of revisions or addenda
- Approved methods for communication of medical information

Summary

This chapter presents three major ideas. First, it presents and explores government's role in HIT. Government intervention in business processes can be justified if markets fail in their role of allocating scarce resources. Understanding why government gets involved assists healthcare and HIT leaders in responding to legislation and anticipating future actions. In healthcare, there are compelling reasons for government intervention, including a weak business case for information technology investment by providers, system fragmentation and lack of interoperability, and regulatory restrictions from fraud-and-abuse standards.

Second, the chapter explores specific legislations—HIPAA, the HITECH Act, and the ACA. These major government legislative and administrative interventions have fundamentally changed HIT. Passed by the US Congress in 1996, HIPAA—particularly two of its components—has a direct impact on healthcare information systems. The administrative simplification provisions of the law are designed to improve efficiency in the healthcare system by establishing uniform, national standards to be used for the electronic transmission of certain financial and administrative transactions. The privacy protection components of HIPAA restrict disclosure of health information to the minimum needed for patient care and administrative support. Patients have gained new rights to access their medical records and to know who has accessed them. HIPAA compliance requires that most healthcare organizations and their software vendors make modifications to computer software to meet the data standards and privacy protection provisions of the law. Changes to business processes and procedures are needed as well. Education and training of employees is particularly important.

The HITECH Act, which is part of the American Recovery and Reinvestment Act of 2009, is designed to facilitate the transition of physicians, hospitals, and other healthcare providers to full users of EHR. Through Medicare and Medicaid reimbursement, the HITECH Act offers financial incentives for adoption and meaningful use of EHR. The HITECH Act established the Office of the National Coordinator for Health Information Technology to foster the electronic exchange and use of health information as well as to enforce health information privacy and security. The ACA is intended to decrease the number of uninsured by introducing incentives and insurance-coverage regulations for both employers and the general population. It also seeks to improve health outcomes and insurance eligibility by eliminating exclusions for preexisting conditions.

Healthcare information systems contain sensitive information. Policies and procedures are needed to protect the confidentiality of information about patients, employees, finances, and organizational strategies. This information is contained in patient care systems, public health systems, and medical research systems. While benefits of public health and medical research systems sometimes conflict with threats to individual privacy, federal and state governments have asserted that providers have a legal and moral obligation to protect patients' rights to privacy. Consequently, all of the laws passed at the federal, state, and local levels of government are aimed at protecting medical information privacy while improving the delivery and outcomes of care.

Finally, the chapter explores HIT leadership roles. The external environment and the government have direct, indirect, and substantial roles in healthcare operations. HIT leaders must understand those roles today and anticipate roles in the future. This section presents an action plan for HIT leadership. In response to HIPAA and other HIT-related legislations—and for ethical reasons as well—healthcare organizations and HIT leadership need enterprisewide standards and policies to maintain data security and protect the confidentiality of certain information. A comprehensive information security program requires disaster protection and recovery procedures as well as procedures for limiting access to certain information stored in computer databases.

Web Resources

A number of organizations (through their websites) provide more information on the topics discussed in this chapter:

- American National Standards Institute (www.ansi.org)
- Center for Democracy & Technology, Health Privacy (www.healthprivacy.org)
- Data Interchange Standards Association (www.disa.org)
- IRM International (www.irminternational.com/rptcard.html), a checklist for disaster recovery
- National Committee on Vital and Health Statistics (http://ncvhs.hhs.gov/index.htm)
- National Uniform Claim Committee (www.nucc.org)
- US Department of Health & Human Services:
  - Office of Civil Rights (www.hhs.gov/ocr/office/news/index.html) offers news releases announcing all of the major settlements of privacy and security breaches.
  - HealthCare.gov (www.healthcare.gov) provides information on evolving health insurance options available.
  - Centers for Medicare & Medicaid Services (www.cms.gov) points to detailed information about CMS's core programs and to research and data of value to HIT professionals. General HIPAA information can be found here: www.cms.gov/Regulations-and-Guidance /HIPAA-Administrative-Simplification/HIPAAGenInfo/index.html. Details of the EHR Incentive Programs are on www.cms.gov /Regulations-and-Guidance/Legislation/EHRIncentivePrograms /index.html.
- Workgroup for Electronic Data Interchange (www.wedi.org)

Discussion Questions

1. Discuss the effects of government involvement in two other industries. Compare the differences and similarities of these industries with the healthcare field.
2. Discuss the impacts of a breach to healthcare information systems, especially the financial and privacy impacts.
3. What is HIPAA? Why was it passed? What are the potential benefits to healthcare organizations to be gained by compliance with HIPAA standards? What are the potential drawbacks?

4. What is the HITECH Act? Why was it passed? What are the potential benefits to healthcare organizations to be gained by responding to the Act's incentives? What are the potential drawbacks?

5. What is the ACA? Why was it passed? What are the potential benefits to healthcare organizations to be gained as ACA features become implemented? What are the potential threats from the ACA?

6. Discuss some of the potential conflicts between a patient's right to privacy and information needed for public health and medical research.

7. There are several implications to the use of provider and employer identification. Please discuss the positive and negative implications.

8. Why are the transaction and code set standards important? What is their value to healthcare?

9. What concepts are important to information security policies and procedures? What effect does HIPAA have on healthcare organizations' policies and procedures? Are there any other laws that may affect them?

10. What concepts are important to disaster recovery policies and procedures? What effect does HIPAA have on those policies and procedures? Are there any other laws that may affect them?

11. Is it important to an organization to have a workgroup that focuses on determining the effects of government legislation? Please discuss your rationale.

12. What components should be included in a plan for protecting information privacy and confidentiality?

LEADERSHIP: THE CASE OF THE HEALTHCARE CIO

Learning Objectives

1. List job duties and analyze functional responsibilities of senior healthcare leadership and the chief information officer (CIO).
2. Identify key knowledge, skills, and abilities of the CIO position.
3. Describe the alternative paths to leadership of healthcare information technology (HIT).
4. Prepare and assess an organizational chart for the HIT department or area of a healthcare organization.
5. Illustrate future challenges faced by healthcare CIOs.

Overview

This chapter discusses the leadership, human resources, and management expertise required to make effective use of information and the healthcare information technology (HIT) infrastructure in healthcare organizations. In past editions of this book, this chapter was located at the end. Moving the chapter to the front of the book reflects both the increased complexity of information management in today's healthcare delivery environment and the important role that HIT leadership plays in that environment. Senior management of HIT departments must now plan for and implement systems to meet today's information needs (which have administrative and clinical applications), anticipate tomorrow's information needs, and ensure a smooth transition between current and future systems and technologies. While doing so, these leaders confront rapidly evolving hardware and software capabilities and ever-changing government interventions—both of which shift the rules that influence the collection, transmission, storage, retrieval, and dissemination of healthcare information.

Senior leadership cannot hope to master all or even most of these complex HIT tasks. They must, however, understand the associated challenges in sufficient detail to effectively manage technology and clinical content experts. Consequently, this chapter details the functional responsibilities of chief information officers (CIOs); the organization, staffing, and budgeting of the HIT department; and the organizational challenge of outsourcing or multisourcing HIT functions. It concludes with a brief examination of future trends related to the role of the CIO and the HIT leadership team.

Today's HIT Management

Determining what area of leadership is responsible for the management of information technology in the healthcare organization has always been a key responsibility of the CEO and the governing board. Historically, many healthcare organizations assigned information management responsibility to the chief financial officer (CFO), reflecting the high priority the organization reserved for accurate and timely financial information generally and patient billing particularly. The administrative functions were well served in the early days of HIT.

Because of the increasing importance of clinical information systems, the regulatory reporting requirements, and the use of information in strategic planning and decision support, most healthcare organizations now assign the responsibility for information management and communications to a separate executive-level position—the CIO. This shift has led to the publication of a host of books concentrating on the CIO and its evolving roles (e.g., Broadbent and Kitzis 2005; Smaltz et al. 2005a).

The Senior Management Role

A discussion of the roles that HIT management plays begins with the active engagement of the senior executives in the organization. In a study of organizations that successfully managed information technologies, Weill and Ross (2004) identify ten characteristics that these successful organizations have in common; Exhibit 4.1 summarizes these ten traits.

Many of the characteristics on this list contribute to the success of organizational information technology endeavors, and this list reinforces the important role of the CIO and other senior leaders. Governance design (item 1) must focus on organizational objectives and performance goals rather than simply on considerations of HIT's internal operations. Senior executives must design, lead, and regularly review HIT governance. Similarly, in effective organizations, senior management must get involved (item 3) not only in strategic decisions but also in technology decisions that have strategic implications. More than just involvement, good HIT governance requires leaders to make choices (item 4). Conflicting goals have become the norm in complex organizations and, if not handled appropriately, may lead to various problems within the institution.

EXHIBIT 4.1
Ten Charac-
teristics
Common to
Successful
HIT
Governance

1. Actively design governance
2. Know when to redesign
3. Involve senior managers
4. Make choices
5. Clarify the exception-handling process
6. Provide the right incentives
7. Assign ownership [of] and accountability for information technology governance
8. Design governance at multiple organizational levels
9. Provide transparency and education
10. Implement common mechanisms across the six key assets

SOURCE: From *IT Governance: How Top Performers Manage IT Decision Rights for Superior Results* by P. Weill and J. Ross, Harvard Business School Press, 2004. Reprinted with permission.

At a fundamental level, successful HIT governance must provide the right incentives and rewards (item 6) within the organization and assign ownership/accountability for the function (item 7). In healthcare, incentives are important to foster synergy between and among operating units. Likewise, accountability for HIT design, implementation, and performance must be firmly assigned at the CEO, CIO, or board committee level. Weill and Ross (2004) recommend that the board or CEO hold the CIO accountable for HIT governance and define and implement clear, measureable success metrics as part of the CIO's performance appraisal. With these considerations, the selection of the CIO leader is vital. Because excellent information technology performance depends on all organizational components working together smoothly, those who are accountable for these components must possess a broad view of the organization; that is, no leader can protect her turf. Organizational leaders (other than the CIO) must be aware that they, too, contribute to information technology governance, and all must understand the symbiotic relationship between HIT and the organization's overall strategic direction.

While considered relatively novel and obtained from a variety of industries, the ten-item list of success indicators presented in Exhibit 4.1 is not that far removed from the list of traits found historically in healthcare. Austin, Hornberger, and Shmerling (2000), for example, reported on management audits conducted by senior management at ten healthcare organizations. The audits evaluated how well the following seven responsibilities for HIT management were carried out: (1) HIT strategic planning, (2) employment of a user focus in system development, (3) recruiting of competent personnel, (4) system integration, (5) protection of information security and confidentiality, (6) employment of effective project management in system development, and (7) postimplementation evaluation of systems. Virtually all of these responsibilities receive substantial direction from HIT governance. Blitstein (2012) lists seven organizational areas in which HIT management is expected to actively participate or lead: business alignment, project selection/delivery, technology selection, financial management, organizational structure, risk management, and performance measurement.

Building on these ideas is a practice-oriented book aimed at helping CIO leaders achieve success—see Waller, Rubenstrunk, and Hallenbeck 2010. The book identifies seven leadership skills that support the need for CIOs to have management skills as opposed to purely technical skills; these leaders do the following (Waller, Rubenstrunk, and Hallenbeck 2010):

1. *Commit to leadership.* Success depends on the ability of the CIO to fully embody the role people play in success. Consequently, the CIO does not just "talk" the leadership mantra but "walks" or adopts behaviors consistent with leadership.

2. *Lead differently.* The point of this characteristic is to not abandon the core analytical approach to problem solving but to make sure that the current processes are collaborative in nature.

3. *Embrace the "softer" side.* This tired rhetoric has a grain of truth in that leaders should become open, caring, and mentors for others. This may involve empowering those around you to enable them to grow professionally. Key to this are not just words but also actions.

4. *Forge the right relationships.* Because HIT is still largely a people, not a technology, function, the leader must devote time and effort on managing relationships. As discussed later in this chapter, those relationships refer to not just with direct reports but also with other leaders inside the organization as well as vendors/suppliers outside the organization.

5. *Communicate effectively.* What a successful leader says and does are constantly being watched for signs of commitment and direction. The ability to effectively communicate at all times and in all manners is essential.

6. *Inspire others.* Getting people to go the extra mile to meet goals requires more than reminding them to do a good job. A leader must learn to inspire employees and convince them to firmly believe that they are working on something grander than their immediate set of tasks. Working for a greater good is inspiring and seems vital to success.

7. *Build people*. Professional development for your employees serves as the greatest success for the organization. It breeds success in the short run and helps to generate the future leaders of the organization.

To make these traits a reality, a solid and mutually supportive relationship between the CEO and the CIO is essential. According to Charles Emory, CIO of Horizon Blue Cross Blue Shield of New Jersey, "Two-way communication, especially between CIOs and CEOs is particularly critical now . . . with use of the Internet making the results of senior management efforts visible to everyone, inside and outside the organization" (Hagland 2001, 19). The gap between these institutional leaders pervades a host of environments. The challenges arise from poor communication as well as misaligned goals between the organization and information technology, diverse education and training, and basic lack of understanding of the environment each leader faces (Perelman 2007).

Functional Responsibilities of the CIO

Information systems can be useful to management, provided the process for planning, designing, installing, and operating such systems is itself well managed. The CEO and other senior managers of a healthcare organization must assume the responsibility for planning and controlling the development of effective information systems to serve their needs. These tasks cannot be delegated to technical personnel if information processes are to be truly supportive of high-quality patient care and managerial decision making. In today's competitive environment, information is essential for strategic planning, cost and productivity management, continuous quality improvement, and program evaluation purposes. Important senior management responsibilities are summarized in Exhibit 4.2.

The person assuming these responsibilities—increasingly recognized to be the CIO—must have broad corporate and system understanding and also must have the ability to lead teams of technical experts responsible for complex information technology. Reporting directly to the CEO (or chief operating officer [COO] in some large organizations), the CIO has two important duties: (1) to assist the senior management team and governing board in using information effectively to support strategic planning and management and (2) to provide management oversight and coordination of information processing and telecommunications systems throughout the organization.

The functions of the CIO are integral to any healthcare business, irrespective of organizational size and complexity. In a large organization, the CIO should be a full-time position. In a small hospital or clinic, the CIO responsibilities may be assigned to an administrative officer. A small physician

EXHIBIT 4.2
Senior
Management
Responsibilities

- Management must insist on a careful planning process that precedes all major decisions related to the installation of computer equipment or the design of complex information systems. A master plan for information systems development should be created and updated at least once a year. The master plan should be linked to the strategic plan of the healthcare organization and should guide all specific implementation decisions.

- Management must employ a user-driven focus throughout the development process. Active involvement of personnel from all segments of the healthcare organization is essential. This participation should begin with a definition of information requirements before the organization considers acquisition of hardware and software. It should continue through all phases of analysis, design, system evaluation and selection, and implementation.

- Management must take the responsibility for recruiting competent personnel for the design and operation of information systems. Consideration should be given to recruitment of a CIO to serve as a member of the senior management team. When outsourcing is used, careful selection of vendors and contract negotiations with the assistance of legal counsel should precede the award of contracts for software, equipment, or services.

- Managers at the corporate level must establish policies and procedures to ensure integration of data files or interfacing among individual information systems for tracking patient flows, consolidating cost and financial data, monitoring quality of care, and evaluating individual products and services. Interoperability of data among systems is an absolute necessity in complex healthcare organizations, particularly those involving subsidiary units and central corporate management.

- Management personnel at all levels must adhere to legal and ethical obligations to maintain security of information systems and to protect the confidentiality of patients, human resources, and other sensitive information.

- The design of individual computer applications must be carried out by an interdisciplinary project team. Systems analysts and computer programmers will take the lead on technical analysis and design activities. Representatives of user departments should help guide the specification of system requirements and evaluate the technical design plans of the analysts. Management should be involved in all major design projects to ensure congruence with organizational goals and objectives, and it should insist on a user-driven system focus rather than a technology-driven focus.

- Once a project team has been organized, careful systems analysis should precede any implementation decisions. Shortcuts in the systems analysis phase will inevitably lead to problems later in the process.

- Managers must ensure that the preliminary design specifications for computer applications are in harmony with the master plan for information systems development.

- Detailed system specifications must be required before any implementation activities take place. These specifications should be reviewed formally and approved by all user departments and by management before proceeding with the next steps in system development.

(continued)

EXHIBIT 4.2
Senior
Management
Responsibilities
(*continued*)

- Throughout the analysis, design, and implementation phases of a project, management must require careful scheduling of all activities and should receive periodic progress reports as the project proceeds.
- Managers must ensure thorough training of all personnel involved in the implementation phase of the new system.
- No computer application should be put into operation without first carrying out a comprehensive system test. The testing should cover all phases of system operation, including computer programs and procedures, personnel training, user satisfaction, ability of the system to meet original objectives, and accuracy of the initial cost estimates.
- Provisions must always be made for adequate maintenance after an application is operational. Maintenance procedures are essential to correct operational errors, to make system improvements, and to facilitate changes necessitated by shifts in organizational needs.
- Management must make certain that information systems are periodically audited and that all systems are formally evaluated once they are installed and operating normally.

group practice must also assign CIO functions or technical oversight to someone—often the group practice manager or a physician in the practice who has an interest and/or expertise in managing information technology. In short, even if an individual with the CIO title does not exist in the organization, someone must be responsible for making strategic and operational decisions regarding information technology for the enterprise.

The range and scope of specific CIO job responsibilities flow from the senior management duties. The scope can be defined in a number of ways, but the job's common parameters are synthesized from job descriptions and from leading healthcare search firms (including hrVillage.com, Community Clinics Initiative, Witt/Keifer, Healthcare Recruiters International, Heidrick & Struggles, Korn/Ferry International, and Tyler & Company). The range and scope generally include the following:

- Enterprisewide planning
- Leadership
- Management oversight
- Human resources management
- Financial management

Notice from this list that technical expertise is not mentioned as a separate responsibility. While the successful CIO cannot be ignorant of healthcare information systems and communication systems, he does not generally become directly involved in the details of software development or hardware design. At the same time, some degree of technical competence is crucial for the CIO to effectively manage an organization's HIT functions. Generally, the CIO must provide a vision for healthcare technology for the organization and leadership for developing and implementing HIT initiatives throughout the institution—from the boardroom to the clinical suites and in between. Many HIT initiatives are often designed to improve the cost-effectiveness of clinical and administrative functions, enhance the quality of healthcare services, and support business development. All initiatives assist the organization in navigating the constantly changing, competitive marketplace.

The CIO leads in planning and implementing enterprise information systems to support all aspects of both distributed and centralized clinical and business operations. Exhibit 4.3 provides a select list of knowledge, skills, and abilities of CIOs. Notice that a significant portion of the skill set and demonstrated abilities extends beyond the traditional HIT domain. This does not mean to imply that those with significant technical expertise cannot become the next CIO. Many paths lead to a leadership position in information technology, and technical expertise provides as good a path as any other. However, moving to the C-suite, as the CIO title implies, does require a skill set beyond technical expertise.

Recently, Healthcare Information and Management Systems Society (HIMSS) released a report on the priorities of information technology leaders, information garnered from responses to HIMSS's comprehensive survey. These are the five key priorities for the next two years identified in the survey (HIMSS 2012a, Figure 6):

EXHIBIT 4.3
Select Knowledge, Skills, and Abilities of CIOs

- Collaboration
- Understanding the nature of the health system
- Formulation of HIT components of strategic plan
- HIT strategic business and market planning
- HIT needs analysis
- Organization's HIT situation
- HIT culture
- State-of-industry assessment
- Technology assessment
- Evaluation, adoption, and implementation standards
- HIT policy development

SOURCE: Applied Health Informatics Learning and Assessment (n.d.).

Priority	Percentage of Respondents
1. Achieving meaningful use	38
2. Focusing on clinical systems	15
3. Leveraging information	13
4. Optimizing use of current systems	11
5. Completing ICD-10 conversion	11

This same publication also identified clinical, financial, and information technology infrastructure focus points for 2012 (HIMSS 2012a, figures 7, 8, and 9). Exhibit 4.4 summarizes these findings.

Characteristics of a Successful CIO

The CIO must possess a good understanding of the healthcare environment and clinical care processes, be an experienced manager, and have sufficient understanding of information technology to ensure that HIT is properly planned and implemented. Following are some justifications for these CIO traits:

- As discussed in chapters 2 and 3, the external environment and government policy have a direct impact on HIT. The CIO must monitor

Category	Percentage of Respondents
Clinical	
Fully operational EHR	25
Physician systems	16
CPOE installation	16
Linking clinical systems to quality measures	15
Data warehouse/clinical analytics	9
Financial	
ICD-10 implementation	67
Upgraded patient-billing system	6
Upgraded patient-access system	2
Infrastructure	
Servers/virtual servers	19
Mobile devices	18
Desktops/virtual desktops	16
Security systems	16

EXHIBIT 4.4
HIMSS's Primary Clinical, Financial, and Infrastructure Focus for HIT, 2012

SOURCE: Data from HIMSS (2012a), Figures 7, 8, and 9.

these activities, understand their implications, and prepare information technology and the organization to respond to these trends.

- As part of the executive team, the CIO must understand clinical processes sufficiently to intelligently discuss issues with the organization's chief medical officer (CMO). This implies that a basic anatomy-and-physiology course and familiarity with common medical terminology should be a part of the CIO training.

- Except in small organizations, the HIT function involves an array of individuals with diverse backgrounds. The CIO must be adept at communicating with and motivating this heterogeneous group.

- Technical skills are important for a CIO because the staff responsible for the technical aspects may have limited respect for a leader who is not conversant with actual and potential technical challenges.

In addition, the CIO must ensure that all HIT internal systems work properly. As a simple example, pharmacy systems (whether stand-alone or integrated) must operate continuously; otherwise, the organization will be unable to control dangerous drugs (particularly narcotics) and to manage drug ordering and inventory, drug distribution to patients, storage and retrieval of drug information, construction of patient drug profiles, the organization's formulary, and the generation of charges for billing (see chapters 9 and 10).

CIO success depends on many factors that are both internal and external to the leader's areas of influence. In an article outlining the secrets of success, Kramer (2006) summarized the skills that, according to CIOs who responded to a national survey, contributed to effective governance: business, clinical processes, leadership, administration, and communication skills—in addition to "technical savvy."

According to HIMSS (2012a), six key factors are the responsibility of information technology executives. These are not success factors per se, but they are factors that the CIO must be capable of handling or supporting: value of information technology investments, overall business strategy, business/clinical processes, organizational management improvement, HIT department management, and process change management. Each factor received 83 percent or higher positive responses from HIMSS's survey respondents. Furthermore, survey data obtained by Scottsdale Institute and HIMSS Analytics (2005, Figure 20) suggested that a key element of success for the CIO was a focus on meeting budgets and timelines for projects, although survey respondents recognized (but found less important) the broader goals of exceeding financial or organizational business measurements. Nearly two out of three respondents indicated that success depended in part on the active support of the CEO for HIT projects. The implication here was that even though the CEO does not set the vision or direction of HIT in most cases, the CEO must still actively support the CIO's initiatives.

More important to a successful CIO than specific training is work experience in healthcare. The Scottsdale Institute and HIMSS Analytics (2005, Figure 8) report indicated that most CIOs and directors of information systems who responded to the survey had HIT experience. Fewer than one out of eight CIO respondents got their start in other industries. Nearly a quarter indicated that they had formal management education specific to information systems, and an equal percentage had technical HIT training. More than one-third (38 percent) had business training, and relatively few had clinical origins. In the future, as HIT supports care delivery, it will be important for CIOs to have a clinical and a healthcare management background. Alternatively, the CIO may need a medical information officer to serve on the HIT team as a liaison with clinical healthcare delivery.

Organization of the HIT Department

The organizational structure of the HIT department should be guided by the institution's strategic objectives or plans and HIT strategic plan (see Chapter 5). Thus, the CIO must be aware of where she fits into the broader organizational framework and how best to structure the internal operating responsibilities. With respect to reporting relations, the pervasive nature of HIT management and the key role HIT leaders and managers play in achieving the organization's strategic initiatives suggest that the CIO should report directly to the CEO. Despite this seeming necessity, data from the Scottsdale Institute and HIMSS Analytics (2005, Figure 2) publication suggested that only a little more than a third (37 percent) of CIOs reported to their CEO, and an almost equal percentage (38 percent) reported to the head of finance or the CFO. The remainder of the CIO respondents reported to a COO, a CMO, or another senior executive. Today, however, the CIO has a somewhat different reporting relationship (Gamble 2012). In a recent survey, 38.2 percent of CIO respondents said they report to the CEO, 17.6 percent report to the COO, and 26.4 percent report to the CFO. The remaining 17.8 percent report to the CMO, chief innovation officer, board of directors, or other leaders.

As mentioned, the CIO oversees a broad range of functions, so the organizational chart must be sufficiently complex to fully capture that scope of responsibility. Organizations have not standardized the range of services reporting to the CIO; thus, organizational charts look different from one institution to the next. The size and complexity of tasks to be carried out by a central HIT department are affected by a number of factors, including the following:

- Degree of centralization or distribution of computer systems throughout the organization
- Use of in-house developed systems
- Use of packaged software or contracts with application service providers
- Extent to which functions/tasks are outsourced to contractors

Despite this variety in organizational approaches, a fairly typical HIT department organizational chart for a large hospital or system can be presented (see Exhibit 4.5). In this case, the complexity of the large organization often necessitates a chief medical information officer (CMIO) taking responsibility for the structured relations between HIT and the clinical staff. In 2012, 36 percent of survey respondents indicated that they employ a CMIO (HIMSS 2012a, Figure 14). In a small system, such as a single hospital or medical center, the CMIO function might still exist, but often the organizational chart looks like the one shown in Exhibit 4.6. In this scenario, the information systems operations manager—along with the directors of management engineering, telecommunications, and health information management—reports to the CIO. In large healthcare organizations and systems, these division directors often have substantial staffs, whereas in midsize organizations, a single person might occupy two or three of these functional positions as well as fill other job responsibilities. In small facilities, one staffer might be responsible for all of these functions. No matter who fulfills the position, the CIO and related functions do exist.

EXHIBIT 4.5
Organizational
Chart of an HIT
Department
in a Large
Organization

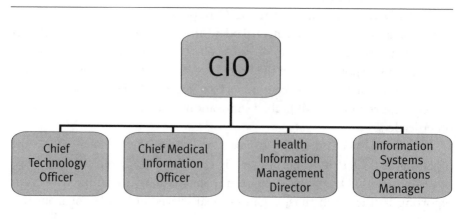

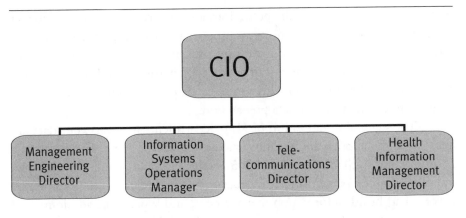

EXHIBIT 4.6
Organizational
Chart of an HIT
Department
in a Small
Organization

Looking further into the organizational structure of the HIT department reveals that, beyond the first level of reporting relations, it has even more layers. Exhibit 4.7 depicts the chart of an information systems operations division. Such a division typically consists of four major components: systems development, software evaluation, user support, and operations. Professional staff members in systems development are responsible for system design and implementation, and the systems development unit is itself organized into three main sections: programming, systems analysis, and systems maintenance. The software evaluation group is responsible for evaluating

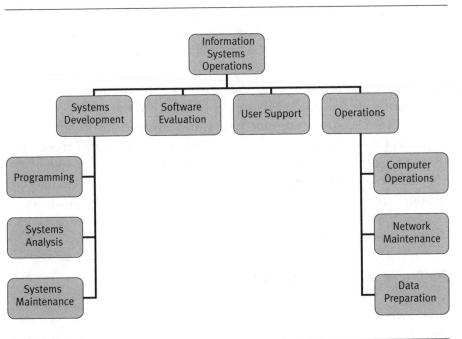

EXHIBIT 4.7
Organizational
Chart of the
Information
Systems Opera-
tions Division

software systems in the health applications area, for reviewing and approving all hardware and software acquisitions proposed by user departments, and for providing technical support on software utilization. The user support unit operates a help desk that users can contact for hardware and software assistance. Finally, the operations division is in charge of computer operations, network maintenance, and data preparation.

The general organization of HIT departments may vary, but data are available that support the specific structure presented here. The Scottsdale Institute and HIMSS Analytics (2005, Figure 7) publication, for example, indicated that 71 percent of HIT departments had telecommunications, 18 percent had health information management, and 9 percent had biomedical engineering staffs. These numbers grew by 2012: HIMSS survey respondents reported that 80 percent of HIT department have telecommunications, 28 percent have health information management, and 22 percent have biomedical engineering (HIMSS 2012a, figure 29).

Aside from this typical organizational structure, two other characteristics are important to note, according to Scottsdale Institute and HIMSS Analytics (2005):

1. Most organizations (85 percent) reported having an HIT steering committee. The role of this committee is to provide strategic direction for information systems decisions. Specifically, it tends to provide strategic approval (89 percent) for HIT decisions, be involved in budgetary decisions (63 percent), and play a role in vendor selection (30 percent). The committee is generally viewed as something that improves HIT operational and strategic effectiveness and that links the HIT department to potential and actual end users; small organizations are less likely to have this linkage function.

2. In many organizations, some HIT staff report to directors of other departments (outside of HIT) and not directly to the CIO. For example, in the Scottsdale Institute and HIMSS Analytics report, 40 percent of survey respondents indicated that none of their staff reported outside of the HIT department, 40 percent had staff reporting to laboratory departments, 35 percent had staff reporting to the radiology department, and 25 percent had staff reporting to the pharmacy department. This complexity necessitates a leadership and governance model that promotes coordination, standards, and efficiency.

Staffing of the HIT Department

Given the organizational structure and responsibilities of the HIT department, each section must be staffed. Selecting the individuals with the necessary skills and expertise is the next task of the CIO. Even the best structure cannot be successful without optimal staffing. Naturally, from the CIO's perspective, matching the skills and expertise of direct reports to their areas of responsibility is most important, but staff selection and assignment as well as other staffing decisions should be based on the design of the HIT unit. Generally, the directors or managers reporting to the CIO should have more technical and operational knowledge, experience, and expertise in their assigned areas than the CIO. Leadership must be able to count on these individuals to plan, design, and implement the best technology solutions for their area. For example, the health information management division should be headed by an experienced and certified registered health information administrator with broad knowledge of information flow and electronic health record (EHR) systems.

As a rule, three levels of personnel must be recruited to staff an HIT department: professional, technical, and clerical. Professional-level staff includes systems analysts and computer programmers. Although finding talented persons who can fill both roles is possible, care must be exercised in not conflating the two positions. Systems analysis requires broad-based skills that computer programmers often do not possess. It is a highly creative process best performed by someone with both technical prowess and organizational insight. Because most systems are complex and involve substantial human–machine interaction, the systems analyst must be able to deal effectively with people and understand how the organization carries out its mission. On the other hand, programmers typically have a narrower orientation and are skilled in the technical tasks of software development and maintenance. Programming requirements are changing. As healthcare organizations move toward the implementation of client/server architecture, network programmers are largely replacing those who used to write and maintain large programs for mainframe computers.

Technical-level personnel operate the computers and maintain the communications network. An experienced technical manager, reporting to the CIO, should head the information systems operations divisions. The manager must have up-to-date knowledge of the technical aspects of systems analysis, computer programming, hardware and software, networks, and systems maintenance, just to name a few responsibilities (see Exhibit 4.7). The manager must be willing to spend the time and effort necessary to stay abreast of the latest trends and upgrades in a rapidly changing field. In addition, the manager must be an experienced financial manager and must be skilled in interpersonal relations. Skilled network managers are highly trained and are often in short supply. The information systems operations supervisor must be both a skilled technician and an effective manager. Similarly, equipment maintenance is handled by technical-level staff. These technicians are typically employed by the vendor and supply periodic preventive maintenance and emergency repairs on call (see the section on outsourcing later in this chapter).

Clerical-level staff members are those who provide administrative support throughout the HIT department. Two primary factors have driven the need for well-trained HIT clerical staff, as is true for most other parts of the organization. First, the monitoring, control, and reporting requirements for HIT have expanded as privacy, security, and other regulatory requirements have become more stringent. Second, HIT leadership and technical staff are now becoming integrated into the broader healthcare system, so clerical staff have had to help these professionals plan, schedule, and support internal and external meetings and initiatives.

The approach to organizing and staffing the HIT department depends on the complexity of the organization. For example, an integrated delivery system composed of multiple facilities is much more complex than a single facility, requiring a larger and more intricate HIT function. Further, as a matter of culture, some systems are highly centralized, with all software development carried out by a corporate information technology staff. In other, less complex systems, more responsibility may be delegated to operational units. Whatever the approach, the organizational structure must facilitate electronic information exchange across the enterprise (DeFord and Porter 2005).

Staffing for HIT has grown rapidly in recent years, a trend that appears will continue in the foreseeable future. Most respondents (61 percent) to the HIMSS (2012a) CIO survey indicated their staffing would grow in the next 12 months. Of the types of staff most in demand, clinical application support was cited by 43 percent of respondents to have the greatest need, followed by network and architecture support (22 percent). Other growth areas include clinical informatics (20 percent), system integration (17 percent), IT security (14 percent), and clinical transformation (13 percent). In total, 32 percent of respondents indicated no change in their HIT staffing in the coming year, and only 5 percent indicated a likely decrease in staffing.

Budgeting the HIT Department

Budgets for HIT are increasing, but they remain low both in absolute terms and relative to similar spending in other industries (Salkever 2004). In a 2006 HIMSS survey, 54 percent of respondents indicated that their organization spent 2.5 percent or less of their operating budget on HIT, and 14 percent indicated that they spent more than 3.5 percent on HIT. In the same survey, more than 70 percent of CIOs indicated that their HIT spending would increase in the coming year (HIMSS 2006a); this corresponded closely with responses in the HIMSS surveys from previous years. In the 2012 survey, 56 percent of respondents indicated that their operating budgets would *definitely* increase and 19 percent forecasted that their operating budgets would

probably increase (HIMSS 2012a, Figure 30). The four top reasons for budget growth were overall IT systems growth (68 percent), additional staffing
needs (57 percent), overall budget increases (43 percent), and compliance
with regulatory changes (43 percent) (HIMSS 2012a, Figure 31). These
are in contrast to reasons given by survey respondents in the past—namely,
growth in the number of systems and technologies (80 percent), alignment
between the long-term HIT and organizational strategic plans (48 percent),
and an overall budget increase (41 percent) (HIMSS 2006a).

The budget increases for HIT are likely to continue as workforce
shortages drive labor costs up and as technology advancements lead to more
opportunities for expanded and enhanced services. Despite the emphasis on
hardware and software, however, labor costs continue to be the key driver
of HIT costs. Exhibit 4.8 presents the average and median salaries for CIOs
overall, for CIOs in various work settings, for CIOs with different educational training, and for CIOs working in different regions of the country. As

Category	Average Salary, 2012
Overall	$208,417
Type of Organization	
CIO—Multihospital/IDN	$254,054
CIO—Standalone hospital	$178,786
CIO—Academic health center	$243,229
CIO—Hospital/clinic	$187,410
CIO—Critical access hospital	$125,573
Education/Degree	
MD	$306,000
PhD	$230,714
Master's degree	$213,705
Bachelor's degree	$194,473
Associate's degree	$175,250
High school diploma	$140,675
Region	
Pacific	$232,181
New England	$217,533
East South Central	$213,341
East North Central	$212,118
Middle Atlantic	$211,959
West North Central	$209,412
Mountain	$191,076
South Atlantic	$186,802
West South Central	$186,429

EXHIBIT 4.8
Salary for CIO
by Type of
Organization,
Education, and
Region, 2012

SOURCE: Data from CHIME (2013).

shown in the exhibit, the "average" CIO in all settings made about $208,000 in 2012—up from $151,000 in 2006 (CHIME 2013; HIMSS 2006b). The size and complexity of the organization influenced CIO salary in 2012: CIOs in multihospital systems made more than $254,000, CIOs in stand-alone hospitals made $179,000, and CIOs in critical access hospitals made $126,000. Similarly, education and geographic location had an effect on a CIO's average salary. A CIO with an MD made $306,000 on average, while one with a high school diploma earned $141,000. CIOs living and working in the Pacific region (Washington, Oregon, California, Alaska, and Hawaii) were paid an average of $232,000 per year, while those located in the West South Central Region (Texas, Oklahoma, Arkansas, and Louisiana) received a $186,000 annual salary.

Outsourcing and Multisourcing HIT Functions

Many healthcare organizations are considering outsourcing portions of their HIT functions as an alternative to in-house staffing. The decision to out-source entails purchasing (or *buy*) the services from an external vendor or a contractor rather than hiring the staff and producing (or *make*) the service in-house. This make–buy decision must be seriously considered as the complexity of HIT increases. Traditionally, the term *outsourcing* has been associated with a contract for facilities management. More recently, however, the term is used in a broader context to denote contracting with the best-qualified company to meet a specific information systems objective. This may involve *multisourcing* to a number of different vendors as well as outsourcing to a single vendor.

Some of the major potential benefits of outsourcing include the following:

1. Reduction of in-house staffing requirements
2. Smaller investment in capital equipment
3. More flexibility in meeting changing requirements and adopting new technology
4. Reduction in the time required to implement new applications
5. More predictable cost structure, particularly if fixed-price contracting is employed

Outsourcing is not without potential dangers and risks to the organization and to the CIO leading the outsourcing initiatives; they include the following:

1. Heavy dependence on vendors, with the possibility that a critical contractor might go bankrupt or change business direction
2. High costs associated with vendor fees and profit structure
3. Employment of contractors who do not understand the operation and culture of healthcare organizations

Hensley (1997) describes some of the principles to follow in outsourcing. He emphasizes the importance of weighing the cultural fit with the vendor; suggests that outsourcing be part of a long-term strategy (not just a quick fix); and recommends good reference checking, looking for staying power among vendors being considered. Further, Hensley states that healthcare organizations should not outsource the things they do best, should not become obsessed with short-term savings, and should not negotiate such favorable terms in a contract that a business partner is put out of business.

Waymack (2000) offers the following four suggestions for selecting outsourcing firms:

1. Seek long-term commitments, because the costs of switching vendors can be substantial.
2. Require relevant experience with the specific service to be outsourced.
3. Develop performance measures for selection on the basis of the services to be outsourced.
4. Do not base evaluation solely on the lowest bid.

From the broader business perspective, many back-office functions are commonly outsourced. For example, Hali (2007) reports that more than two of three firms engage in some form of business process outsourcing. His study examined accounts receivable specifically and found five key arguments for outsourcing:

1. *Bottom line.* Contrary to the general expectation, outsourcing does not reduce costs but may generate increased recoveries. This is the primary reason to outsource accounts receivable.
2. *Expertise.* Because an outsourcing firm's core business is the function for which it is hired/contracted to do, its staff members have great expertise in that specific function and the organization that hires the firm is likely to achieve excellence.
3. *Technology.* Similarly, the outsourcing firm employs the most current technology, which often leads to better outcomes. Because this technology typically requires substantial investment, the firm has technology-based cost advantages.

4. *Consistency.* A dedicated staff in the outsourcing firm follows up on invoices in a timely and professional manner.
5. *Core business focus.* By outsourcing an important but noncore business or process, the organization is free to concentrate on its core business.

Similarly, Menachemi and colleagues (2005) report systematically on the nature and extent of outsourcing by urban or rural status, ownership (not-for-profit or for-profit), organization size, system affiliation, CIO reporting relationship, and information technology strategy value. They also report outsourcing rates for a number of specific HIT functions in six broad categories. These categories, along with examples of function and reported outsourcing rates, are as follows:

1. Development/integration: applications development, 11.3 percent
2. Staffing: CIO, 14.4 percent
3. Operations/management: personal computer support, 15.5 percent
4. Employee support and training: help desk, 6.2 percent
5. Applications and services: transcriptions, 51.5 percent
6. Web-related: e-business, 4.1 percent

A survey by Waller, Rubenstrunk, and Hallenbeck (2010) reveals the top three reasons for outsourcing HIT services, according to survey respondents:

1. Expertise of vendor (90 percent)
2. Cost savings (63 percent)
3. New service (9 percent)

In addition, between 27 percent and 34 percent of respondents indicated that they outsource EMR, patient surveys, and the help desk function. *Modern Healthcare* magazine conducts an outsourcing survey as well. The top outsourcing firms, based on size of the client base, reported a 13 percent gain in the number of clients in 2011 (Kutscher 2012). However, information technology ranked seventh in terms of money spent by organizations on outsourcing.

Many examples of outsourcing can be found, all with direct application to a particular type of information technology. Specific examples of successful outsourcing experiences are numerous, but they generally come from the testimonials posted on vendor websites. However, one organization that received recognition was Mercy Hospital in Chicago. Mercy outsourced an array of information systems to a vendor, leading HIMSS to recognize the hospital's efforts to modernize its medical information systems (Mercy Hospital 2009). Similarly, Jefferson Regional Medical Center in Pittsburgh worked with Siemens Medical Solutions to fulfill its strategic goal of bringing "medical excellence closer to home" (Siemens Medical Solutions 2005, 1). For Jefferson, this goal meant reducing costs and enhancing its quality reputation. Information technology was targeted as the vehicle to implement the goal, and the decision to outsource HIT was integral to achieving it. Jefferson employed a CIO to manage the Siemens outsourcing relationship. Their joint vision was that HIT should always deliver appropriate technology and resources to meet the hospital's strategic goals.

This outsourcing collaboration yielded many positive results, some of which are as follows:

- The decision support and managed care recovery unit recovered $1 million in revenue in 16 months through the use of Siemens's Contract Management System.
- This unit recovered an additional $400,000 in charges in 16 months by correcting clinical documentation issues concerning comorbidity conditions prior to patient discharge.
- Jefferson's accounting department worked with HIT to automate employee time reporting and management to reduce payroll department staff by half while improving manager online reporting capacity.

This successful outsourcing experience led to plans for other joint efforts, including providing personal digital assistants (PDAs) for physicians that would allow physicians to access patient information from their PDAs throughout the hospital.

Results of the CIO portion of the *Seventeenth Annual HIMSS Leadership Survey* indicated that 38 percent of the organizations responding to the survey outsourced the development and maintenance of their websites, 33 percent outsourced dictation and transcription services, 19 percent outsourced applications development, 19 percent outsourced project management, 18 percent outsourced both the help desk function and database management, and 17 percent outsourced telecommunications (HIMSS 2006a). Interestingly, these numbers were similar to those in previous years, except that outsourcing personal computer support, network operations support, and technical support did not make the 2006 list, and dictation and transcription was new to the outsourcing list in 2006. Twenty-nine percent of respondents indicated that they did not outsource any HIT functions.

Evolving Role of the Senior HIT Executive

Looking into the future of HIT and the role of the HIT executive is an exercise filled with uncertainty. A number of analysts have carefully considered the role that advancements in HIT are likely to have on the organization of health delivery entities. Brynjolfsson and Hitt (2000) and Oliner and Sichel (2000), among others, examine the relationship of technology and productivity growth. They find that organizational change is needed to capture the potential to which computers and other technology offer support. Without fundamental changes in the ability of managers to "invent new processes, procedures and organizational structures that leverage this capability" (Brynjolfsson and Hitt 2000, 24), the gains from increased HIT spending may not be realized. The CIO is at the center of the changing role of HIT and its potential impact on healthcare delivery.

In the 2005 HIMSS *Annual Report of the US Hospital IT Market*, the following key challenges emerged:

- Underinvestment in HIT
- Need to replace technologies and applications
- Interoperability of applications and systems
- Integration of ambulatory systems
- HIT financial accountability

By 2012, participants in the *23rd Annual HIMSS Leadership Survey* listed a more future-oriented set of priorities (HIMSS 2012a):

- *Achieving meaningful use.* In 2012, 38 percent of respondents identified that achieving meaningful use for their institution is their principal priority. This percentage is somewhat lower than that for 2011, but it indicates that this challenge continues to be a major concern for HIT leaders. Twenty-six percent of respondents reported having accomplished Stage 1 of meaningful use, and almost half expect to complete attestation during 2012; another 17 percent have plans in place for 2013.
- *Developing clinical systems.* These systems refer to EHR, e-prescribing, and computerized physician order entry (CPOE). In total, 15 percent of respondents indicated that development of these systems is a priority.
- *Leveraging information.* Cited by 13 percent of respondents, the effective use of clinical and administrative data for decision making is the third priority. Together, data mining, evidenced-based medicine, and

clinical decision support techniques have increased in importance for
HIT leadership.

- *Optimizing current systems.* Making the best use of as well as effectively
  operating the systems currently installed is a concern for 12 percent of
  respondents. The proliferation of applications in particular raises questions about how to get these features and functions to work in an optimal fashion as intended and to deliver the best results.

- *Preparing for ICD-10.* This priority was cited by 11 percent of respondents. It communicates the need to complete the preparation for the
  conversion to the ICD-10 clinical coding system.

Specific business issues faced by senior executives in healthcare HIT
have remained essentially the same from year to year in recent years. In 2006,
the HIMSS survey indicated that customer satisfaction, Medicare cutbacks,
reducing medical errors, and cost pressures were the four top business priorities of information technology executives; all of these priorities were also at or
near the top in the 2005 survey. New to the 2006 survey was a fifth concern:
interoperability. By 2012, 40 percent of the HIMSS survey respondents cited
healthcare reform as the top priority, and 23 percent named policy mandates
(often related to reform). The next two concerns were financial considerations (cited by 14 percent) and health information exchange (cited by 5
percent) (HIMSS 2012a, Figure 11).

The Expanded CIO Role

In discussing the changing role of healthcare CIOs, Wood (2000, 81) states,
"in the past, chief information officers were responsible for nothing else but
assuring a constant flow of information. Today, they are being asked to do a
great deal more. From E-business to E-health strategy, the chief information
officer is the focal point of an organization's ability to leverage new technology." The CIO role has expanded since Wood made this statement, with the
explosion of concern about healthcare quality, cost pressure, efficiency concerns due to labor shortages, and other constraints. CIOs have emphasized
their strategic role rather than their technical management role (Morrissey
1996). The complicating and often unmentioned point is that the CIO
position is usually not the first job that a person holds out of college. Most
CIOs started their career in intermediate-level positions and, if successful,
rose to the CIO position. The initial jobs can be in the information systems/
information technology areas or can be outside of this domain entirely. CIOs
may come from medicine, nursing, or other clinical/administrative areas. The
prior jobs, especially in information systems/information technology, held by
a candidate for a CIO role do require the individual to have technical or data
management skills to be successful. In other words, a CIO does not need the

technical skills to perform the CIO job but may be required to have those skills and experiences to get that executive position.

Realize that today's CIO no longer just manages one of many operating units within a healthcare organization. The person also must look beyond HIT and engage in significant strategic thinking on behalf of the unit as well as the entire organization. The broad classifications of CIO activities serve or are accountable to the following three distinct interest groups:

1. *Upward.* The CEO and/or the board rely on the CIO to assist in strategic and operational planning for the organization as a whole by supporting enterprisewide planning. This is a future-looking role, which is, by nature, strategic. However, they also require the CIO to effectively manage data quality, security, privacy, and integrity to comply with a growing array of government regulations, such as the Sarbanes-Oxley Act of 2002, Health Insurance Portability and Accountability Act of 1996 as modified by the Health Information Technology for Economic and Clinical Health (HITECH) Act of 2009, and the Patient Protection and Affordable Care Act of 2010.

2. *Horizontally.* Executive leaders throughout the hospital—such as the CFO, CMO, and chief nursing officer—also rely on and work closely with the CIO to improve their respective department's data collection, storage, analysis, and reporting.

3. *Internally.* The CIO must be able to effectively manage the information technology business unit.

The Scottsdale Institute and HIMSS Analytics (2005) report suggested that less than half of respondents to a survey indicated that the CIO was facilitating HIT-related discussions with the board. More often, the report stated, the CEO or another senior executive had responsibility for board discussions related to information technology. This trend is not consistent or incongruent with the growing role and responsibility of the CIO today, and it (partly) contributes to the uncertainty of the future of the CIO. For example, the Sarbanes-Oxley Act reporting requirements may have shifted the responsibility of data integrity away from the CIO and back to the CFO. With that responsibility, CFOs may want to control the data warehousing and data management functions more closely. Furthermore, Schwartz (2005) suggested that the CIO as a title will disappear; in the future, functions under the CIO's domain may report to the CFO.

In addition, greater board involvement in information technology is likely. In 2005, 56 percent of healthcare organization boards approved budgets, and only 39 percent approved specific systems projects (Scottsdale Institute and HIMSS Analytics 2005). Given the central role of HIT systems in influencing healthcare quality and organizational competitiveness, boards will likely be more involved in HIT decisions in the future.

Today, the future remains uncertain; thus, the CIO and other HIT leaders must maintain vigilance to ensure continued success. Many key issues must be considered, and HIMSS Analytics (2012a) and other publications offer a guide to regularly monitoring a few of the current priorities:

- *Revenue cycle management.* A number of features on the horizon will affect this vital organizational function. Examples of those that pose significant demands on HIT include recovery audit contractor requirements for key audit data, bundled payment and value-based purchasing, patient eligibility and authorization transactions for accountable care organizations, and ICD-10 encoding upgrades.
- *Healthcare information exchanges (HIEs).* These are a buzzword now, although their existence seems to not have a strong business case. They require coordination for smooth transfer to and from unrelated organizations that pose major threats. In 2012, 55 percent of surveyed leaders indicated that they participate in an HIE (HIMSS 2012a, Figure 18).
- *Patient Protection and Affordable Care Act.* This legislation poses a host of challenges, the most important of which is great uncertainty. The US Supreme Court helped move it forward to some extent, by ruling that the act is fundamentally constitutional because the most contentious portion of the law—the individual mandate—is a tax. After all, the federal government has the authority to tax. However, the Supreme Court ruled that the federal government cannot force states to expand Medicaid coverage to 133 percent of the poverty level as the legislation proposed. This ruling enables individual states to opt out of Medicaid expansion if they so chose. As such, state participation in this aspect of the act varies.
- *Interoperability.* Discussed later in the chapter, interoperability is still a dream because of the lack of standards. The implications are that standards are likely to add demands on HIT leadership.

Priorities for Application Development

Reduction of medical errors and enhancement of patient safety will continue to be "hot issues" among government agencies and private consumer organizations. To that end, the Leapfrog Group (2002), a consortium of major purchasers of healthcare, expanded its efforts to reduce preventable medical mistakes. Chapter 9 addresses computerized physician order entry as a technique to reduce medication errors in hospitals. Emphasis on the development of computer-based records will continue and will likely be placed on information systems that can support evidence-based medicine and disease management programs.

Communications between patients and providers, facilitated by the Internet, will expand in the next ten years. Armed with information obtained online, patients will participate more fully in decisions about their care. Home-based monitoring systems will become more common and will help to reduce the need for repeated outpatient visits and to delay or defer the need for inpatient care.

Reemphasis on the use of HIT for strategic decision support is likely in the next few years as well. This topic received considerable attention in the early 1990s but was sidetracked by data-conversion concerns in anticipation of the year 2000 (Y2K hype) and then further put off as components of the Health Insurance Portability and Accountability Act were implemented.

System Communications and Interfaces

Developing efficient communications among and between computer applications on an enterprisewide basis continues to be problematic for many healthcare organizations. As mentioned earlier in this chapter, management audits conducted by senior managers in ten major healthcare organizations revealed that "most organizations reported concern about this issue [system integration] and stated that they were working toward a solution" (Austin, Hornberger, and Shmerling 2000, 235).

Some organizations continue to have problems in obtaining meaningful data from transaction-processing systems to use in decision support and management studies. More emphasis on process reengineering during systems analysis and selection could help to improve the situation. This ongoing problem has now been clearly identified and labeled as *interoperability*. As seen in Chapter 1, to improve, care delivery systems must work together within and across organizations. HIMSS Analytics (2005) adopted a definition of interoperability as the ability of HIT to work together within and across organizational boundaries to advance the effective delivery of healthcare for individuals and communities. Naturally, this is complex in concept and application. The National Alliance for Health Information Technology (2007) endorsed four levels of interoperability with different technical specifications and containing varied organizational implications, as defined by Walker and colleagues (2005):

1. *Nonelectronic data.* Sharing information does not include any use of information technology and thus relies on conventional phone service.

2. *Machine-transportable data.* Sharing information uses generally available information technology, but that information has not necessarily been standardized and thus cannot be manipulated. This transmission relies on fax transmission or sharing of portable document format (or PDF) files only.

3. *Machine-organizable data.* Sharing information uses electronic information technology, but the messages are generally not fully standardized. Data received must be modified by programs (interfaces) that help the receiver understand the data's meaning. This transmission might consist of sharing of files stored in incompatible formats.

4. *Machine-interpretable data.* Sharing information uses electronic information technology, but the information has been fully standardized in terms of format and vocabulary. This transmission might include coded information from a lab to the receiver's EMR.

Because of this interest, investigators are looking to assess the value of information exchange, which depends on interoperability. The Center for Information Technology Leadership assessed the expected net value of electronic data transactions using the New York State HIE model. It concentrated on measuring the value from clinical encounters among hospitals, medical group practices, and other providers and among major payers, laboratories, pharmacies, and other key stakeholders. The model assumes a full transition to computer-linked data exchange of standardized information, and the measurement was conducted over a ten-year implementation period. The center estimated a net value of electronic data transactions of 3.3 percent of total health expenditures in the state in 2003—or about $4.54 billion (Hook et al. 2006).

At this point, the challenge of interoperability—at least for hospitals—appears to have declined. Only 4 percent of respondents to the HIMSS 2012 survey reported that interoperability is a barrier to implementing systems (HIMSS 2012a, Figure 12), making interoperability the ninth item on a list of barriers for HIT leaders.

Advances in Technology

Technology will continue to improve and will offer new opportunities for healthcare organizations during the next ten years. The most frequently identified technologies cited by respondents to a HIMSS Analytics (2005) survey were sign-on/identity management technology, barcoding technology, speech recognition, and PDAs. By the 2012 HIMSS survey, a question about advances in technology was not even addressed. The HITECH Act has changed the landscape of CIO priorities, making adoption of EHR and implementation of systems to meet meaningful use requirements the central focus. The 2012 survey included specific issues related to the HITECH Act, such as meaningful use, HIE, and information privacy and security. Although the emerging technologies mentioned in the 2005 survey have not gone away, they are deemed less pressing by HIT leaders who are dedicating their efforts to current demands. For the CIO and other HIT leaders, the prospect of mastering existing technologies—much less forecasting the next innovation—remains overwhelming. Successful leaders will need to maintain a high level of awareness, be flexible to adapt and adopt, and become continuous learners.

Other Challenges

The evolving role of the CIO will face myriad challenges in the near future. In addition to those discussed above, survey information suggests the following key priorities to consider (HIMSS 2012a):

- *Security concerns.* Internal breaches of security continue to be the primary security concern, with 13 percent of HIT leadership experiencing a security breach in the last six months and 22 percent in the previous year.
- *Remote access to online patient information.* HIT leadership reported that 97 percent of physicians, 60 percent of nurses, 59 percent of other clinical professionals, and 67 percent of nonclinical staff have access to patient information online. In addition, 23 percent reported that patients in their organization have this access.
- *Meaningful use.* Few (26 percent) CIOs claimed they have already attested to Stage 1 meaningful use, and by the end of 2012, another 49 percent expected to attest.

Summary

This chapter discusses the leadership, human resources, and management expertise required to make effective use of HIT infrastructure in healthcare organizations. The organizational position of the CIO has evolved over the years and is now a separate, executive-level role. This elevation is due to the growing importance of clinical systems, regulatory reporting requirements, and the use of information in strategic planning and decision support.

Today, the CIO generally reports directly to the CEO, primarily assists the senior leadership team in using information effectively, and provides management of information processing and telecommunications in the organization. The required skills of the CIO include enterprisewide planning, leadership, management oversight, human resource management, and financial management.

The HIT department's organization has also evolved over the years. Generally, managers in management engineering, information systems operations, communications, and health information management report directly to the CIO. However, this department varies widely by size and complexity of the organization. In large, complex organizations, the chief technology officer and chief medical information officer roles may exist. Most HIT departments have a steering committee to assist in providing strategic direction. One added complexity of the CIO role is that many organizations have information systems staff members who report to operational units outside of the HIT department.

The evolving role of HIT will force the CIO to work upward with the CEO and board, horizontally with other hospital leaders, and internally to manage the HIT business unit. The functions and roles outlined for HIT leadership exist even in small organizations that do not have individuals with those assigned tasks. The functions must be managed in small institutions as in large organizations, but individuals with other non-HIT roles often assume the responsibilities for these functions.

Key priorities for application development in the coming years include systems communications and interfaces, advances in technology, security concerns, and website use.

Web Resources

A number of organizations (through their websites) provide more information on the topics discussed in this chapter:

- American College of Healthcare Information Administrators (ACHIA; www.aameda.org/Colleges/ACHIA/healthcareinformation.html). A subunit of the American Academy of Medical Administrators, ACHIA is a personal membership organization for information managers with special focus on continuing education and research in healthcare information administration.
- American Health Information Management Association (AHIMA; www.ahima.org). AHIMA is a personal membership organization of information professionals who specialize in the utilization and management of clinical information.
- American Medical Informatics Association (AMIA; www.amia.org). The term *medical informatics* is used to describe the science of

storage, retrieval, and optimal use of biomedical information for problem solving and medical decision making. AMIA is a personal membership organization of professionals interested in computer applications in biomedicine.

- Applied Health Informatics Learning and Assessment (www.nihi.ca/hi). This comprehensive website details the competencies necessary for CIOs and other HIT leadership. Here, you can view the challenge faced by the CIO or other leader, a detail of the micro roles necessary to meet that challenge, an assessment of the importance of this challenge/role, and even suggestions for how to gain the experience necessary for the role. See www.nihi.ca/hi/ahimacroroles.php?id=1&Menu ItemID=5.

- College of Healthcare Information Management Executives (CHIME; www.cio-chime.org). CHIME is a personal membership organization of CIOs in the healthcare field. CHIME provides professional development and networking opportunities for its members.

- Healthcare Information and Management Systems Society (HIMSS; www.himss.org). HIMSS is a personal membership organization representing professionals in clinical systems, information systems, management engineering, and telecommunications. HIMSS provides professional development opportunities to its members through publications and educational programs.

- Health Information Technology and Quality Improvement, Health Resources and Services Administration, US Department of Health and Human Services (www.hrsa.gov/healthit/index.html). This is a rich website for information, fundamental data, research studies, and manpower assessments related to HIT.

Discussion Questions

1. Why is healthcare/clinical experience more important for healthcare CIOs today than in past years?
2. What factors can increase the size and complexity of the HIT organizational structure?
3. An HIT steering committee is used in most healthcare organizations to make strategic and budgetary decisions. Do you consider the steering committee to be a good design? Why or why not?
4. Why is demand increasing for HIT staffing?

5. Compare the roles/functions and the average salary of a CIO with that of other HIT personnel. Are the roles complementary or substitutes? Can you justify the salary differences?

6. Do the benefits of outsourcing outweigh the risks? Order the highly ranked outsourced services from riskiest to least risky, and explain your rationale for the decision.

7. Based on the changing roles of CIOs, do you agree or disagree with Schwartz (2005) that the role of CIO will disappear?

8. Why is system integration such an important topic in HIT?

9. Several priorities for application development are listed in the chapter. Can HIT assist in any other important priorities?

HIT GOVERNANCE AND DECISION RIGHTS

Learning Objectives

1. Explain why healthcare information technology (HIT) strategic planning has become more important for healthcare organizations.
2. Summarize the five major components of HIT governance.
3. Describe the major elements of a healthcare organization's planning effort.
4. Assess the major elements of an HIT strategic plan.
5. Describe systems theory, and explain why it is vital to HIT governance and planning.

Overview

The competitive advantage that successful healthcare information technology (HIT) governance may bestow has become the center of much discussion and even some debate. Smaltz, Carpenter, and Saltz (2007) and others (Broadbent and Kitzis 2005; Glaser 2002; Weill and Ross 2004) conclude that effective governance and expanding decision rights, inherent in HIT leadership, are essential for organizational success. The discussion of what *governance* and *decision rights* mean and how these concepts have evolved in healthcare organizations is a major portion of this chapter. Such emphasis on governance does not imply that the more traditional HIT strategic planning is either unimportant or out of date. Planning is still vital and is an important part of HIT governance.

Today, more so than in the past, successful HIT governance and planning must address challenges from outside HIT operations. Broad questions that need to be addressed include these: What is HIT governance? How does the governance model differ from historical HIT strategic planning? What changes must be made in organizations to transform HIT functions to a corporate asset?

This chapter presents an overview of HIT governance and strategic planning in healthcare organizations from the perspective of an integrated governance model. Topics covered are the background of governance and planning, including their purpose and components; organizing an HIT strategic planning effort; the importance of system integration; the basics of systems theory; and management control and decision support systems.

Background of HIT Governance and Strategic Planning

Information systems in many healthcare organizations evolved piecemeal, rather than from a carefully controlled planning process. Specific requirements for capturing, storing, and retrieving data when needed were developed on an ad hoc basis as new programs and services were added. As a result, the same data were captured repetitively, files were duplicated, and information was not always available when needed. Analysts recognized that if an HIT planning process was not in place, priorities for developing individual computer applications were often established by the exigencies of the moment.

The broader corporate perspective suggests *governance* is the way in which owners and managers of an organization manage the *agency problem*—the fundamental conflict of interest imposed by delegating operational authority to managers who do not own the resources managed (Denis 2001). Managers want to keep their job of running the business and thus may become risk averse in their decisions to minimize the chance that they will have a bad outcome that would cost them their employment. This risk aversion does not maximize returns to the owners. The owners want to make sure the business operates in such a way as to maximize its *well-being*, which means long-run profit in the business world and quality, reputation, or size for healthcare organizations. In any event, the challenge facing the owners or the governing board is how best to ensure that management makes the right decisions. Two solutions to this agency problem are bonding and monitoring.

Bonding is developing contracts that reward managerial behavior that leads to positive outcomes or penalize managerial behavior that leads to negative outcomes; incentive-based compensation is one method of bonding. *Monitoring*, on the other hand, refers to owners closely observing managerial behavior to ensure managers behave as desired. Both bonding and monitoring strategies have costs. The complexity of the HIT functions being managed are so great that monitoring has a minimal chance of being successful. Likewise, the weak link between the activities of the HIT leaders and the outcomes that owners desire make bonding strategies questionable. These strategies are made even more problematic during periods of rapid change. Specifying contracts and monitoring activity pose challenges in a changing environment.

HIT priorities have changed to focus on integration of systems across multiple facilities, automation of patient records, and improved decision support for clinicians and managers. Achieving these complex objectives requires a careful planning process to develop a functional, scalable, and flexible information architecture that facilitates data exchange and provides users real-time, remote access to information from any location.

HIT *strategic planning* is the process of identifying and assigning priorities to the applications of information technology to assist an organization in executing its business plans and achieving its strategic goals and objectives. This historical definition, which might have been seen as many as ten years ago, does not sound much different from the definition of HIT governance. Despite the similarities between the two definitions, there are subtle differences with regard to the importance of the external focus of HIT orientation. Many have analyzed HIT governance issues from theoretical and applied perspectives, and much conceptual work has been done—one of which led to the development of Conceptual Framework for IT Governance (Brown and Grant 2005). The Conceptual Framework is a logical structure for assessing and classifying previous efforts to understand HIT decision making as either related to governance (centralized versus decentralized decision framework) or a form of contingency analysis (why and how decisions are made in an organization). Menning and Carpenter (2005) provide a comprehensive review of the healthcare HIT governance alternatives in place, summarize the roles of governance, describe what works in healthcare, and list some potential impediments or pitfalls to avoid. This study is done from the perspective of the experienced HIT leader. One of the few empirical investigations examines in detail how two very different organizations built and sustained an effective governance structure (Smaltz, Carpenter, and Saltz 2007). They conclude that governance effectiveness may depend in part on attaining five domains of governance—strategic alignment, risk management, resource management, performance management, and value delivery. These domains are essentially the same as those found by Menning and Carpenter (2005), and they have remained in place in more current assessments, such as that by Haseley and Brucker (2012), or used in a slightly different format, such as by Herman, Scalzi, and Kropf (2011). Finally, Weill and Ross (2004) present the characteristics of successful HIT governance (which are discussed as components of HIT leadership in Chapter 4).

The importance of HIT strategic planning has increased as healthcare organizations have grown in size and complexity and as information technology has become increasingly sophisticated. Aside from assigning management to coordinate an orderly planning process, HIT governance also requires managers to expand their reach beyond HIT operations to ensure that information technology is used to effectively support the strategic priorities of the organization (Herman, Scalzi, and Kropf 2011; Menning and Carpenter 2005; Weill and Ross 2004). For example, discussions among and about chief information officers (CIOs) often center on topics such as mergers, acquisitions and divestitures, and other strategic options for the organization (as opposed to internal operational issues and new technology). The *23rd Annual HIMSS Leadership Survey* reveals that improving quality outcomes (according to 38 percent of respondents) and reducing medical errors (according to 22 percent of respondents) are the top patient care areas that CIOs believe could be affected by HIT (HIMSS 2012a, Figure 13). This is just one example of how challenges outside of formal HIT operations occupy the attention of CIOs today.

In 2001, Gabler pointed out that governing boards and senior managers of healthcare organizations were increasingly concerned about the business value of investments in information technology and wanted assurances that information systems would deliver strategic benefits to the enterprise. Today, as a continuing response to demands that emerged a decade earlier, HIT strategic planning has assumed a higher priority.

Purpose and Components

HIT governance helps the organization make business decisions accurately and in a timely manner. With that benefit in mind, many have attempted to define the purpose and scope of HIT governance (e.g., Broadbent and Kitzis 2005; Lutchen and Collins 2005; Sambamurthy and Zmud 1999; Weill and Ross 2004). Although they reached no strict agreement, these analysts issued conclusions with mostly subtle differences. Haseley and Brucker (2012) present a compelling case for strict HIT governance review criteria. Following the IT Process Institute's guidelines, they propose five domains or focus areas that purport to have meaning to all HIT processes (Haseley and Brucker 2012, 56):

> *Strategic alignment*—Maximize opportunities for the business use of IT while providing transparency and assurance that IT objectives are being achieved. This includes defining the IT value proposition, determining the linkage between business and IT plans and increasing managerial effectiveness.
>
> *Risk management*—Address legal and regulatory compliance needs and understand and manage key operation risks. This includes determining risk appetite and tolerance, assessing IT risk awareness and identifying risk exposures.
>
> *Resource management*—Appropriately align IT capabilities with business needs, including optimizing IT resources, optimizing knowledge and aligning capabilities.

Performance measurement—Utilize real-time data to continuously improve IT delivery. Approaches include measuring strategy implementation, reporting and the application of operational and strategic metrics.

Value delivery—Optimize return on IT investments by executing on the IT value proposition, meeting business requirements and verifying the integrity and accuracy of information.

The domains listed above do not translate directly to the operational needs of HIT leadership. If you synthesize the information from Menning and Carpenter (2005); Smaltz, Carpenter, and Saltz (2007); and Herman, Scalzi, and Kropf (2011), you find the primary operational components of HIT governance necessary to achieve the key domains. These operational components are listed in Exhibit 5.1 and discussed in more detail in the following sections.

Consistent (and Consistently Applied) HIT Strategy

HIT should support the strategic goals, objectives, and priorities of the organization it serves. As healthcare organizations have become more sophisticated, they use information more effectively to strategically position themselves in the environment in which they operate (Austin, Trimm, and Sobczak 1995, 27; Shortliffe 2005).

As mentioned, hospitals and other healthcare organizations historically employed information technology to support day-to-day operations. Increasingly, healthcare managers are recognizing the role of information systems in increasing market share, supporting quality assessment and improvement, and adding value to the organization. To accomplish these strategic objectives, the HIT plan must be consistently applied across the multiple operating units of an organization. Creating consistent applications in an environment that has grown piecemeal and that consists of employees who do not report directly to the CIO presents a challenge.

---

1. Consistently applied HIT strategy
2. Alignment of HIT strategy with organizational strategy
3. Well-developed HIT infrastructure, architecture, and policies
4. Well-managed HIT project priorities and investments in HIT infrastructure
5. Documented HIT value or benefits to enhance accountability

EXHIBIT 5.1
Components of
HIT Governance

Demonstrating how the HIT strategic planning trend has evolved is the way it has grown and has been given its due over the years. In 1996, 35 percent of the respondents to the *Seventh Annual HIMSS Leadership Survey* indicated that their organizations did not have an HIT strategic plan (HIMSS 1996). By January 2002, that number went down, with only 8 percent of the responding organizations admitting that they lacked such a plan (HIMSS 2002). By 2005, the question of having an HIT strategic plan in place was left out of that year's survey and was replaced by a question of whether the plan was an integrated component of the organization's overall strategic plan (46 percent responded yes) or was integrated in content but stood as a separate plan (44 percent responded yes) (Scottsdale Institute and HIMSS Analytics 2005). In 2012, 48 percent of respondents to the *23rd Annual HIMSS Leadership Survey* indicated that their HIT strategic plan was a component of the organizational strategic plan, while 37 percent of respondents reported that the two plans were separate but integrated in content. Only 7 percent of respondents indicated that the HIT plan was not aligned, and 7 percent reported that the organization did not have an HIT strategic IT plan (HIMSS 2012a, Figure 19).

Alignment of HIT Strategy with Organizational Strategy

The HIT strategic plan must be closely aligned with the strategic plan of the organization. The issue of alignment has been an integral part of the HIT planning mantra for years (see Ward and Griffiths 1996; Wilson 1989). Aligning HIT strategy with the overall organizational strategy requires (1) a consistently applied HIT plan and (2) the recognition by HIT leadership of the importance of the interrelationships among HIT, the rest of the organization, and the external environment. Moreover, Stacey and Skinner (2005) argue that alignment involves three essential elements for success. First, an alignment of purpose must be in place. HIT leadership and organizational leadership must agree that they are trying to achieve the same ends. Second, both sets of leaders must agree to work jointly to develop goals and tactics to meet those ends. Third, they must agree to share the responsibility and accountability for achieving the ends. In the words of Stacey and Skinner (2005, 41), "we're in this together."

Because business objectives change over time, the HIT plan should be reviewed frequently to ensure it remains in alignment with current organizational strategy. Implementing an aligned plan is much more difficult than stating the need for alignment. To assist leaders in achieving strategic alignment, the following six questions must be addressed by the CIO and organizational leadership together from the perspective of the organization:

1. What does the organization do?

2. Who does the organization do it to or for?
3. Where does the organization do it?
4. When does the organization do it?
5. Why does the organization do it?
6. How does the organization do it?

Well-Developed HIT Infrastructure, Architecture, and Policies

Healthcare organizations must make choices and set priorities for their information systems. The plan should identify the major types of information required to support strategic objectives and establish priorities for installation of specific computer applications, the architecture on which the systems function, and the detailed rules that drive HIT operations.

To meet strategic objectives and develop high-priority applications, the healthcare organization must develop blueprints for its HIT infrastructure. This involves making decisions about hardware configuration (architecture), network communications, degree of centralization or decentralization of computing facilities, and types of computer software required to support the network.

The Healthcare Information Management Systems Society (HIMSS) attempts to determine current and future HIT use and adoption through its annual leadership survey. HIMSS has found that use has not varied much during the first decade (2001–2010) of the twenty-first century. For example, the 2005 survey identified the same four information technologies as reported in the 2002 survey:

1. High-speed networks
2. Intranets
3. Wireless information systems
4. Client/server systems

By the 2012 survey, however, the emphasis has changed somewhat. Infrastructure has become the focus, which includes (HIMSS 2012a, Figure 9):

- Servers/virtual servers (according to 19 percent of respondents)
- Mobile devices (18 percent)
- Desktops/virtual desktops (16 percent)
- Security systems (16 percent)
- Storage and backup (8 percent)
- Wired/wireless networks (7 percent)
- Cloud computing (3 percent)
- Telemedicine (2 percent)

After the infrastructure and architecture are developed, the HIT steering committee (see that discussion later in this chapter) should oversee the development of a set of enterprisewide policies that govern the design, acquisition, and operation of information systems throughout the organization. Important policies needed by every organization include data security policies; data definition standards; policies governing the acquisition of hardware, software, and telecommunications network equipment; and policies on use of the Internet.

Data Standardization

As discussed, system integration is an important element of HIT strategic planning in healthcare organizations. Most computer applications must include the ability to share information with other systems. For example, a laboratory results-reporting system must be able to transfer information for storage in the computerized medical records system operated by the organization.

Electronic data exchange cannot occur without some level of standardization of data structures used in computer applications. For this reason, healthcare organizations should consider developing a *data dictionary*—a tool or list that specifies or defines the format of each data element and the coding system (if any) associated with that element. For example, the data dictionary might define the data element "date of birth" as follows:

Date of birth—Eight-digit numeric field with three subfields:
> Month—two digits ranging from 01 to 12
> Day—two digits ranging from 01 to 31
> Year—four digits ranging from 1850 to 2100

In this example, notice that the range of the subfield for year is designed to accommodate historical records of patients with birth dates that go backward to the mid-nineteenth century and forward to the end of the twenty-first century.

In addition to data compatibility among information systems within the organization, there is a growing need to facilitate extra organizational exchange of information among health systems, government and private insurance companies, medical supply and equipment vendors, and other entities. A number of projects have been initiated to develop voluntary, industrywide standards for electronic data interchange in the healthcare field. Examples of these projects include the following:

- The American National Standards Institute (ANSI; www.ansi.org) X.12 Group works on specifications for transactions involving the processing of health insurance claims.

- The Health Industry Business Communication Council (www.hibcc.org/about-hibcc/governance-board/) works to provide common coding of supplies, materials, and equipment.
- Health Level Seven (HL7, version 3; www.hl7.org) is a standard for healthcare electronic data transmission.
- The Healthcare Information Technology Standards Panel (HITSP; www.hitsp.org) received a contract from the US Department of Health & Human Services to support a new collaborative effort to harmonize HIT standards.

The HL7 project was initiated in 1987. It is a voluntary effort of healthcare providers, hardware and software vendors, payers, consultants, government groups, and professional organizations with the goal of developing a cost-effective approach to system connectivity. Its purpose is to develop standards for clinical and administrative data. As with other standard-developing organizations certified by ANSI, HL7 develops messaging specifications that enable organizations to exchange clinical and administrative data; it has been working on improving these specifications since 1987. Version 3 of HL7 embodies a new approach that addresses many of the weaknesses of earlier versions and encompasses messaging, component specifications, structured document architecture, and more. Even earlier versions provided a coherent set of standards for messages, component interfaces, and documents that all users can embrace (Beeler 2001).

The federal government has continued to support the creation and adoption of HL7 and other data exchange standards. As a part of the presidential initiative on consolidated health informatics, the departments of Health & Human Services, Defense, and Veterans Affairs announced the adoption of HL7 messaging standards along with prescription drug, imaging, and other standards in 2003 (Presidential Initiatives 2006). These standards enable the federal agencies to share information and improve coordination of care. Similarly, in 2004, five additional standards related to information exchange were announced (Presidential Initiatives 2006).

In addition to these voluntary efforts at industrywide data standardization are the mandatory electronic data standards and standard transaction formats for claims processing, which were established by the Health Insurance Portability and Accountability Act (HIPAA) of 1996. Providers are required to follow these standards to receive reimbursement from Medicare, Medicaid, and other health insurers. As a means of addressing growing mandatory standards, "HITSP [brings] together a wide range of stakeholders to identify, select, and harmonize standards for communicating data throughout the healthcare spectrum," (ANSI 2005). Under a contract from the Department of Health & Human Services and the sponsorship of ANSI, HIMSS, the Advanced Technology Institute, and Booz Allen Hamilton (a strategic partner), HITSP attempts "to accelerate the adoption of health information technology and the secure portability of health information across the United States" (AHRQ 2005; HIMSS 2005b). The purpose of HITSP is to develop a generally accepted "set of standards specifically to enable and support 'widespread interoperability, accurate use, access, privacy and security of shared health information'" (ANSI 2005; HIMSS 2005b). HITSP is designed to function with public and private partnerships that have the potential to access much of the healthcare community. If successful in getting healthcare software developers and users to adopt these standards, it will buoy the Nationwide Health Information Network initiative for the United States called for by President George W. Bush by Executive Order #13335, which established the Office of the National Coordinator for Health Information Technology (ONCHIT).

The challenge of achieving data standards to enable organizations to share data internally and externally is a work in progress. Mostly concerned with the external challenge, the ONCHIT has continually updated information regarding the status, requirements, and progress of moving toward health data standardization. The Office of the Director of Science and Technology is a valuable starting point for keeping current (see www.health it.gov/policy-researchers-implementers/desk-chief-science-officer). While constantly changing, common information initiatives include the following:

- Federal Health Architecture (www.healthit.gov/policy-researchers -implementers/federal-health-architecture-fha) seeks to coordinate data exchange and reporting requirements across federal agencies responsible for delivery and support of healthcare.
- Interoperability Portfolio (www.healthit.gov/policy-researchers -implementers/interoperability-portfolio) is the central repository of current standards development and setting.
- Standards Acceleration (www.healthit.gov/policy-researchers -implementers/standards-acceleration) works to ensure that a functional infrastructure is in place to support the adoption of HIT throughout the country.
- International Health IT Standards aim to assemble the planning and coordination being done with providers and systems abroad so that US HIT standards are not at odds or incompatible with HIT systems from other countries.

Despite these ongoing efforts, data standards still present major challenges. Panangala and Jansen (2013) published an assessment of the potential for the Department of Defense and the Veterans Health Administration to merge health information across active service and retired service member systems. They suggest that significant challenges exist such that the original goal of creating a single medical record for all service-connected personnel is being replaced by improved interoperability between the systems. Furthermore, health information exchanges (HIEs) are not progressing as quickly or easily as hoped (Kellerman and Jones 2013). The reason the HIE has been stalled is not exclusively due to data standards, but Kellerman and Jones's analysis indicates that a major impediment is the failure to specify a standard structure and format of data exchanged or the definition of the terms used.

As part of the HIT strategic planning process, the steering committee should study requirements for data interchange, including HIPAA mandates, and should develop a policy on data standardization for the organization. For example, many hospitals and integrated delivery systems (IDSs) are specifying that all software purchased from vendors must meet an industry standard protocol such as HL7.

Hardware and Software Standards

Healthcare organizations need to develop a number of technical policies related to information systems. Most of these are highly technical and should be drafted by the CIO or the director of information systems operations. However, the HIT steering committee should oversee the creation of a broad set of policies related to the acquisition of computer hardware, software, and network communications equipment for the organization.

The steering committee must determine whether the organization will require central review and approval of all computer hardware and software purchases. As the costs of personal computers and related software packages have come down, their purchase now falls within the budgetary authority of individual organizational units. However, some compelling reasons exist for requiring central review and approval, regardless of cost, including the following:

1. Central review and approval helps ensure compatibility with enterprise-wide data standards, such as HL7.
2. Central review and approval of personal computer purchases can ensure that data terminals and workstations use a common operating system, such as Windows.
3. Central review and purchasing of generalized software provides cost advantages through the acquisition of site licenses for multiple users of common packages (e.g., word processing, spreadsheets, database management).
4. Central review and approval ensures that hardware and software are of a type that can receive technical support and maintenance from the HIT staff.

5. Central review and approval can help prevent illegal use of unlicensed software within the organization.

In addition, the HIT steering committee should approve the network communications plan for the enterprise. A variety of network configurations are possible, and the network plan must be compatible with the overall HIT development plan for the organization.

Well-Managed HIT Project Priorities and Investments in HIT Infrastructure

The HIT function must also effectively oversee the purchase and implementation of HIT infrastructure consistent with the needs of the organization. The specialized knowledge and skills of HIT staff and the growing complexity of the underlying technology make this overseer role vital to the success of HIT operations. The use of technology has made information available and accessible to clinical and administrative staff across the organization, but the infrastructure on which software and other applications operate in the systems through which data are transmitted remains the domain of HIT. While end users are vital considerations in the priority-setting process, governance of HIT requires HIT leadership to effectively manage the priorities among alternative investment options (Menning and Carpenter 2005). This management includes items directly from the HIT strategic plan; for example, as outlined by Stacey and Skinner (2005, 44), a hospital had to change all of its human resources, finance, patient accounting, and other support services information systems to enable integration with the rest of the health system and investments that arise episodically (a good example was Y2K considerations; see Wilson and McPherson [2002]).

Documented HIT Value or Benefits to Enhance Accountability

The final purpose of HIT strategic planning is to provide data for estimating the budget and resources required to meet the objectives and priorities established through the planning process. Planning is the basis for developing operating and capital budgets for HIT in the organization. The importance of this purpose has increased as CIOs report the need to obtain value from HIT (Glaser and Garets 2005). Turisco (2000, 13) called for value management in justifying HIT investments: "There is a growing demand for ensuring that . . . HIT investment practices and processes not only justify the large cash outlays, but track and realize the value. . . . Values can only be realized through measurable business changes supported by the business units." The Center for Information Technology Leadership published a number of articles arguing that greater documentation of HIT value is essential (e.g., Johnston, Pan, and Middleton 2002). This "call to the field" identifies three dimensions from which to derive HIT value: financial, clinical, and organizational. With this direction, a host of studies have emerged to address all or some of these dimensions (see Buntin et al. 2011; Encinosa and Bae 2011; Menachemi et al. 2006; Rahimi and Vimarlund 2007). The financial return on these investments is addressed in more detail in Chapter 13.

The financial dimension is the most obvious source of value, consisting of cost reductions, revenue enhancements, and productivity gains. Clinical enhancements seek evidence of HIT's impact on service delivery (e.g., adherence to protocols) and clinical outcome indicators. Organizational enhancements include stakeholder satisfaction improvements and risk reduction. In all cases, Johnston, Pan, and Middleton's (2002, 1) fundamental point is that healthcare executives currently must rely on "anecdote, inference, and opinion to make critical HIT decisions." The evidence is still mixed, but some studies show the value of HIT when applied to specific technologies such as computerized physician order entry (CPOE) (e.g., Johnston et al. 2003; Koppel et al. 2005: Yu et al. 2009) and information exchange and interoperability (e.g., Walker et al. 2005). In addition, positive results have been observed when applied in small group practices (Miller et al. 2005) and among primary care physicians (Pizziferri et al. 2005) and when tangible and intangible financial benefits are examined (Simon and Simon 2006). At this point, diverse research has not yet achieved a consensus on the financial or clinical value of HIT.

Organizing an HIT Strategic Planning Effort

The development of information systems in a modern healthcare organization is a complex task involving major capital expenditures and significant staff commitments if the systems are to function properly. Developing a consistent, integrated master plan for information systems is essential. To exclude this critical planning activity would be analogous to beginning a trip without knowing precisely the destination, the method of transportation, the route or directions to the destination, the time frame of arrival or departure, and the budget or allowance for the trip. While we would not do this as individuals, organizations continue to move directly into the acquisition of computer systems without any kind of master plan. This section provides guidelines for those organizations that have yet to create, organize for, or implement an HIT strategic plan.

General Approach

The CEO should take direct responsibility for organizing the planning effort. As discussed, appropriate governance creates an environment in which the board of trustees assigns responsibility, authority, and accountability to the

CEO; thus, the impetus for action rests with the CEO. Many structures have been proposed for this planning effort, ranging from highly centralized to informal discussions between the CEO and the CIO (Menning and Carpenter 2005). Naturally, the level of sophistication of this structure depends on the size and complexity of the organization and the nature of the environment in which it operates.

Generally, because the CEO often does not have the expertise or time to develop the HIT plan, an HIT steering committee should be formed with representatives from major units of the organization that contribute to and benefit from HIT functions. This committee should include representatives from senior management; the medical staff; and nursing, finance, human resources, planning and marketing, facilities, clinical support services, and information technology functions. The committee should be directed by a senior manager—preferably the CIO if such a position has been established. HIT strategic planning is primarily a managerial, not a technical, duty. A suggested organizational chart for the planning effort is shown in Exhibit 5.2. The HIT steering committee usually has subcommittees that manage discrete aspects of the steering committee's responsibilities. Specific tasks of subcommittees differ according to local needs, but the following are the three components that subcommittees typically address:

1. *Priorities for new and replacement systems.* The identification and planning for new and, importantly, replacement applications serve to determine the scope of user needs.
2. *Specifications for information technology infrastructure.* Technology infrastructure specifications must be created by the most technically proficient members of the steering committee.
3. *Capital and operating budgeting.* The budget group is essential to keeping the scale and scope of technology needs under control.

Steering committee composition includes senior staff in HIT as well as representatives from the key constituencies across the organization. Additional personnel from the organization and technical consultants can be appointed members of specific subcommittees as needed. The chairs of the subcommittees usually come from the steering committee.

Consideration also should be given to use of outside consultants if additional technical expertise is needed in the planning process. Except for the largest, most organizations cannot employ all of the specialized technical expertise necessary to make quality, informed decision about information technology. Consequently, hiring these experts is a necessity, but consultants should be chosen carefully. They should possess technical knowledge of systems analysis and computer systems and should be well informed about

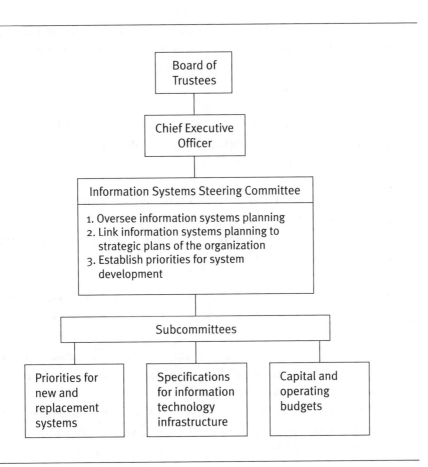

EXHIBIT 5.2
Suggested Organizational Chart for HIT Strategic Planning

healthcare organizations. Consultants must be independent practitioners—not associated with any equipment manufacturer or firm that sells software. When hiring independent consultants, executives must be sure that the consultants have no bias or stand to benefit from the decisions made, especially in cases when the organization lacks the in-house expertise to validate consultants' recommendations. Finally, consultants should be familiar with the latest technological developments but must be able to resist the temptation to push for applications that are too close to the leading edge.

Lohman (1996) suggested that the following factors be considered in selecting an information systems consultant; this advice is still valid more than 15 years after publication:

- *Independence and objectivity.* The consultant should exclusively focus on the interests of the client.
- *Healthcare expertise.* The consultant should have an understanding of healthcare business and clinical issues.

- *Resources.* The consultant should have sufficient breadth and depth of resources to complete the assignment without "on-the-job training."
- *Effective personality.* The consultant should have an appropriate mix of character traits and skills.

Advice abounds regarding how to select consultants in general and HIT consultants in particular. For example, Goedert (2004) provides the following tips, all of which apply to almost any situation:

- *Do your homework.* Research your needs and the experience that each prospective firm brings to the table.
- *Pick the team.* Once you narrow the search, get background information on the actual consultants who will be working with you on the project.
- *Build trust.* A long-term consulting engagement is built on mutual trust and respect. If not, you will spend your time monitoring and wondering.
- *Define the job.* Make sure that you are clear about the scale and scope of the job being contracted. Job creep and unclear expectations can arise if you are unsure of your goals.
- *Watch for bias.* Consultants have built-in bias as does everyone, but often this involves operational directions or vendor affiliation. These are not always bad but need to be recognized up front.

EMRapproved.com (2012) recommends healthcare leaders to ask a potential HIT consultant the following questions:

Do you have any certifications or support experience in healthcare specific technology?

What do you know about HIPAA compliance?

How familiar are you with EMR/EHR/PM solutions?

Do you have any experience with or access to Medical Device connectivity?

What do you know about electronic vs. paper medical workflow?

Consultants should be used as sources of technical information and as facilitators of the planning process; they should not be employed to do the planning. Planning must be the responsibility of knowledgeable managers and users of information within the organization itself. Consultants can be of most assistance by advising those on the steering committee of the functionality specifications of the technology or systems being considered and the system-level consequences of an action or decision. Before using a consultant's "off the shelf" planning product, ensure that the planning methodology is compatible with the organization's culture and strategic priorities.

Boyd (2005) presents an interesting set of reasons for and against outsourcing HIT. Although his discussion is more in the context of outsourcing fundamental HIT functions, the reasoning applies in the case of hiring consultants to advise the steering committee. Simply put, organizations should outsource to take advantage of the capacity and expertise of the external resource and reduce the fixed costs of having added expertise in-house.

The CEO should ensure that staff members participating on the steering committee are provided sufficient "release time" from their normal duties so that they can participate fully in the planning efforts. Release-time estimates should be drawn up in advance, and formal written notification of this time should be provided to all involved. Senior management and the board of trustees should be prepared to allow a significant number of the institution's staff to carry out this important task.

As stated, the CIO should chair the steering committee, if the CIO position has been established. Reporting directly to the CEO or COO, the CIO serves two important functions: (1) assist the senior management team and governing board in using information to support strategic planning and management and (2) provide management oversight and coordination of information systems and telecommunications throughout the organization. See Chapter 4 for a full description of the role of the CIO.

Elements of an HIT Strategic Plan

Exhibit 5.3 lists seven major elements that should be included in the HIT strategic plan, each of which is discussed in this section.

Statement of Corporate/Institutional Goals and Objectives

The HIT strategic plan should begin with a review and concise statement of major organizational goals and objectives for the three- to five-year planning period. HIT goals and objectives should be aligned with the strategic objectives of the organization. For example, if reduction of medical errors is a major priority, then this goal should be reflected in the priorities for HIT development, paying particular attention to medical records, clinical protocols, clinical decision support systems, and incident reporting. If diversification and expansion of the market service base are strategic objectives, then information systems should focus on utilization analysis and forecasting, analysis of changes in the demographic profile of the service market, and analysis of resource requirements for new service development. If an urban

EXHIBIT 5.3
Elements of the
HIT Strategic
Plan

1. Statement of corporate/institutional goals and objectives
2. Statement of HIT goals and objectives
    a. Management information needs
    b. Critical success factors
    c. Information priorities
3. Priorities for the applications portfolio
    a. Clinical
    b. Management/administrative
    c. Electronic networking and e-health
    d. Strategic decision support
4. Specification of overall HIT architecture and infrastructure
    a. Level of distribution
    b. Network architecture
    c. Data location (central data warehouse to total data distribution)
    d. Integration via Internet
    e. Database security and control requirements
5. Software development plan
    a. Commercial packages
    b. In-house development
    c. Contract software development
    d. Application service providers
    e. Combinations of the above
6. HIT management and staffing plan
    a. Central information systems staffing and control
    b. Limited central staffing in support of department-level HIT staff
    c. Outsourcing
    d. Combinations of the above
7. Statement of resource requirements
    a. Capital budget (e.g., for hardware, software, network communication equipment)
    b. Operating budget (e.g., for personnel, supplies, consultants, training)

medical center has placed priority on expansion of ambulatory care services, but HIT priorities continue to focus on inpatient services, then the organization has a serious problem of goal displacement.

Critical success factors are often used in defining information requirements and HIT goals during the planning process (Rockart 1979; Ward and Griffiths 1996). Variations on the approach have been adopted. Kuperman and colleagues (2006) used a "requirements-driven" approach for quality improvement, identifying data warehousing and clinical encounter documentation as the critical factors that would lead to improved patient quality. Similarly, Johnson (2005) used a continuous cycle of assessment, prioritization, and scheduling to optimally allocate scarce HIT resources. Senior management must define these requirements for HIT, but executives often have difficulty with specifying needs for information. By pointing out the critical areas in which things must go right for the organization to flourish, senior managers assist the HIT planning team in determining information requirements and setting priorities for system development. Effectively communicating goals among the C-suite officers of the organization is critical to success.

Statement of HIT Goals and Objectives

Objectives should be as specific as possible and should flow from a review of strategic priorities and an analysis of deficiencies and gaps in current information processes. The CIO and other members of the steering committee should consult a good text or how-to book on strategic planning at this stage so that goals and objectives are well specified (Swayne, Duncan, and Ginter 2005). Avoid general statements of objectives such as "information systems for Metropolitan Health System should be designed to improve the quality of care and increase the efficiency of system operations." Such statements are self-evident and nonfunctional as far as planning is concerned. Rather, a detailed list of objectives should be established that will provide specific targets against which future progress can be measured and systems can be evaluated. Examples of specific objectives might include the following:

- Information systems for the health plan should be designed such that all records from the master patient index file are available online to all physicians in the plan.
- Information systems for the clinic should be designed such that all diagnostic test results are available online within two hours after the tests have been completed.
- Information systems should be designed such that information on inpatient and outpatient activity by major diagnostic categories is reported to corporate management on a monthly basis, with reports indicating the health system's share of the total services provided in the market area.
- Disease-management protocols for the ten highest-volume chronic conditions should be available online and should be used to provide automatic reminders to all physicians practicing in the hospital.
- If the organization is a university-affiliated health system, expand the university's current information infrastructure to optimally meet the ongoing needs of the institution in the areas of research, education, patient care, and community service.
- Support the institution's information technology users through the formation of a service center.

These goals and objectives then provide the pool from which the organization must derive its set of key priorities.

Priorities for the Applications Portfolio

Healthcare organizations cannot acquire all the systems they need in any given year. The statements of corporate and HIT objectives aid the steering committee in preparing a priority list of individual computer applications to be acquired. The applications priority list, in turn, is essential in planning how limited resources can be used to have the greatest impact on strategic priorities. Chapter 8 provides a comprehensive discussion of application opportunities.

The applications list should consider the needs of all major functional areas of the healthcare organization, such as finance, human resources, resource utilization and scheduling, materials management, facilities and project management, and office automation. Both new and replacement systems should be considered, and the need for major changes to existing systems should be reviewed as well. Applications should be rank ordered in the recommended sequence for implementation, and items on the applications priority list should be linked to specific organizational strategies. If an HIT steering committee determines that financial control is the most pressing organizational problem, the development of a new financial information system might assume highest priority.

Many healthcare organizations have initiated programs of business process reengineering to achieve operational efficiency through dramatic improvement in core processes used in the organization. The pay-for-performance movement sponsored by government and business has raised the urgency of process improvement (Rosenthal et al. 2006). This broad movement makes clear not only the importance of HIT but also the involvement of all components of the delivery systems (Petersen et al. 2006). Many of these reengineering projects involve development of new information systems, and these should be considered by the HIT steering committee in developing the applications priority list.

After the priority list has been completed, the steering committee should report preliminary results back to the CEO and board of trustees. The statement of objectives and priority list should be carefully reviewed and modified as necessary to make sure that together they reflect the positions of senior management and the board.

Specification of Overall HIT Architecture and Infrastructure

Specification of overall systems architecture is a critical task in the planning process. Chapter 6 provides an overview of HIT architecture and infrastructure. In short, the plan must specify an overall architecture and infrastructure, including the following:

1. *The degree to which computing is centralized or decentralized throughout the organization.* Opinions differ about the degree to which computing should be centralized or decentralized in healthcare organizations (DeFord and Porter 2005). Carr (2003) argues that HIT no longer matters in obtaining a competitive advantage for healthcare organizations. The reason is that information technology is such an integral part of all aspects of healthcare delivery that no one organization benefits more than its competitors from having extensive information technology. DeFord and Porter (2005) argue convincingly, however, that information technology infrastructure as one part of overall HIT is still valuable and benefits from centralization. In their opinion, centralized information technology does the following:

   - Reduces variability
   - Improves security
   - Reduces human resource requirements
   - Enhances flexibility
   - Reduces procurement costs
   - Reduces total cost of ownership
   - Improves end-user satisfaction
   - More effectively and efficiently aligns HIT to business needs

   Proponents of decentralization, on the other hand, claim that decentralization places control of information systems back where they belong—in the hands of users. It fosters innovation in system design and develops increased user interest and support. Local flexibility is maintained, and the frustrations of lengthy programming and processing backlogs at a central facility are avoided.

2. *The network architecture that specifies how computers and workstations are linked together through communication lines and network servers.* Chapter 6 includes a detailed description of alternative network architecture configurations, including the following:

   - Terminal–host system
   - Client/server computing
   - File/server architecture
   - Peer network
   - Grid and cloud computing

   Data distribution plans help determine which type of network architecture should be employed by the healthcare organization. Alternatives range from creation of large, centralized (enterprisewide) data warehouses to complete distribution of data in which each organizational unit on the network maintains its own database.

3. *The manner in which data are stored and distributed throughout the organization, including database security and control requirements.*

Many healthcare organizations, particularly IDSs, have moved toward a combination of approaches to data distribution. For example, the IDS might develop a centralized data warehouse containing a master patient index and computerized records for all patients in the system. Individual organizations within the IDS (e.g., hospitals, ambulatory care centers) might maintain their own data files for patient appointments, employee records, inventory control, budgeting, and financial management. The telecommunications network supporting the system is designed to facilitate electronic exchange of information so that patient records are accessible at all treatment sites and financial information can be transmitted to corporate offices on a periodic basis. In addition to describing the network architecture, the plan should specify how the infrastructure supports related activities such as audio, video, and wireless communications; document imaging; and radiographic imaging.

4. *The manner by which individual applications are linked so that they can exchange information.* Interoperability is discussed fully in Chapter 2, but briefly it is a key strategic consideration that affects all clinical and administrative components of the delivery system.

Regardless of the approach followed for data distribution and system integration, data standards are required. Data security and protection of information confidentiality are discussed in Chapter 3. The subcommittee that reviews HIT architecture and infrastructure must include competent technical staff and/or consultants working closely with representatives of management, the medical staff, and other major HIT users.

Software Development Plan

The HIT strategic plan should specify procedures for software development. In the early days of healthcare computing (1960s to 1980s), most hospitals and other healthcare organizations employed a staff of computer analysts and programmers to develop computer applications in-house. Today, most healthcare organizations rely primarily on software packages purchased from commercial vendors. A wide array of software products is available; see, for example, the annual resource guide published by *Health Management Technology* magazine (which is available online at www.healthmgttech.com). This source presents a vast listing of companies, including a brief description of the company, its product categories, and contact information.

Use of application service providers (ASPs) is another alternative for software acquisition that has grown in popularity among healthcare organizations. An ASP is a firm that contracts with a healthcare organization on a subscription basis to provide access to and use of applications on an off-site server (Monohan 2001). Many large healthcare organizations and IDSs use combinations of these software development options. Commercial software may be combined with tailor-made programs developed by in-house staff, particularly programs that support database management and electronic communications across the network. ASPs may be used for selected applications by smaller units affiliated with the enterprise.

HIT Management and Staffing Plan

The HIT strategic plan should specify the management structure for information systems. Most healthcare organizations still employ an in-house staff for information system operation and management, even if all or most software is purchased from commercial vendors or leased from ASPs.

Decisions must be made on the extent to which technical personnel are centralized or distributed among the major user departments of the organization. An increasing number of organizations are outsourcing all or some of their information-processing functions to contractors who provide on-site system implementation and management services.

Centralized staffing offers the advantages of economies of scale and reduction in the number of technical personnel to be employed. Decentralized staffing brings systems management closer to the user and offers the potential for increased support and user involvement in system development and operation.

Outsourcing HIT functions allows the healthcare organization to get out of the information technology business through contracting with experts in the field. However, the costs of outsourcing may be high and may tend to generate too much distance between users and technical systems specialists.

Statement of Resource Requirements

The final element of the HIT plan identifies the resources required to carry out the plan. The capital budget should include five- to ten-year projections for the cost of computer hardware, network and telecommunications equipment, and software. The operating budget includes costs for personnel, supplies and materials, consultants, training programs, and other recurring expenses. Both budgets should be updated annually, and the timing of their preparation should be coordinated with the overall organizational budget cycle.

Although the information technology budgets of healthcare organizations lag those of other information-intensive industries, the *23rd Annual HIMSS Leadership Survey* reports that budgets are increasing in an attempt to keep pace with developing technology. Seventy-five percent of the survey respondents indicated that their budgets definitely or probably would increase in the current year, and only 7 percent expected their budgets to decrease (HIMSS 2012a).

The planning process is the subject of many other books, but to round out our discussion here, we provide a generic planning methodology adapted from Glaser (2002) in Exhibit 5.4. This plan starts with the necessary gathering of information to review existing organizational strategies with senior management and middle management. The goal is to identify information systems needs by contrasting existing resources with the requirements that will meet users' expressed needs. Glaser suggests that much of the information gathering should be done by external consultants.

Once the gap between needs and capabilities is determined, the next step is to delineate information systems alternatives. These alternatives will require key implementation steps to be specified, followed by estimates of resource requirements and timelines for implementation. Finally, the full plan with recommendations is presented to management.

EXHIBIT 5.4
Generic HIT
Strategic
Planning
Methodology

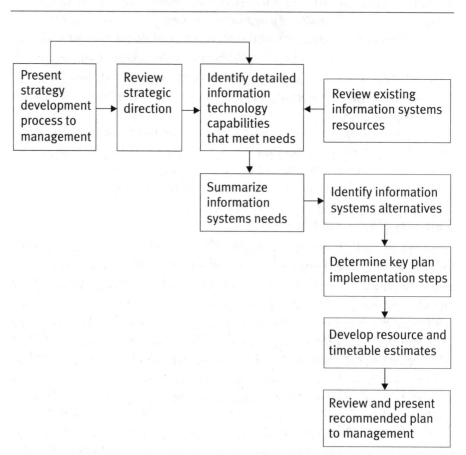

SOURCE: Glaser (2002). Adapted with permission of John Wiley & Sons, Hoboken, New Jersey.

Review and Approval of the HIT Strategic Plan

The HIT plan should include an overall schedule, detailing the target dates for implementation. Although cost estimates and target dates are preliminary at this point, they assist management and board members in evaluating the magnitude of organizational commitments required to implement the recommended set of alternatives.

After the HIT steering committee has approved the plan, it should be presented to executive management and the governing board for their review and approval prior to implementation. The written plan should be submitted to management in advance of a formal presentation and discussion session.

As with any plan, the HIT strategic plan must be a dynamic instrument that is reviewed periodically and updated regularly. At least once a year, the steering committee should review progress in meeting the original criteria set forth in the plan, and the plan should be changed as necessary. This review process is essential for the steering committee to monitor progress in completing goals (or any related barriers) and to report that status to HIT leadership. If problems arise or should the environment change dramatically, the committee may put forward a suggestion that the organization change strategic direction.

End-User Computing

A problem that many healthcare organizations face is what to do about dissatisfaction among organizational units whose information systems needs are not identified as priorities in the HIT strategic plan. End-user computing strategies offer one potential solution to this problem.

Many employees have become sophisticated in their computer use. Powerful personal computers with user-friendly software and user-oriented programming tools have helped to facilitate end-user computing in that they no longer require the services or resources of the central HIT department.

End-user computing most often involves use of departmental software packages purchased from vendors (e.g., laboratory, pharmacy, radiology systems) or leased from an ASP. In some cases, computer-literate users may write programs to meet specialized needs in their departments. For example, end users at an outpatient clinic in a large medical center may create and maintain a database of companies that provide medical supplies for the clinic.

End-user computing offers the potential to expand the base of HIT development and overcome issues that arise when a low priority is assigned to certain applications that are nevertheless viewed as important to units within the organization. End-user computing must be approached cautiously, however. Most activities in healthcare organizations are interrelated, and computer applications must be able to exchange information for efficient operations (see the next section on standards and policies). If a departmental system can stand alone, management might authorize acquisition, provided that department funds are available and the system is developed in accordance with the HIT strategic plan and enterprisewide standards and policies. If the system needs to exchange information with other units of the organization, central control and planning is needed before the end-user department is authorized to acquire the system. *Data compatibility*—use of common codes and data definitions for electronic information exchange across the organization—should be mandatory (see the following section).

HIT Strategic Planning for IDSs

IDSs must consider the need for integration of information systems across institutions as well as within individual organizational units. Such integration is particularly critical in vertically integrated organizations, where patients may progress and seek treatment at various organizational units such as clinics, surgical centers, acute care hospitals, substance abuse centers, and skilled nursing facilities. Information systems must be patient centered to aggregate data from the various medical care units and track patients throughout the healthcare delivery organization. At the same time, corporate system management must recognize that different types of facilities (e.g., hospitals, ambulatory care centers and clinics, nursing homes, home health agencies) have their own distinct information requirements. Corporate policy must provide mechanisms for specialized information systems to meet the needs of individual units.

Information systems for an IDS must be able to provide comparative financial data for management to efficiently allocate resources to individual units. Such a capability is especially critical when healthcare costs are paid on a capitation basis. Corporate management will need to carefully monitor how patient care dollars are being spent across units for actuarial risk analysis. The IDS also needs special information for the purposes of market research and analysis of competitor services. Physician performance in various components of the system must be monitored as well.

At the technical level, information systems for an IDS may require standardization of coding and data definition for all organizational units— for example, a common chart of accounts for financial reporting. If such an approach is not feasible, then complex data conversion tables are required to facilitate electronic data exchange. To serve corporate management information needs and operational support requirements of each medical care unit, IDSs need to strike a balance between centralized data management and local control of data processing.

In recent years, hospitals have merged to form corporate systems, medical centers have acquired community hospitals and brought them into their organizations, and some corporate systems have sold or divested some of their existing facilities. These mergers and changes in ownership can create special problems with respect to information systems at the individual facilities.

If the corporate system has highly centralized information processing through a corporate data center and acquires a new facility, it needs to draft a special HIT plan to bring the new unit into the central system while allowing it to continue to use its current hardware and software to support ongoing operations. If computing within the corporate system is decentralized at the facility level, the newly acquired facility may not have compatible hardware and/or software with other units of the enterprise. Conversion programs may be required to convert data from these legacy systems to meet corporate reporting requirements. Unique information-processing problems usually result from these mergers, acquisitions, and joint ventures. Management at both the corporate and institutional levels must be prepared to address these problems as the plans for organizational change are developed.

Data Warehouses

Many health systems are developing data warehouses to serve the needs of facilities within their systems. Breen and Rodrigues (2001, 87) present a case study on development of a data warehouse and conclude, "Successful implementation of a data warehouse involves a corporate treasure hunt—identifying and cataloging data. It involves data ownership, data integrity, and business process analysis to determine what the data are, who owns them, how reliable they are, and how they are processed."

The Cleveland Clinic, based in Ohio, has extended its efforts to report quality indicators by using its administrative and clinical data repository of patient data to aggregate and report physician indicators of quality. In its settings, advanced practice nurses (APNs) provide primary care to patients in the ambulatory setting, but the data are traditionally linked to the primary care provider and not to the nurse. The extension is to link patient information assembled via its electronic health record to the APN managing the patient. In this way, quality outcomes can be reported for this vital provider group, demonstrating APNs' contribution to patient care (Kapoor et al. 2006).

Even the federal government has developed the data warehouse concept for collection, storage, and dissemination of the vast quantity of healthcare data it manages. For example, the website of the National Center for Health Statistics, part of the Centers for Disease Control and Prevention (see http://healthindicators.gov/) has information on the Health Indicators Warehouse. This repository enables users to select vast quantities of health information by topic (e.g., health behavior, disabilities), geography (e.g., state), or initiative (e.g., Healthy People 2020, County Health Indicators). Similarly, the Healthcare Data Warehousing Association (http://hdwa.org/hdwa/home/) was created to facilitate the use of health data to control costs, improve quality, and improve patient satisfaction and quality.

Importance of System Integration

The What

Certain background concepts are important to an understanding of the effective application of information technology in healthcare organizations. These concepts include general systems theory, which is the basis of the key principles of management related to the development and operation of information systems, including the need for change management in adapting systems to the organizational culture.

Systems Theory

Systems theory is the foundation on which the development of information systems is based. Healthcare managers should have a general understanding of this theory to determine how information systems function in their organizations, particularly in using information for management control. Scientists have completed considerable research on systems and how they function in all phases of society. Interest in *general systems theory* developed in the post–World War II period. Initial research efforts were focused primarily on the physical sciences, with the study of strategic military weapons systems, systems for space exploration, and automated systems of all kinds to reduce manual labor and improve the overall quality of life.

In the 1960s, attention shifted to the application of systems theory to the social sciences, including organizational theory and management. Although much of this work is highly theoretical and of interest to those involved primarily in research, some general discussion of systems theory is a useful background for understanding management control systems in healthcare delivery and for setting forth principles of information systems analysis and design.

The systems approach is important because it concentrates on examining a process in its entirety, rather than focusing on the parts, and relates the parts to each other to achieve total system goals. Management control requires that performance be compared against expectations and that feedback be used to adjust the system when performance goals are not being met.

Systems analysis is a fundamental tool for the design and development of information systems. It is the process of studying organizational operations and determining information systems requirements for a given application. Systems analysis employs concepts from general systems theory in analyzing inputs, processes, outputs, and feedback in defining requirements for an information system. The remainder of this section presents a general overview of systems theory and its application in healthcare organizations.

A variety of systems compose the functioning of healthcare organizations. These systems can be categorized into three groups: mechanical systems, human systems, and human–machine systems. *Mechanical systems* are an integral part of the physical plant, serving such purposes as heating and cooling; monitoring temperature, pressure, and humidity; and supplying chilled and heated water. Most of the essential functions of a healthcare organization are carried out through *human systems*—organized relationships among patients, physicians, employees, family members of patients, and others. Many of these human systems are formally defined. For example, nursing care is provided in accordance with a scheduled set of predetermined protocols and procedures, and nursing service personnel are trained and supervised in the proper execution of this system of care. Many things also happen through informal relationships, which often become well defined and known to those in the organization. Thus, certain activities get accomplished by "knowing the right person" or sending informal signals to key individuals about actions that need to be taken. Because of the development of modern information technology, many systems fall into the third category of *human–machine systems*. These are formally defined systems in which human effort is assisted by various kinds of automated equipment. For example, computer systems have been developed to continuously monitor the vital signs of critically ill patients in intensive care units of hospitals or medical centers.

HIT falls into the second and third categories of this simple taxonomy; that is, information systems are either human systems or human–machine systems designed to support operations. Information systems that operate without any type of machine processing of data are referred to as *manual systems*. Although much of this book deals with computer-aided information processing, most of the principles set forth here—particularly those dealing with systems analysis and design—apply equally to the manual systems for information processing.

A healthcare organization can be described in a systems context as well. Exhibit 5.5 is a systems diagram for a healthcare organization; it shows the relationships among and between various inputs and environmental factors as these factors influence the provision of services to the community. In this context, mechanical, human, and human–machine systems constitute elements (or subsystems) of the conversion process (discussed later).

Certain basic concepts explain what systems are and how they function:

Systems Characteristics

- *A system must have unity or integrity.* A system must be viewed as an entity in its own right; it has a unity of purpose—the accomplishment of a goal or function. A system must have an identity and must have

EXHIBIT 5.5
The Healthcare Organization as a System

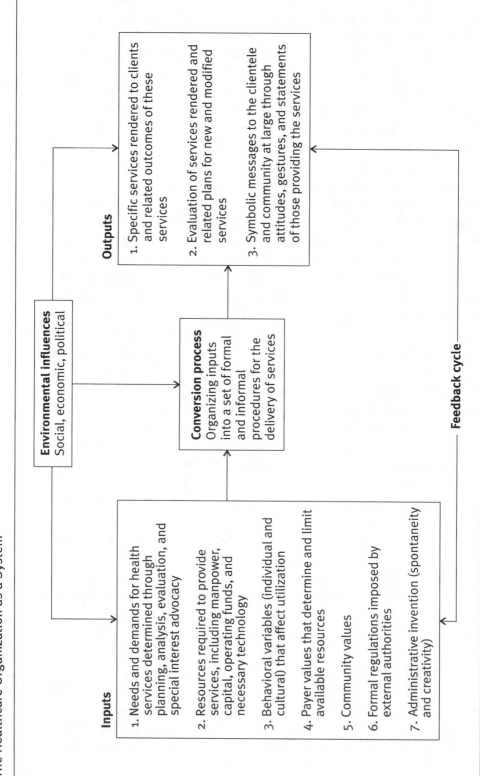

Environmental influences
Social, economic, political

Inputs

1. Needs and demands for health services determined through planning, analysis, evaluation, and special interest advocacy

2. Resources required to provide services, including manpower, capital, operating funds, and necessary technology

3. Behavioral variables (individual and cultural) that affect utilization

4. Payer values that determine and limit available resources

5. Community values

6. Formal regulations imposed by external authorities

7. Administrative invention (spontaneity and creativity)

Conversion process
Organizing inputs into a set of formal and informal procedures for the delivery of services

Outputs

1. Specific services rendered to clients and related outcomes of these services

2. Evaluation of services rendered and related plans for new and modified services

3. Symbolic messages to the clientele and community at large through attitudes, gestures, and statements of those providing the services

Feedback cycle

describable boundaries that allow it to be defined without reference to external events or objects.

- *Systems at work in healthcare organizations are, mostly, very complex.* The intricate web of complex relationships that constitute most social systems often makes describing the simple cause-and-effect relationships among individual system components difficult. System complexity is often described as a byproduct of a system being more than the sum of its parts.

- *Complex systems are further defined by their hierarchical structure.* Large systems in healthcare organizations can be divided into several subsystems, and these subsystems in turn are subject to further subdivision in a nested format. For example, the patient care component of an IDS is composed of several subsystems—diagnostic, therapeutic, rehabilitative, and so forth. Each of these subsystems can be further delineated by a series of smaller systems. The network of systems and subsystems of a patient care system has a nested structure (see Exhibit 5.6).

- *Although most organizational systems are dynamic and subject to frequent change, they nonetheless must possess some stability and equilibrium.* The

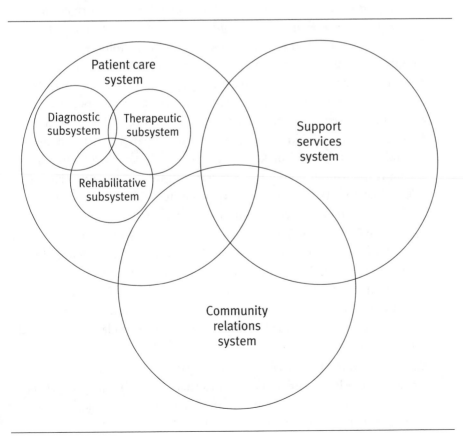

EXHIBIT 5.6
Healthcare Organization Systems Network

system must continue to function in the face of changing requirements and changing external environment in which it operates. To accomplish this, procedures must be sufficiently generalized to accommodate a variety of situations that could develop. Complex systems must be self-adapting and must include control functions that are continuous and automatic. When the system can no longer adapt to changing requirements or external environment, it no longer functions as a system and signifies that a breakdown has occurred.

- *Systems can be either deterministic or probabilistic.* In a deterministic system, the component parts function according to completely predictable or definable relationships. Most mechanical systems are deterministic. On the other hand, a human systems or human–machine systems (including an information system) is probabilistic because all of its relationships cannot be perfectly predicted. In healthcare organizations, for example, most clinical systems are subject to fairly extreme fluctuations in the quantity and nature of the demand for patient services. Systems theory, then, provides a perspective—a way of viewing not just the parts and not just the whole but the spectrum of relationships of the parts in the context of the entire system's unity of purpose.

- *The simplest of all systems consists of three essential components: one or more inputs, a conversion process, and one or more outputs* (see Exhibit 5.7). Consider, for example, the appointment-scheduling process of an ambulatory care center as a simple system. *Inputs* to the system consist of appointment requests from patients; physician schedules; and clinic resources, including personnel, treatment rooms, and supporting materials. The *conversion process* comprises a set of actions: the scheduling clerks collect information from patients, match patient requirements to available time slots, and make appointments. The *output* of this simple system is the patient scheduled for service in the clinic. Note that the output becomes the input for several other functional systems of the clinic, such as medical records and patient accounting.

- *Most systems involve feedback. Feedback* is a process by which one or more items of output information feeds back into and influences future inputs (see Exhibit 5.8). In the previous example, feedback is in the form of adjusted information on the number of time slots available as the patient is scheduled for service in the clinic. In other words, each time an appointment is made, input data on times available are revised and updated.

- *Systems are either open or closed.* A *closed system* is completely self-contained and is not influenced by external events. In an *open system*, the components of the system exchange materials, energies, or information with their environment (see Exhibit 5.9); that is, an open system

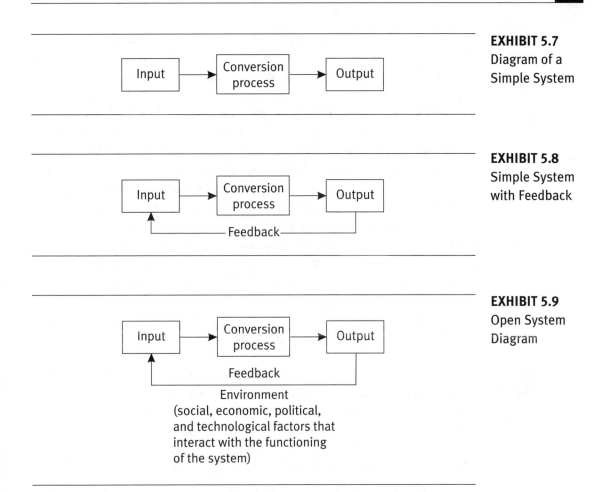

EXHIBIT 5.7
Diagram of a
Simple System

EXHIBIT 5.8
Simple System
with Feedback

EXHIBIT 5.9
Open System
Diagram

influences and is influenced by the environment in which it operates. All closed systems eventually die (cease to function as a system). Only open systems that adjust to the environment can survive as systems in the long term.

Healthcare systems, with the exception of certain purely mechanical systems in the physical plant, fall into the category of open systems. Human or human–machine systems in healthcare organizations are influenced by a variety of environmental factors (sometimes referred to as *exogenous factors* or variables) that are important to consider in understanding how a system functions. These environmental factors fall into four broad categories: social, economic, political, and physical.

Environmental Factors in Open Systems

Healthcare systems are influenced by *social factors*—characteristics of individuals and groups of people involved in the transactions that organizations undertake. Social factors affect patient behavior and patterns of utilization of services. Informal patterns of behavior develop among employees, and these have definite effects on the way operating systems function. The organizational roles played by physicians and other health professionals interact with the formal functioning of healthcare systems. Social factors are important determinants of system functioning, and systems analysts need to be well versed in the art of human-factors engineering when designing systems.

A second major category is *economic factors*. Systems are directly dependent on the availability of resources, and fluctuations in the local and national economy influence both demand and resources. It is well known, for example, that patients often defer elective procedures during a recession. Healthcare systems are also affected by *political factors*, the third category. A variety of special interest groups place competing demands on healthcare organizations, and systems are influenced by both community politics and organizational politics. These political realities must be considered in the analysis and design of any system for the institution. The *physical factor* constitutes the fourth and final category that affects organizational systems. This tangible environment refers to the amount of space available and the way in which system components relate physically to each other.

Cybernetic System A cybernetic system is also known as self-regulating (Weiner 1954). Feedback in a cybernetic system is controlled to adjust the future functioning of the system within a predetermined set of standards. The following are added to the system components to enable automatic control:

1. A sensor continuously gathers data on system outputs.
2. Data from the sensor are fed into a monitor to continuously match the quantity or quality (or both) of performance with the standards—predetermined expectations of system performance.
3. Error signals from the monitor are sent to a control unit, whose purpose is to automatically modify inputs and conversion processes to bring the functioning of the system back into control.

The most often cited example of a cybernetic system is a thermostat for the automatic heating and cooling of a building. The sensor unit continuously measures ambient temperature and sends signals to the monitor, which compares the current temperature with the preset standards. Through the control process, automatic correction signals are sent back to the heating and cooling units to keep their temperature within control limits.

Management Control and Decision Support Systems

Organized systems in healthcare organizations should be designed as cybernetic systems, which have built-in formal management controls. The inputs include the demand for services by patients and their representatives (e.g., family members) and the resources required to provide the services (e.g., labor, materials, capital, technology). The conversion process consists of actions taken by employees and other clinicians aided by formal procedures, informal patterns of functioning, equipment, and management. The outputs include the services rendered and the specific outcomes or impact of the services provided.

Management control in a cybernetic system is presented in Exhibit 5.10. The sensor continuously gathers data on the quantity, quality, and other characteristics of the services rendered as well as the resources consumed in the provision of these services. Data from the sensor (i.e., management reports) are monitored against the established standards of quantity (production and service goals), quality of care, efficiency of the service process, and patient outcomes. When standards are not met, a control process is activated to initiate necessary changes and improvements. The control process contains several components, including education and training of personnel, community or public education, reengineering of the care process, personnel changes to improve service, employee incentives, disciplinary action, and many others.

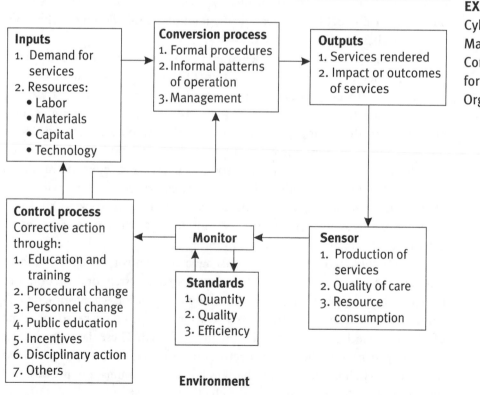

EXHIBIT 5.10
Cybernetic Management Control System for a Healthcare Organization

A key component in management control systems is the establishment of standards for performance and quality control. This is not an easy task and requires considerable effort and thoughtful planning from managers and professional personnel practicing in or employed by the healthcare organization. Standards can be developed or emerge in a number of ways. First, the administrative or medical authority in the institution may take the lead in the process. Second, the standards may be the result of negotiations and subsequent agreement between employees and supervisors. Third, the organization may conduct empirical studies of previous performance, using industrial engineering techniques, to determine the best standards to follow. Fourth, in certain areas of operation, standards are mandated by external regulations, legal requirements, or accrediting agencies. Whatever the approach to or circumstances of establishing standards, healthcare organizations must realize standards are essential to effective management control. Standards prevent management control from operating on an ad hoc basis, and they require careful management planning, continual review and revision, and frequent reinforcement through incorporation into the formal employee reward system.

Consider as an example the operation of a centralized clinical laboratory in an IDS that can be described as a cybernetic system with planned controls built into the system for quality assurance and performance-control purposes. Exhibit 5.11 is a schematic diagram of the functioning of the laboratory in cybernetic system terms.

System inputs include scheduled demand (i.e., laboratory tests planned, ordered, and scheduled in advance) and unscheduled demand (i.e., tests required to be processed on an emergency, or stat, basis). Resource inputs include technical personnel in the laboratory, materials and equipment used in the testing process, and related technology. The conversion process consists of those formal and informal organizational actions related to collecting specimens; conducting laboratory tests; and reporting results to appropriate points in the hospitals, outpatient clinics, and other service units of the IDS. System outputs include the test reports sent back to clinicians ordering the tests, charges for services transmitted to the patient accounting department for billing purposes, and various statistical reports.

Cybernetic components for management control are also included. The sensor component is the management reporting system of the laboratory by which data on the number of tests conducted by various categories, quality control data, and records of resources consumed (including personnel time of laboratory technicians) are collected and recorded. These data are used by laboratory managers who monitor actual performance against predetermined standards, including those established by The Joint Commission, professional standards of quality established by the chief pathologist and medical staff, and

EXHIBIT 5.11
Clinical
Laboratory as
a Cybernetic
System

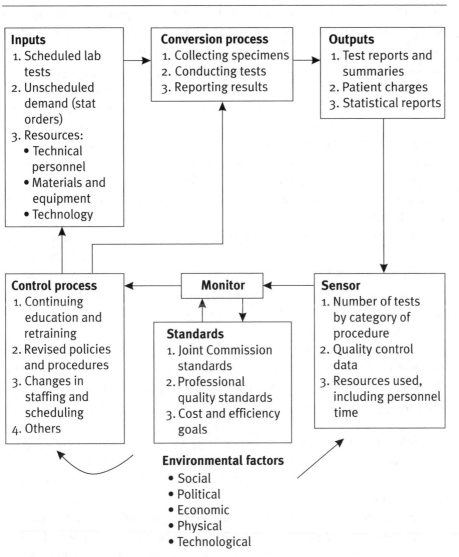

cost and efficiency (productivity) goals established jointly by the administrative and medical personnel in the organization. When standards are not met, corrective actions are initiated, including activation of continuing education and retraining; revision of operating policies and procedures, including recalibration of test equipment if necessary; and change in staffing patterns and scheduling. The laboratory operates overall as an open system influenced by several contextual or environmental factors, including the physical environment of the laboratory facility, current economic conditions of the IDS, social and political factors related to personnel interaction in the laboratory, and advancement of technology.

Useful Information for Management Control

Any management control system is information dependent. Information requirements permeate the system diagrams presented in the preceding exhibits. For healthcare programs to be properly managed, information is needed about each of the major system components.

Input information must be collected to monitor continuously both scheduled and unscheduled demand as well as the resources consumed in the provision of services. Operational procedures must be constantly observed through information on exceptions, error rates, system malfunctions, and similar performance measures on a management-by-exception basis. Output information on the quantity and quality of services rendered must be matched with information on related outcomes of the specific services provided. In addition, the effective manager must keep in close contact with the environment in which her department or institution functions. Environmental information—such as demographic characteristics of the service population, previous utilization patterns, services offered by other organizations, and recent changes in community values—is essential to this task. An effective information system is designed with these kinds of management information needs in mind.

What, then, are the attributes of information that is useful for management control in the delivery of healthcare? Some of the more important characteristics of effective management information are listed in Exhibit 5.12 and explained as follows:

- *Information must contain information, not just raw data.* Data must be intelligently processed in accordance with predesigned plans before they become information useful to management or operating personnel.
- *Information must be relevant to the purposes for which it is to be used and must be sufficiently sensitive.* This kind of information provides discrimination and meaningful comparisons for operating managers. Many information systems provide data that are so aggregated that they provide no meaningful indicators for management planning or control purposes. Overall hospital cost per patient day is a good example. By contrast, separating costs into fixed and variable components and allocating variable costs by diagnostic groupings and level of care provide more useful information to management.
- *Information must be unbiased.* This means information must not be collected or analyzed in such a way that it meets self-fulfilling prophecies.
- *Information should be comprehensive.* In this way, all elements or components of a system are visible to those responsible for administering that system.

EXHIBIT 5.12
Characteristics of Useful Management Information

- Information—not data—driven
- Relevant and sensitive
- Unbiased
- Comprehensive
- Timely
- Action oriented
- Uniform (for comparative purposes)
- Performance targeted
- Cost-effective

- *Information must be timely.* It must be presented to users in advance of the time when decisions or actions are required. Many information systems produce beautifully prepared reports that are completely useless because of their failure to meet operational time requirements.
- *Information should be action oriented.* It should be designed to aid the manager directly in the decision process rather than merely present passive facts about current operations. For example, information from an inventory control and materials management system should include direct indicators of when specific items need to be reordered rather than just data on current numbers in stock.
- *Information systems should have the goal of producing uniform reports.* This way, performance indicators can be compared over time—both internally against previous performance and externally against the experience of similar organizations or competitors.
- *Information must be performance targeted.* It must be designed and collected in reference to predetermined organizational goals and objectives.
- *Information should be cost-effective.* The anticipated benefits of having the information available should be worth the costs of collecting and processing that information.

The Why

Why is system integration one of the most important objectives of HIT strategic planning? Healthcare delivery involves a wide range of providers. Much of that care used to be given primarily in a hospital or in a physician's office, but today, care is provided in many settings by many providers. Getting these diverse groups to coordinate care is a challenge because of geographic and organizational separation. For optimum care, these organizations must become highly interconnected.

The foremost challenge in realizing this highly interconnected ideal is getting the disparate units in the organization to communicate with one another and share clinical information. To make diagnostic and treatment decisions, clinicians need information that is generated by several different departments (e.g., radiology, pathology). Mixing of clinical and financial information is essential for effective management and strategic decision support.

Internal communication and sharing of information is only half the battle, however. The concept of system integration has expanded from the need to connect internally to the need to connect externally—across organizations (Markle Foundation 2004). Healthcare organizations need to link to outside institutions or providers for both business and regulatory reasons. The federal government's mandate for interoperability has raised the urgency for system integration and has led to the establishment of the Certification Commission for Health Information Technology (CCHIT). CCHIT is charged with creating standards of communication for healthcare organizations, and the idea behind such government standards is to force vendors to develop software that meets interoperability requirements. In addition, connectivity must include the organization's business partners and all other providers in an integrated delivery network. For example, Exhibit 5.13 presents a schematic diagram of the information requirements for a truly integrated healthcare delivery system (Markle Foundation 2012).

Oas (2001) states that system integration has been slow in coming to healthcare. Information systems developed in the 1980s focused on billing and business office functions. Most of these systems contained limited clinical information. In the 1990s, emphasis shifted to automation of clinical processes and provision of access to clinical data to individuals across the enterprise. Seamless integration and information sharing are essential in today's environment. However, much has yet to be done to achieve this. Former CCHIT chair Mark Leavitt indicated that providers in the healthcare field have limited ability for any two-member entities to exchange information (Robeznieks 2006b), and the current CCHIT chair, Karen Bell (2012), implies that this exchange ability is still limited. CCHIT is in the process of developing certification standards to enable reliable exchange of information across multiple entities.

Achieving system integration requires careful front-end planning prior to the selection and acquisition of computer hardware and software. The technical aspects of data and software integration are discussed in chapters 9 and 10. The planning processes described in this chapter are essential in ensuring that systems are connected for information sharing across the organization.

EXHIBIT 5.13
Information Requirements for an Interconnected Network

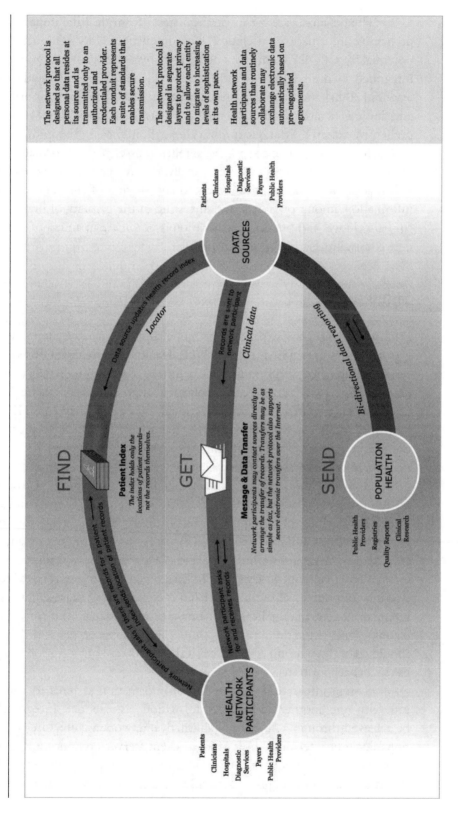

SOURCE: Figure 3.13: ©2012, Markle Foundation. This was originally published as part of the *Markle Connecting for Health Common Framework: Resources for Implementing Private and Secure Health Information Exchange.* Reprinted with permission.

The business case for integration stems from the vital impact of comprehensive information on clinical and administrative decision making. The potential for CPOE to reduce medical errors rests firmly on HIT capacity and integrated medical, nursing, and pharmacy systems (see Hillestad and colleagues [2005] and Johnston and colleagues [2003] for general discussions and findings regarding CPOE as well as Yu and colleagues [2009] for a comprehensive review). Strategic growth through fully using the joint inpatient, ambulatory, and physician practices relies on seamless information flows among and between these entities. Finally, the movement to regional health information networks requires access to and sharing of clinical and financial information among organizations. Investing in the capacity of organizations to share clinical and financial information is occurring in an era of significant cost constraints for healthcare and HIT.

Summary

HIT governance has expanded in scope and importance along with the growth of the integrative role of HIT. Healthcare organizations that successfully implement HIT must have a governance structure that effectively (1) develops (and consistently applies) a consistent HIT strategic plan; (2) aligns HIT strategy with organizational strategy; (3) develops HIT infrastructure, architecture, and policies; (4) sets and manages HIT project priorities and investments in HIT infrastructure; and (5) documents HIT value or benefits to enhance accountability.

A successful HIT strategic plan includes (1) a statement of corporate/institutional goals and objectives; (2) a statement of HIT goals and objectives; (3) priorities for the applications portfolio; (4) specification of overall HIT architecture and infrastructure; (5) a software development plan; (6) an HIT management and staffing plan; and (7) a statement of resource requirements. The planning process should be guided by an enterprisewide HIT steering committee, whose membership is composed of representatives from senior management, medical staff, nursing staff, finance, human resources, planning and marketing, facilities, and clinical support services. The CIO should chair the steering committee (if the healthcare organization has established a chair position).

System integration—the ability of information systems to communicate with one another and share information—is essential. Integration can be achieved through a number of alternative network architecture configurations, including terminal–host system, client/server computing, file/server architecture, peer network, and grid and cloud computing. In addition, the strategic planning process should include the development of major institutional policies related to HIT. The steering committee should oversee policies related to data security, privacy, and confidentiality; data standardization; acquisition of hardware, software, and telecommunications network equipment throughout the enterprise; and use of the Internet.

An understanding of general systems theory is useful in designing and developing management control systems and in obtaining the kinds of information required to enable such control systems to function effectively. Healthcare systems are open systems, and as such they are influenced by the environment in which they function and exchange information within that environment. Key environmental factors include social, economic, political, and physical that influence system performance. Healthcare systems are also considered cybernetic systems if they include formally planned components that introduce automatic control into the systems. Cybernetic components include sensors to continuously gather data on current system functioning; monitors to compare these data against predetermined standards; and control elements to change inputs or process (or both) when system functioning is out of control. Management control systems in healthcare organizations can be designed according to the principles of cybernetic systems.

Healthcare delivery viewed in a systems context is information dependent. Effective information for management control purposes has several important characteristics, including dependence on information (not data), relevance and sensitivity, objectivity, comprehensiveness, timeliness, action orientation, uniformity, performance targeting, and cost-effectiveness. Good information systems are developed with these characteristics constantly on the minds of those charged with their design and implementation.

Web Resources

A number of organizations (through their websites) provide more information on the topics discussed in this chapter:

- American National Standards Institute (ANSI; www.ansi.org). ANSI's X.12 Group works on specifications for transactions involving the processing of health insurance claims.
- Centers for Disease Control and Prevention, National Center for Health Statistics (http://healthindicators.gov/). This is a federal government source for data warehousing.
- CharlesRiver Advisors (www.charlesriveradvisors.com/). This group consults on a wide variety of HIT issues and specializes in helping organizations assess, select, and implement appropriate technologies.

- Dearborn Advisors (www.dearbornadvisors.com/). This group consults with organizations to deliver clinical HIT.
- Environmental Protection Agency (EPA; www.epa.gov/enviro). See EPA's Envirofit, another federal government–maintained source for data warehousing.
- *Health Management Technology* magazine (www.healthmgttech.com). This publication contains a vast array of vendors organized by function.
- HL7 (www.hl7.org). HL7 is a standard for healthcare electronic data transmission.
- The Joint Commission (www.jointcommission.org). This accreditation organization provides guidelines for information management planning and broader strategic planning as a part of its overall accreditation standards (by subscription).

For diverse examples of HIT strategic plans, including guidelines and templates available from associations and vendors, see the following:

- Advanta Health Partners strategic plan: www.advantapartners.com /projects/project9_itsd.html
- Centers for Disease Control strategic plan: www.cdc.gov/od/ocio /docs/CDC_IT_Strategic_Plan_2012_2016.pdf
- Indiana University School of Medicine: http://technology.iusm.iu.edu /iusm-strategic-plan/
- Stanford University Medical Center: http://medstrategicplan.stanford. edu/retreat03/IRT.ppt
- University of Utah strategic plan: www.healthcare.utah.edu/technology /itsPlan/2010%20UUHC%20ITSP%20Full%20Version.pdf

Discussion Questions

1. With the change in the definition of HIT governance, why is the external focus of HIT orientation important?
2. What factors should be considered when developing a consistent HIT strategy?
3. Should the HIT strategy be developed with the HIT department in mind and then aligned with the organizational strategy, or should the HIT strategy be developed with the organizational strategy in mind? Why?
4. Why is data standardization becoming increasingly important in healthcare?

5. Several reasons for central review and approval of software and hardware standards are presented in the chapter. In what other ways could central review and approval assist the organization?

6. What factors/concepts should be included in a master plan for information systems development?

7. What would be the functions of the members of the HIT steering committee, such as senior management, medical, nursing, finance, human resources, facilities, and clinical support services staff? Why is having all these organizational areas represented on the steering committee important?

8. There are several reasons to prefer centralized computing over decentralized computing, and vice versa. Which would you prefer, and why?

9. What are your opinions on end-user computing? What are its advantages and disadvantages?

10. What is the importance of data warehouses or clinical data repositories?

11. Give five examples of simple systems, and include the input(s), conversion process, and output(s) in your answer. Ensure that some feedback is included in your examples.

12. Why do closed systems eventually die, while open systems continue to be upgraded and modified?

13. Find examples of the use of cybernetic systems in healthcare, other than the examples provided in the chapter.

14. What challenges does system integration present between and among healthcare organizations? What are the solutions to these problems?

OPERATIONAL EFFECTIVENESS

6

HIT ARCHITECTURE
AND INFRASTRUCTURE

Learning Objectives

1. Define and use in context the technical terms related to information technology architecture.
2. Distinguish between the hardware and software elements of an information system, and provide illustrative examples.
3. Identify the elements of a computer network, and give examples of various network structures.
4. Distinguish among operating systems, utility programs, and application software.
5. Discuss basic telecommunication concepts.

Overview

As many healthcare executives will happily attest, managing information resources and using information effectively do not require an in-depth knowledge of computer technology. However, managers and leaders in information-intensive organizations do need a basic understanding of the physical and logical structures of information systems and their various components. Such an understanding is of particular importance when the manager is part of a cross-disciplinary team—along with physicians and other clinicians, financial experts, and technology specialists—charged with the responsibility for defining the health enterprise information system needs, negotiating system contracts, or implementing new applications to support patient care and business operations. To be an effective member of this team, the manager must not be intimidated by technical computing concepts or technology jargon. At a minimum, broad-based knowledge about the various hardware and software elements of an information system as well as system design and configuration principles is needed. As done for any other investment decision, thoughtful, knowledge-based consideration must be given to selecting the physical components of the enterprise information system.

The physical components and devices configured into an information system are known collectively as *hardware*. Computer hardware spans incredibly broad spectrums of size and function. Some devices are small enough to be held in and manipulated with one hand and may be used for data capture or for data processing. A large segment of the general population enjoys personal computing with such devices as notebook or desktop computers and even multifunction telephones, and these products have applications in healthcare organizations as well. Many diagnostic machines are computers that analyze clinical samples, process data, and produce reports. At the upper extreme of the spectra are large and powerful supercomputers. Size, function, and sophistication of data-storage devices vary—from thumb drives (which can be smaller than an adult's thumb) to high-resolution, high-volume storage for diagnostic images. In addition to the plethora of products and devices currently available, computer hardware technology changes at such a rapid pace that keeping up with cutting-edge technology is difficult even for the information systems specialist, let alone the healthcare manager.

Computer hardware is useless without programming or application software, which provides the device's functionality. Applications to support healthcare enterprise computing are addressed later in the chapter. A key point for this chapter is that software and hardware decisions must be made in tandem; one cannot be considered independently of the other. Healthcare managers need an understanding of basic software concepts to be knowledgeable participants in the complex processes of selecting, implementing, and testing software to maximize the value of their healthcare information technology (HIT) investments. Knowledge needs include an understanding of the functionality of clinical, business, and communication application software; an awareness of the distinction between integrated and interfaced systems; a recognition of the role of system management software; and a general comprehension about programming languages and language translators.

This chapter discusses the devices, programs, and communication networks that combine to form a computer-based information system. This is not an exhaustive treatment comparable with that found in computer science texts. Rather, this is an overview that provides the healthcare manager with appropriate background knowledge to understand the various elements of an information system and how they may be configured to achieve desired functionality to support the enterprise's clinical service delivery and associated business processes. The fundamentals discussed in this chapter are designed to make the manager feel comfortable participating in the selection, implementation, and evaluation of HIT systems.

Computer Hardware

A *computer* is an electronic, digital device characterized by its ability to store a set of instructions—known as a *program*, and the data on which the instructions will operate. The Electronic Numerical Integrator and Calculator (ENIAC), completed in 1946 at the University of Pennsylvania, Philadelphia, was the first computing device built in the United States (Rosen 1969). ENIAC launched what has since become known as the first generation of computer hardware, consisting of devices that used vacuum tubes. Today, the computer world has evolved to the fourth generation of hardware, which employs microprocessor technology, and is exploring the fifth generation of parallel processing and artificial intelligence. One impressive facet of this evolution has been that, as technical capacity has increased, the size of the processor has decreased. Fortunately, mass production has reduced the cost of personal computing devices for public purchase. In a span of about 30 years, ENIAC's enormous vacuum tubes gave way to the second and third computer generations' transistors and integrated circuitry and then to the presently employed microprocessor (microchip). A user can now hold in one hand a device that has more computing power than did early computers that required a large, controlled-environment room. Further, that small device is so easy to use, children as young as four or five quickly learn to manipulate the device and use it as a toy or as a tool. Since the advent of microprocessing technology in the early 1970s, computers have become omnipresent in society, enjoyed both for entertainment and work. In fact, a large segment of the current workforce has no memory of life or work without computers.

Although this hardware evolution has been impressive in terms of design and functionality, the basic schematic of a computer remains the same. Exhibit 6.1 depicts the six major components of a computer system. Simplistically, a computing system comprises the central processing unit, primary storage, secondary storage, input devices, output devices, and communications devices. The communications devices create connections that enable the computer to interact with other computers, either within or outside the organization. The ability to connect multiple devices that work collaboratively to complete a work process gives rise to the concepts of networking and telecommunications.

Central Processing Unit

The central processing unit (CPU), where the actual "computing" takes place, consists of three major subcomponents: the arithmetic/logic unit (ALU), the control unit, and the registers. The speed and power of the CPU greatly influence the computer's capabilities. As noted previously, each generation of computer technology has increased the processing capability but

EXHIBIT 6.1
Major Compo-
nents of a
Computer
System

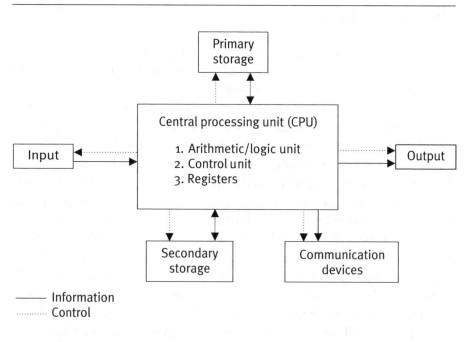

reduced the size of the processing component. An important by-product of processor evolution has been the increased speed of processing.

The basic computational and comparison capabilities of the computer lie in the ALU, which has the ability to perform arithmetic functions at high speeds. The ALU also can perform the logical operation of comparison of both numeric and character (nonnumeric) data. The ALU's speed is an important performance characteristic, particularly in applications that involve a large number of arithmetic operations. Examples of such applications include image processing, interpretation of electrocardiogram (EKG) data, and statistical analysis of very large sets of data.

Processing instructions are communicated to the CPU in a structured language, which has evolved over time from binary code (0, 1) to instructions resembling spoken language. However, no matter what programming language is used to communicate a problem to the computer, the problem description ultimately is converted to a series of binary machine instructions stored in primary storage. The control unit orchestrates the sequential processing of these machine instructions by coordinating retrieval of the data to be manipulated, retrieval and application of processing instructions, and storage and/or output of the results.

When program instructions or data are transferred from primary storage to the CPU for processing, they are held in a high-speed memory area within the CPU known as *registers*. Enhancing the computer's performance is possible by increasing the number of operations performed within the CPU's registers and minimizing the number of accesses to data stored in memory.

Primary Storage

Primary storage refers to "internal" memory, where data to be processed are stored for access by the CPU. The capacity and speed of the primary storage greatly affect the computer system's performance, and, fortunately, the cost of this component has lessened greatly since the early designs. Read-only memory (ROM) is used to store sets of instructions for special tasks such as the computer start-up process. Data cannot be written to this storage area by the user, but the existing readable data are retained even when the machine is turned off.

Random access memory (RAM), the largest volume of the types of primary data storage, houses data and processing instructions in specified locations that can be accessed in any order (i.e., random access). The contents of RAM are volatile, meaning the data are deleted when the computer is powered off. Cache memory stores selected redundant data to be quickly accessible for high-speed processing. Although most cache storage is cleared when the computer is powered off, some data stored in cache for specific applications, or for data access tracking, may be retained. Users of personal computing devices may associate the need to "clear their cache" periodically with this concept.

Secondary Storage

It is not possible for a computer system to have sufficient primary storage to accommodate all the information maintained and used in the many healthcare information system applications required. In fact, few individuals are able to manage their personal computing needs with primary storage alone. Secondary storage devices include a variety of devices and media designed to maintain small or large quantities of data. The speed with which data are entered into and retrieved from secondary storage devices is an important specification within the overall system. However, the ability to ensure the security of these devices and media is of paramount importance.

Healthcare enterprises, and even individuals, need large capacity, non-volatile storage media from which desired information can be obtained as necessary. Most personal computer (PC) users, as well as large information systems managers, employ a variety of storage media. The "best" medium is the one that meets the users' needs for access efficiency, data integrity, and security. Exhibit 6.2 provides a summary of commonly used secondary storage media and some key attributes of each.

Data and information storage poses several extremely important issues in healthcare information systems. Key among these issues are storage

EXHIBIT 6.2
Examples
of Secondary
Storage Media

Medium	Description	Advantage(s)	Disadvantage(s)
Magnetic tape	Data are recorded as magnetized "spots" on tape.	Large amounts of data can be stored at low cost; relatively stable medium	Older medium; slow speed; sequential access only
Magnetic disk	Data are recorded as magnetized spots on rigid (hard) or flexible (floppy) disks. Hard disks consist of stacks of "platters" sealed in dust-proof cases and may be internal to the CPU or an external peripheral device. Floppy disks are small (3.5"), removable, and may zip files to increase storage capacity.	Hard disks can store large amount of data in small physical space; floppy disks are very inexpensive	Floppy disk storage volume is relatively small; disks are insecure and easily damaged or lost; medium is essentially obsolete
Optical disk	Data are burned onto a rigid plastic disk with a laser device. Examples include compact disk (CD) and digital versatile (or video) disk (DVD), both of which may be read-only recordable or rewritable.	Can store large amount of data on small disk; disks are inexpensive and convenient to use	Disks are easily damaged or lost; portable media pose security issues
Optical or laser card	This resembles a plastic credit card. Data are permanently written to card with laser, and data can be added, but not erased. It could be useful for personal health record.	Large memory capacity; permanent data storage	Requires special reader; easily lost; portable media pose security issues
Smart card	This resembles a plastic credit card but has embedded computer chip to store and process information.	Convenient; good memory capacity	Requires special reader; easily lost; portable media pose security issues
Portable hard drive	This is an external (peripheral) hard drive often used to back up data in other storage or to store digital photographs, music, or movies.	Available in many physical sizes and storage capacities; relatively inexpensive	Portable media pose security issues
USB flash drive (thumb drive)	This is a small circuit board encased in metal or plastic that interfaces with the computer via the USB port.	Very small, highly portable storage; inexpensive	Memory cells eventually fail; easily lost; portable media pose security issues

volume, physical security, disaster recovery, and expansion planning. These points are discussed briefly here, but the savvy manager will use a just-in-time approach to explore these issues in further detail when the need to apply these concepts is job-relevant.

Storage Volume

The actual secondary storage required for captured and archived data in a healthcare enterprise is massive, and the associated costs are a significant component of the total HIT cost equation. How much literal storage is required for a given application is dependent on the type(s) of data captured, access and retrieval requirements, retention requirements, and volume of data captured. For example, are data in text or nontext format? The size of image and other nontext files is a significant contributor to the total volume of archival storage space required, as nontext data require significantly more storage space than text data do (*Journal of AHIMA* 2011).

Many other questions must be posed to inform decisions about storage needs. For diagnostic images, how many procedures are performed in a year? How many years must original images be maintained? Must the diagnostic image and the clinical interpretation be maintained in the same "file"? Must previous diagnostic data be accessible for comparison with current diagnostic tests? Must the data be accessible in real time for an extended period, or can the data be archived quickly with minimal access requirements? These and other questions are paramount to establishing system data storage requirements.

In addition to nonvolatile storage options, cache storage requirements for components that store certain types of data, such as diagnostic images for viewing and interpretation, must be extensive to enable rapid retrieval of the stored files. When evaluating certain types of systems, cache capacity can become the determining factor in selecting one vendor product over another. For application-specific parameters, such as cache requirements for image viewing, including clinician users on the product evaluation and selection team is extremely important. If a technology solution does not produce quality data that can support clinical decision making, the solution is insufficient. With issues of clinical adequacy, patient safety, and patient satisfaction, product cost is rarely the deciding criterion.

Physical Security

The physical security of data and information storage is essential for compliance with regulatory and legal requirements. One of the most significant legal protections for health information generally, and electronic information specifically, is the Health Insurance Portability and Accountability Act (HIPAA) of 1996 (CMS n.d.[b]), and the modifications to HIPAA made via the Health Information Technology for Economic and Clinical Health

(HITECH) Act of 2009 (HHS n.d.[a]). The HIPAA Privacy Rule references personal health information (PHI), sometimes described as "protected health information" or "individually identifiable health information." PHI is defined as "individually identifiable health information held or transmitted . . . in any form or media, whether electronic, paper, or oral" (HHS n.d.[b]). Because a significant proportion of the data maintained by a healthcare enterprise is classed as PHI, compliance with these security regulations is not a trivial matter.

Disaster Recovery

Not only are healthcare enterprises accountable for protecting all medical and patient identification data maintained and used in the facility, they also must maintain a secure but accessible copy of these data in an off-site location in anticipation that information resources could be damaged or destroyed by a natural or man-made disaster. This obligation effectively doubles the secondary storage requirements mandated by the clinical and administrative operations of the enterprise. Disaster recovery plans and procedures for information resources are discussed in more detail in Chapter 3.

Expansion Planning

It is a certainty, equally as profound as death and taxes, that the required volume of data to be stored by healthcare enterprises will only increase. The corollary of that certainty is that data integrity and security requirements for archived PHI will not lessen. Technology capabilities will continue to evolve, the types of data that can be captured will expand, and the storage media employed will change. All of these changes will occur rapidly. A continuing challenge for information resource managers will be to ensure that previously archived data and information can be migrated to emerging storage media with no loss of data integrity.

Input Devices

The power of an information system can be realized only when data and programs have been entered for processing and information is generated for the user. A number of peripheral devices are available to facilitate the process of entering data into the computer in a variety of formats, including keyboard or touch-screen entry, optical scanning, and voice input. The field has progressed tremendously since the early days of computing, in which keypunched cards served as the exclusive input medium. System designers now select from multiple input options to meet the organization's needs for speed, accuracy, and cost-effectiveness for a given application. A selection of currently employed devices and techniques used to input data are reviewed in Exhibit 6.3.

Device	Description	Advantage(s)	Disadvantage(s)
Keyboard	This contains a panel of "keys," including alphabetic and numeric characters and special function keys.	Familiar, similar to typewriter; inexpensive	Poor keying skills result in data-entry errors; smaller boards on handheld devices may be difficult to use
Pointing device (mouse, rollerball, touch screen)	This is a device that controls the screen cursor; the "pointer" may be a finger or a special device. Functions are activated at cursor location.	Easy to use; rapid data-entry method	Precision in pointing required to avoid data-entry errors
Scanning device (barcode readers, optical mark readers	Data are captured by reading differences in light reflection between the mark and the white space.	Rapid data entry; good error control; useful in tracking systems	Limited amount of data captured; fairly limited application
Handwriting recognition device	This is a stylus or other device used to write data on touch-sensitive screen, or it is optical scanning of writing on paper.	Familiar skill, no training required	Handwriting must be intelligible
Voice input technology	User enters data and instructions via a microphone; software program converts spoken language to machine language by digitizing sound waves.	Technical skills not required	Expensive, not widely used; machine must "learn" user's voice pattern and pronunciation; vocabulary must be built

EXHIBIT 6.3
Input Devices

Although the keyboard remains a frequently used input device, healthcare organizations have found that other input devices are especially suitable for specific applications. For example, scanning devices provide an efficient and accurate means for tracking many types of inventory items, locating paper documents, and even identifying patients. Medical supplies, pharmaceuticals, and patient identification bands may be tagged with bar codes or graphical markings that perform several functions when scanned and recognized by the computer software. For example, a medical supply item or drug may be removed from current inventory, charged to a patient's account, and scheduled for inventory replacement with one simple scanning process. Paper documents converted to images for inclusion in an electronic health record typically are indexed for retrieval using a bar code (Dunn 2006). Additionally, the computing skills and time constraints of the staff members who will enter the data may be a consideration in choosing the input approach. Busy clinicians often respond better to data-entry devices that are highly automated rather than to keyboard entry, which requires some skill and perhaps more time than is desirable.

Physicians may order diagnostic tests or medications simply by touching the monitor screen where a list of options is displayed. Scanning handwritten documents may make the information available to more users much sooner than if the document is audio-recorded and transcribed through keyboard entry. Scanned graphical material, such as EKG reports, can be accessed online by users in multiple locations, unlike hard copies stored in a single location, which requires users to travel to the storage location or the document to travel to the user.

Selection of the best input device for a given application should consider both efficiency and accuracy criteria. While speed of input provides user convenience, which is important to time-pressured clinicians, speed should not be gained at the expense of data quality, patient safety, and information confidentiality. Clinicians must be able to trust the accuracy of electronic data, and the quality and resolution of captured images must be adequate for visual recognition and interpretation of clinical data.

In the early phases of healthcare computing (pre-networked systems), data entry typically occurred at centralized locations, such as nursing stations or dictation rooms. Today, information systems are designed to facilitate data capture at the point of care, such as the patient's bedside or in other diagnostic or treatment areas. Often, data are captured concurrently with patient examination and treatment (point of care), through voice recorders or digitally enhanced diagnostic devices. Data also may be entered using computer workstations in or near the patient's room or by using a portable or handheld device. Thin client (dumb terminal) devices often are used in point-of-care locations to reduce initial hardware costs and the costs of continuing support and maintenance. A thin client device essentially serves the user as an access portal to the computer or storage device that houses the needed data or serves as the data processor. The user can input new data through the thin client and access existing data from the thin client's archived location, but any actual data processing or archiving is performed on a remote system. The thin client has no computing capability of its own.

Output Devices

The actual work performed by the computer system is of little value until it is produced (output) in a usable format accessible to the user, such as in print or as a screen image, digitally for additional processing, or in audio or spoken form. An important goal of the information technology industry is to make both entry and retrieval as simple as possible. Accurate, comprehensive data are required to produce the information that clinical and administrative decision makers need, and the ability to access the information at the time it is needed is crucial.

Types of output of particular value to healthcare managers include visual displays, printed documents, and audio (including voice) output. The oldest and still most widely used form of displaying output from an information system is a *video display terminal* (VDT). Typically called a monitor, the VDT has evolved from small monochrome screens into large, high-resolution liquid crystal displays (LCDs). These sophisticated monitors can display images at resolutions high enough to support clinical diagnosis and treatment. Where processing devices have evolved to smaller sizes, monitors have moved in the opposite direction. LCD monitors come in more than a dozen sizes and vary in resolution and pixel density. Two or more monitors can be connected to a single computer to allow simultaneous viewing of data from multiple applications. Although most users prefer larger, higher-resolution monitors, purchasing decisions should be based in part on the applications to be used on the system and the data to be displayed on the monitor. For example, monitors to be used for image display need higher resolution than do monitors used for text processing. Individuals who are coding medical diagnoses and procedures may need multiple monitors, or very large split-screen monitors, to access multiple applications simultaneously. If the processing output is intended to meet the needs of a mobile user, the built-in monitor in a smart phone or other handheld device serves that purpose.

Printers, too, have developed extensively from the early impact devices that were similar to typewriters, except they printed on track-fed continuous paper rolls. Today's color laser printers are capable of reproducing artwork, photographs, and detailed diagnostic images. These machines can print on a variety of sizes and multiple grades of paper and cardstock. Photocopying machines now multitask, given that printers and high-resolution printers are available for lease or purchase at acceptable costs. In fact, for many low-end printers, the cost of color ink cartridges compared with printer cost may cause a user to question whether the printer is the disposable item. Key printer characteristics to consider in lease/purchase decisions include memory capacity, print resolution, and print speed. Networking and wireless technology enable a single printer to service multiple computers and the many users who may share access to those computers. Thus, as with monitors, decisions about printer selection can be based on users and applications served rather than on cost alone.

As technology has enabled digitization of sound with good quality, audio output has become a more viable option in clinical technology applications. When digital text is converted to understandable speech by voice synthesis, an ordinary telephone can be used to access healthcare information. For example, a physician needing a patient's diagnostic test results could use a telephone to call the laboratory or radiology system and hear the results read by a voice synthesizer. Clinicians also can listen to body sounds, such as breathing or heartbeat, from distant locations. This capability allows expert consultation without patient travel or monitoring of home-bound patients with chronic conditions.

Computer Software

The hardware components of even the most powerful supercomputer cannot by themselves produce output that is of value to the healthcare manager because they need a detailed set of instructions that describe, step by step, the tasks that must be performed to achieve a desired objective. This detailed set of instructions is known as a *program*, and programs are collectively referred to as *software*.

Although for many people software is equated with applications—either general purpose or function specific—computer software also includes operating systems, utilities, programming languages, software development tools, and language translators. The healthcare manager must consider many factors in choosing computer software. Among them are the number of existing and potential users, required hardware configurations, security considerations, anticipated future growth in computer applications, and functional requirements for individual applications.

Software issues are important for healthcare managers to understand for a number of reasons. First, although most healthcare organizations do little in-house development of software, the manager must be a knowledgeable participant in software acquisition. Managers must acknowledge that the quality of available software is variable, and in some cases software purchased at significant expense fails to meet expectations. Perhaps knowledgeable and informed managers participating in the evaluation, acquisition, and implementation of software will help ensure that installed systems meet their organizations' needs.

Second, all software must be appropriately licensed. It is relatively easy for someone to copy software for personal use or to load a single-license program on multiple machines without any thought of impropriety. Users may want to install personal applications on facility computers. While these issues can be controlled to a large degree by system security configurations, policies should be in place that emphasize the organization's strong stance on exclusive use of legally licensed software and facility ownership.

Third, managers should be aware of the rapid evolution of software versions. Operating systems and application software are constantly being revised. Sometimes, users will campaign to upgrade a software package solely to have the most current version, even when the current version meets their needs. In other cases, the vendor might actually cease to support a given version, thereby forcing the user to upgrade. Again, knowledgeable participation by the manager is valuable in making upgrade decisions.

Finally, and perhaps most important in the current technology environment, the manager must understand the challenges created by the need for interfaces that link disparate software packages and system components. Upgrading one module of an interfaced system may require extensive modification of the interface as well. Increasingly, there is a need to connect facility applications with those hosted by other providers in the continuum of care or with enterprise partners. A simple example is the electronic transfer of a patient prescription to an external pharmacy, a procedure that may contribute to patient satisfaction.

Application Software

From the users' perspective, the most important category of software is application software. After all, this is the software that accomplishes the useful tasks that justify the purchase of the information system. A general overview of application software is provided here, and the topic is covered in greater detail in chapters 8 and 9.

Application software can be further classified as general purpose or application specific. Many computer programs provide an environment in which a user can solve a particular *class* of problems rather than a single, narrowly defined problem. Examples include word processors, desktop publishing software, spreadsheet software, statistical packages, database management/break software, presentation graphics software, and web browsers. These types of programs are known as *general purpose* application software, and it is generally purchased as a suite of integrated, menu-driven module programs. Microsoft Office is a common example of this type of software and is used for personal computing and in business and healthcare organizations.

Application-specific software is a computer program designed to solve a single, specifically defined problem. A good example is a payroll program, which is developed to accumulate labor hours, compute deductions, process payroll disbursements, post summaries to the general ledger, and complete forms required by federal and state governments. In the current environment, these programs frequently include electronic transfer of funds from the enterprise's operating bank account to the employees' personal accounts.

Numerous vendors offer an array of application-specific software aimed at the healthcare industry. *Healthcare Informatics,* a print and online technology journal, publishes a resource guide of information technology companies, products, services, and associations. The online database (www .healthcare-informatics.com) may be searched by product category or by vendor.

Healthcare organizations have the option of developing application-specific software in-house or purchasing (or leasing) a vendor-designed application and installing it on their computer system. However, the process is not as simple as it might sound. Each approach has its advantages and disadvantages. With in-house development, the software can be tailored specifically to the organization's needs, and changes are generally easier to make when necessary. Purchased or leased software, by comparison, is generally less expensive, takes less time to get running, and requires fewer in-house computer personnel. However, any changes to the program must be negotiated with the vendor. A third approach—modifying an existing package—attempts to integrate the advantages of the first two alternatives, but it is not without its own set of problems.

In the early years of healthcare computing, in-house development of application software was a favorite choice of many healthcare organizations. Today, most software is purchased or leased. The high cost of specialized software has led some organizations to contract with application service providers (ASPs) that provide needed computing services via a network connection. The ASP may provide a single application, such as billing, or a full range of computing services. This second option might be particularly attractive for a small physician practice. Outsourced computing is not without risks, however, and managers must be savvy when negotiating contracts. Two key issues to include in contract negotiations are (1) data ownership and (2) return of data should the relationship be terminated (Dolan 2006).

Most healthcare managers have concluded that they are in the business of providing healthcare services, not developing software. However, they must still be knowledgeable participants in the process of purchasing or leasing software. In addition, involving key users in software purchasing decisions is very important, especially when major systems are being acquired. Other factors that must be considered when choosing application software are the required staffing and equipment resources, the cost of maintenance, the complexity of the operations being automated, the number of potential users, and data security issues.

Integrated System Versus Interfaced System

Two general approaches are available for acquiring and implementing application software in a healthcare organization. In the first approach, all modules required to satisfy the organization's computing needs are identified and purchased from a single vendor. Typically, these modules will have been designed to work with one another so that data transfer among modules proceeds smoothly. This type of system is known as an *integrated* information system. Epic (www.epic.com), Cerner (www.cerner.com), and Siemens Healthcare (www.medical.siemens.com) are well-known vendors of integrated healthcare system solutions for all types of organizations. Some vendors of integrated products offer solutions for specific facility types, such as the ICHS DiagnoSYS product for behavioral health (www.ihealthcs.com).

By contrast, each of the required modules could be purchased from the vendor thought to be the leader in that particular application area—or one that offers a unique feature valued by the enterprise. In some cases, the decision might reflect the personal bias of influential members of a particular department in the organization. In any event, although a given module might work well for its particular application area, connecting the module to other modules for data sharing could be problematic. For example, the data contained in one module could be incompatible with the data format of other modules. The data formats or the vocabulary used could differ between the two systems. Something as simple as the way a date is recorded (e.g., 01–31–13 versus 2013–01–31) can prevent data from transferring or being matched correctly. Often, the solution is the development of an *interface*, which acts as a bridge between the two modules and which, for example, translates the data format into one that the receiving module can handle.

The use of an interfaced approach is made simpler if the modules composing the interfaced system have all been developed in accordance with a standard that makes data formats compatible. The American National Standards Institute, the National Information Standards Organization, and the Organization for the Advancement of Structured Information Standards are examples of organizations and consortia working toward consensus standards for information products and services. Compliance with accepted industry standards is an important criterion to apply when evaluating vendors' products.

Advantages of an integrated system include compatibility among the modules and the need to have only a single source for system support and maintenance. On the other hand, interfaced systems that allow users to choose the leading system for a given module can sometimes result in lower costs by leveraging one vendor against another, which obviates the need to replace all existing modules when updates are considered.

System Management Software

System management software is the group of programs that manage the resources of a computer system and perform a variety of routine processing tasks. Unlike the role of application software, the function of system management software typically is not obvious to the user. Thus, many computer users are unaware of the important functions being performed by the operating system and by utility programs.

Operating System

Operating system serves as the interface between the human user and the computer, managing the functioning of the software and hardware. The operating system incorporates a graphical user interface (GUI), which uses icons (graphical symbols on the monitor screen) to represent available operating system commands. The user simply clicks on a given icon with the computer's mouse or other pointing device to invoke the desired command. The advent of GUI made computing accessible to the general public, as a user did not have to be skilled in delivering text commands to the processor in a structured language.

The complexity of the operating system and the scope of services that it must provide depend on the complexity of the computing environment in which the operating system is installed. An environment that allows only one user to run one program at a time possesses the least complexity and places the fewest demands on the operating system. Examples include the early mainframe computers and the early PCs, which could not support multiple applications simultaneously.

The computing power of a device is more effectively exercised when multiple tasks can be run by either a single user or by multiple users. In such an environment, known as *multitasking*, the operating system plays a more essential role in assigning processing priorities, memory access, and file management tasks. Multiple users must be able to perform a variety of tasks with no perceptible slowing of processing time. Today's typical computer user could be preparing a report with a word processor, basing the report on data being extracted from a spreadsheet, copying key points into a presentation format, researching concepts on the Internet, and monitoring e-mail all at the same time. All these applications can run simultaneously and produce data in real time. As noted previously, much of the current workforce has no memory of a computing environment where such multitasking could not occur.

Utility Program

Utility program is software, often incorporated into the operating system, that performs generalized data processing, computational functions, or system maintenance functions. These functions are not specific to any particular computer application. They offer general utility and support to a variety of information-processing tasks, including functions of the operating system as well as application programs. Examples of utility programs include virus scan programs, screen savers, and encryption programs. Many of these programs may be set to operate routinely, such as scanning all incoming e-mail files for a virus before placing the message in the user's inbox, or automatic shift to a screensaver following a specified period of inactivity. Some utility programs require the user to initiate the program's action, such as a disk defragmentation operation that reconnects file components that have become scattered in multiple disk locations.

Programming Language

All software—application, system, or utility—consists of a detailed set of instructions describing the specific steps the computer is to perform. These instructions must be communicated to the computer in a specific *programming language*. When a spreadsheet user enters a formula for an arithmetic computation in a particular cell on the spreadsheet, that user is actually writing a program statement.

Although the typical healthcare manager will make limited use of programming languages as little in-house program development is done, a few brief comments can illustrate some key points. Despite the number and type of programming languages in existence, the objective of all languages from the user's perspective is simple. The overarching goal is to communicate with the computer in some prescribed format so that useful output can be generated. Whereas skilled programmers may find reward in creating complex code, for the nonprogrammer user, the satisfaction of this communication process lies in the output created, not in the communication process itself.

When computers were first developed, instructions were specified in *machine language*—strings of zeros and ones that a computer is capable of understanding. The progression of programming languages can be tracked through successive *generations*, with each generation improving the computer–human interface. The evolutionary goal is to achieve *natural language* input, whereby the user is able to give commands to a computer as easily as communicating with another person. A translator program would convert natural language statements into the binary number commands intelligible to the computer. The technology necessary to recognize the spoken words, interpret their content, transform them into a set of procedures, and translate this sequence into machine commands is complex and has not been perfected. Voice-recognition applications are available for business or personal use, but acceptance for medical applications is not widespread. TopTen-Reviews (n.d.; see www.toptenreviews.com), which conducted a review of several voice recognition products available to consumers, lists the following factors as most important in evaluating a voice-recognition program:

- Features—such as voice training, customizable commands, and accent support
- Commands—specifically the ability to engage other applications by voice command
- Dictation—transcription of spoken language using a text editor
- Accuracy—ability of the program to transcribe all kinds of words accurately
- Ease of use—intuitive commands and menus

Networking and Communications

Today's clinicians and managers require information from a variety of sources outside of, as well as within, their organizations. When geographically separated healthcare delivery units are combined to form a healthcare enterprise or an integrated delivery system, sharing information among the system's components becomes increasingly challenging. Communicating electronically with organizations and strategic partners that are not a legal component of the enterprise organization adds further complexity to the issue. The implementation of computer networks and the use of communication channels and protocols help these organizations manage their information flow.

The technology associated with data communication systems and computer networks is relatively complex, involving the expertise of communications engineers, computer hardware specialists, and software professionals. While these functional experts assume responsibility for the design and installation of this technology, the healthcare manager must assume responsibility for overseeing these activities and making sure that the organization's information needs are met.

As is true in the areas of hardware and software, the manager will need sufficient understanding (working knowledge) of networking and communications concepts to work intelligently with the functional experts in these fields. The following discussion is meant neither to be exhaustive nor to make the healthcare manager a networking or communications expert but to present an introductory overview of these subjects. Again, more comprehensive study at the time this knowledge is needed should be a priority.

Computer Network
Early applications of computers in hospitals, as in many other industries, began with financial applications such as billing, payroll, and general

accounting. These programs typically were run on a large mainframe computer located in the organization's data-processing department. In some cases, the organization might have chosen to have its computing performed by an outside vendor of data-processing services. The input data for these early programs were contained in handwritten documents or simplistic paper forms such as charge slips, invoices, or time and attendance sheets. Most of the time, the data had to be *keypunched* or manually entered for processing. The output consisted of standardized printed reports that were distributed to the appropriate users.

The demise of the mainframe approach to healthcare computing can be attributed to two key developments in the computing industry: (1) the introduction of software systems designed to perform specific functions and (2) the introduction of the microprocessors and the PC. Special function applications for departments such as pharmacy, radiology, and laboratory systems frequently were run on minicomputers (mid-range computers smaller than mainframes) that could be located within close proximity of the department using the system. Using a PC, managers were able to analyze a variety of operational and financial data themselves. They were no longer dependent on the data-processing department to run special reports, which often had an unacceptable time delay, as special reports were generated after routine processing had been completed. Without the ability of the computer to multitask, processing priority had to be established for individual job orders.

As department managers purchased minicomputer-based systems and other managers became increasingly dependent on personal computing, they soon realized the utility of the various programs was not optimal if they operated as independent, stand-alone modules. In fact, a high level of interdependence needed to exist among these programs. For example, the laboratory, pharmacy, and radiology systems all needed information captured by the admitting system. Similarly, many of the management reports generated on PCs were derived from data abstracted from a printed report generated by a mainframe financial application. From perspectives of efficiency and data quality, the ideal situation is to capture data once and then distribute the data to every application that uses the data to perform its assigned processing tasks.

Stand-alone systems are particularly problematic in a healthcare system because data on a given patient might be found in a number of locations, and a single diagnostic service might serve widely separated patient care locations. Data must flow across a large area, and managers often require input from many sources to arrive at a solution to a problem. Clearly, disparate systems throughout the organization (and even beyond) need to be connected to facilitate the exchange of data and the sharing of information resources. *Interoperability* is the term typically applied to the capability of elements of an information system or network to communicate and exchange information (Heubusch 2006). Full interoperability cannot be achieved without industry standards. Most healthcare organizations, particularly larger ones, purchase HIT products from more than one vendor that must serve users in locations throughout the organization. Without extensive standardization, particularly in communication media and protocols, connecting the system elements is a difficult and expensive venture.

The linkages needed to facilitate data exchange and sharing of resources are accomplished through the construction of a network. When all components of the network are located within relatively close proximity to one another—perhaps within a single facility—generally the network is referred to as a *local area network* (LAN). A network that extends into a broad geographic area is referred to as a *wide area network* (WAN). The actual connections between the network components may be constructed through physical wires or cables, or achieved without "hard wiring" (i.e., wireless) by transmitting data using radio wave or microwave technologies and communication satellites. In addition to public access media, communication lines for an extended network may be leased from a private network provider. When the provider offers services beyond allowing traffic on the leased line, it may be referred to as a *value added network*. In effect, wireless computing has extended possible network area to global. Global area network capability is extremely important to corporate enterprises with service locations distributed nationally or internationally, and it also serves well the individuals in our mobile society. An illness or injury that occurs during travel may be better managed clinically if the treating provider has access to previous medical information.

Ways of Distributing the Processing Function

One basis for classifying networks is the way in which the processing functions are distributed among the devices composing the network. Four configurations are in common use, ranging from a *centralized* computing environment, in which the processing functions are concentrated in a single device, to a *decentralized* environment, in which these functions are split, or distributed, among all of the users on the network. Decentralized networks typically create greater managerial challenges, a fact that is particularly relevant for the healthcare manager.

Terminal–Host System

In the most centralized computing environment, dating back to the 1960s, users work at devices known as *terminals*. Early terminals had no processing capability and were often known as *dumb terminals*. Today, a PC is used to mimic, or emulate, a terminal. The terminal is connected to a large central *host computer*, typically a mainframe. The important feature of this computing environment is that all computing takes place on the host system. A more current descriptive term is *thin client*, which continues to mean that little computing work is done at the workstation. This terminal–host configuration is depicted in Exhibit 6.4.

Depending on the level of sophistication of the program running on the host machine, the terminals allow users to perform a variety of functions, including the following:

- Entering a set of data for a program to be run at some later time in batch mode—that is, as part of a sequential stream of programs from several users. For example, staff at patient care units may enter select

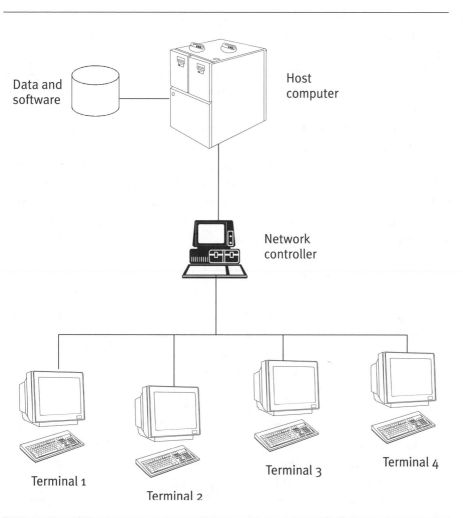

EXHIBIT 6.4
Terminal–Host
Configuration

data about the patients in their unit that are aggregated with patient data from all other care units for end-of-shift or daily reporting.

- Real-time processing of a program immediately after entering data and/or programming commands. Staff may enter current patient vital signs and immediately receive an updated graphical display that shows the patient's vital signs as a trend over a specified period of time.
- Responding to a query in real time. As a patient is processed for inpatient admission or current outpatient service, the patient's outstanding account balance can be determined.

The terminal–host configuration enables *remote job entry* (RJE), where terminals might be located at considerable distance from the host machine. Thus, an organization that outsources a processing function can transmit the source data to the vendor's processing center. Several major companies have specialized in providing computing services to healthcare organizations on an RJE basis. Alternatively, remote data entry into the enterprise system is an option. One example of remote entry is diagnostic coding. Professional coders may work in remote locations, even in their homes, and transmit coded data to the enterprise system for inclusion in the electronic health record system.

The terminal–host configuration provides strong data security when the data flow is unidirectional (i.e., users can enter raw data but cannot access processed information). The ability to restrict data and information access on a need-to-know basis is crucial but faces complexities in implementation. While the technical element is fairly straightforward, managing the human element is more challenging. Well-defined administrative policies must be established and consistently enforced.

Client/Server Computing

Users of dumb terminals connected to a host computer easily recognized the advantage that would result from their terminals having computing capability. Data could be edited, preliminary computations could be made, and other processing could be done that did not require the power of the host machine. This early conceptualization was predictive of today's client/server computing configuration, which is characterized by less centralization than is possible with a terminal–host installation (see Exhibit 6.5).

Client/server architecture divides applications into two components: (1) client, or *front-end* functions, which include the user interface, decision support, and data processing, and (2) server, or *back-end* functions, such as database management, printing, communication, and applications program execution. Special-purpose machines or PCs, minicomputers, or mainframe computers can function as servers, and multiple servers can be used in a

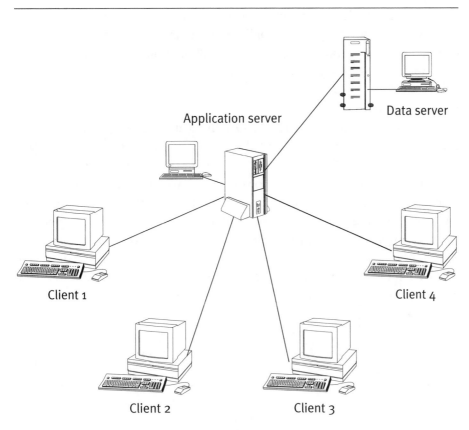

EXHIBIT 6.5
Client/Server
Computing
Configuration

Application server

Data server

Client 1

Client 4

Client 2

Client 3

client/server network. In fact, information technology staff sometimes refer to their network management activities as "working the server farm." Servers often are described internally by the applications they process for clients, such as databases, e-mail, or printing.

The user hardware in this type of network may be thin clients with little processing capability, but in many instances the hardware are PCs that have general purpose software such as Microsoft Office. PCs cost more than thin-client hardware, but they may be more cost-effective because PCs can be used as both server access and independent computing devices. The decision between thin clients and PCs should be based on how the workstation will be used and whether the users need PC capability to perform their jobs. Because access to servers can be granted to users as needed, this configuration offers some data security benefits even when PCs are used as the interface.

The most simplistic configuration is to have all clients connected to a single server that performs all back-end functions. A single server may be functional for very small healthcare organizations, such as a community service organization or an adult daycare center, or for a restricted application in larger organizations that have relatively few users. The next level is to use two servers or more, separating application programs from data storage. This configuration supports faster processing and distribution than does housing both applications and storage on a single server.

File/Server Architecture

Even less centralized than client/server installations is file/server architecture. In a file/server network, a relatively large number of network processors are able to share the data contained in files on the server (see Exhibit 6.6). The actual processing of data, however, is distributed across the network machines. The file server does not perform computing tasks, it stores data and manages rapid retrieval by the workstations where the computing occurs.

Many small LANs are configured with file/server architecture. The file server typically has a large fixed-disk drive with fast disk-access time. The other computers on the network have much more modest fixed-disk drive requirements, but they benefit from fast processors to support their execution of application software.

EXHIBIT 6.6
File/Server
Architecture

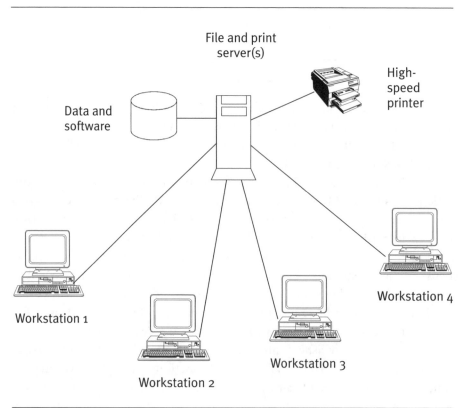

Peer Network

Peer networks represent a decentralized computing environment, in which each computer on the network has either data or some hardware resource that it can make available to the other users on the network. The key distinguishing feature of peer networks is the fact that there is no server, and all of the computers on the network can be used as workstations (see Exhibit 6.7). Key advantages of a peer network are the ease of installation and configuration and the relative low expense compared with those associated with client/server networks. However, peer networks are generally considered suitable only for small installations, as large peer networks may not be secure and are unreliable (Hayden 2001, 93).

Grid and Cloud Computing

Grid computing emerged in the late 1990s as a form of distributed computing. In this model, a "grid," or large number of Internet-connected computers, is used to emulate a supercomputer, capable of managing complex computing and data storage needs for users within an organization, whether real or virtual. Grid computing is deemed most effective for organizations with large amounts of data but few users (Schiff 2010), and it has not received widespread acceptance in healthcare.

The grid concept enabled the cloud computing model, a system that allows users to access computing services and data storage via the Internet

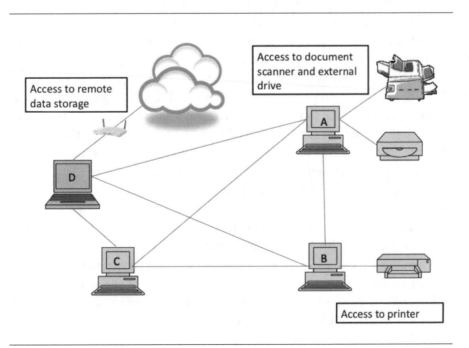

EXHIBIT 6.7
Peer Network Configuration

without concern for the actual physical location of the hardware where the processing or storage occurs. Data transmission using this model is wireless (transmitted over air waves) or "in the clouds." For example, a Google gmail account is accessed via the Internet, but the location of the server holding the e-mail is unknown to the user. An enticing element of cloud computing is that users pay only for the services or storage space actually used, not a monthly or annual service fee, and no capital investment is required for additional computing resources (Mitchell 2009). However, while a student may not particularly care where a term paper is stored, healthcare organizations are accountable for protecting the security and integrity of patient and business data. Cloud computing for healthcare applications requires due diligence in selecting a vendor and ensuring that data are managed in compliance with all applicable regulations.

In addition to using a cloud host for primary storage and computing, healthcare organizations may use the cloud as redundant secondary data storage as part of a disaster plan. If the organization's physical plant is damaged or destroyed through a natural or man-made disaster, information resources are secure for recovery from the cloud host.

Management Issues

As healthcare managers participate with their functional specialists in selecting the appropriate networking configurations for their organization, they must consider several issues. First, while distributing computing capability down to the user level is desirable from an efficiency perspective, in a highly complex and interrelated field such as healthcare, some degree of centralization of the computing and information storage functions is necessary. In addition, the need to support integrated healthcare systems and managed care makes information system integration even more vital.

Second, the network configuration can affect the choice and maintenance of application software. For example, a single "network version" of an application package can be installed on a server accessible to the users on the network, or individual licensed copies of the software can be placed on each user machine. Careful evaluation of the purchase price of the software, software licensing fees, and software maintenance costs as well as hardware costs is of paramount importance.

Healthcare managers are well advised to monitor closely the architecture being designed by their functional specialists to ensure that the information systems function is moving in a direction that appropriately supports the organization's strategic direction. Specification of the overall systems architecture and infrastructure is one step in the strategic development of information systems plans (see Chapter 3).

Network Components

Creating an information network requires the assembly of a variety of hardware and software components. This section presents an overview of these components.

Transmission Media

Early in the process of designing a network, a decision must be made regarding the transmission media to be used. Transmission media, which carry the signal being transmitted from one location to another, include metal wires, which carry electrical signals; fiber-optic cables, which carry optical signals; or air, through which radio waves or microwaves travel. Each transmission medium is discussed in this section.

Wired Media

Wired media consist of one or more strands of metal—frequently copper, which is an excellent conductor of electricity. Data are transmitted along these conductors in the form of changing electrical voltages and may be represented as either a *digital* or *analog* waveform. Digital transmission involves the representation of data with binary digits or bits. Analog transmission represents data by varying the amplitude (height), frequency, and/or phase of a waveform. A key distinction is that analog transmits across a continuous range of values, whereas digital transmissions are discrete. Traditional telephone lines carry signals in an analog format, while integrated services digital network lines, digital subscriber lines (DSL), and the cable in a LAN carry signals digitally. Wired connections are physical, meaning the scope of the network connections is limited to the distance the wiring is extended. Network elements connected by wire cables internal to a building can be extended by connecting a computer in the network through a telephone line to a geographically distant computer. While hardwiring has important positive characteristics in network designs, the physical element severely constrains the scope of the network and imposes significant cost.

Fiber-Optic Media

An optical fiber is made of glass, a much less expensive medium than copper, and can be made in a diameter about the size of a human hair. Data are carried in the fiber-optic medium in the form of light pulses that shine inside the shaft of the fiber to the receiving end. The electrical data signal is used to turn a light source on and off very rapidly. At the receiving end of the cable, an optical detector converts the light signal back to an electrical signal. Fiber-optic cable is thinner and more durable than copper wiring, provides higher bandwidth, and is not subject to electronic eavesdropping.

Radio Media

Unlike copper wire and fiber glass media, radio media use radio waves of different frequencies to transmit data through the air. *Broadcast radio* is used to support some paging devices and cellular technology. *Microwave radio* is capable of higher data rates than broadcast radio and is used in WANs and wireless LANs. However, microwave signals travel only in a straight line, so microwave transmission over long distances requires the use of repeaters or satellites. Microwave transmissions are subject to interference from adverse weather conditions as well as any objects that might interfere with the transmissions' travel from transmitter to receiver. All communication using radio waves is subject to electronic eavesdropping, thus resulting in special security issues that must be addressed.

Transmitter/Receiver

The general process of communication consists of a transmitter sending information (or in some cases raw data) through a transmission medium to a receiver. When two people have a conversation, at a specific point in time the person speaking plays the role of the transmitter and the person listening has the role of the receiver. During the course of the conversation, these roles alternate many times. Similarly, in an information systems network, at any given time one network component acts as a transmitter while a second component acts as a receiver. As with personal conversations, the roles of these components can change frequently. The devices used to connect transmitters and receivers to the transmission media depend on the media type and data format.

Network Interface Controller

A network interface controller (NIC) is a piece of hardware that serves as an adapter to allow a personal computer to connect to a network. The device is sometimes referred to as a *card*, which is a general term for a printed circuit board that can be inserted to add functionality not originally programmed into a computer. The specific interface device required depends on the architecture of the computer and the network communication protocol, such as Ethernet or wi-fi wireless technology. When an NIC is installed, it is also necessary to install appropriate software, known as the *device driver*, which allows the computer to "talk" to the NIC. Finally, note that every NIC is assigned a unique 48-bit number—called *media access control*—that identifies the computer to the network (Hayden 2001).

Modem

A modem (modulator/demodulator) is a device capable of changing signals from one format to another and then back again. Two types are available:

copper based and fiber optic. The copper-based modem converts a device's digital signals to analog signals appropriate for copper media. It can take the form of a card (circuit board) located inside the computer (internal modem) or a separate component connected to, but physically located outside, the computer (external modem). Fiber-optic modems convert a device's digital signals to optical digital signals, which can then be carried over a fiber-optic network. Modems are classified by data transmission speed as bits per second (bps) or baud rate, the frequency of sending a new signal.

Multiplexer

A multiplexer increases the speed of data that can be transmitted over a given bandwidth line by efficiently distributing multiple input signals to available output lines. Several devices (i.e., computer, printer, and scanner) can be connected to a multiplexer. The output of the multiplexer serves as the input to the transmission medium. A multiplexer at the receiving end of the transmission medium separates the signals. Thus, the devices appear to have their own transmission channel when in fact they are sharing the transmission medium. Exhibit 6.8 graphically represents the function of a multiplexer.

Bridge, Gateway, and Router

Data are transmitted across networks as formatted "packets," unlike one-to-one links that send straightforward user data. Packets include addressing information and other instructions as well as user data. Moving the information packets from one network component to another requires the components to employ communication protocols (rules or conventions governing the communication process) and some specific hardware devices and

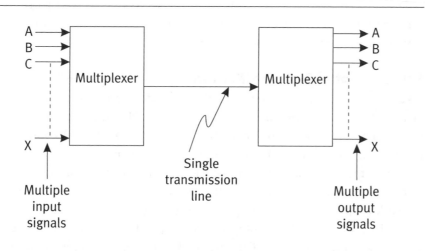

EXHIBIT 6.8
Function of a Multiplexer

programming. A *bridge* is an interface that connects two or more networks that use similar communication protocols. A *gateway* represents the interface that must be created between two networks that use dissimilar protocols to communicate. A gateway allows users to access data and programs outside of their own defined network. Gateways are network entrances and play an important role in the interconnection of the many disparate networks that compose the Internet.

A *router* is a device located at any gateway to manage the data flow between the networks. The router decides, on the basis of its current understanding of the activity state of the networks, which way to send each packet of information flowing on the network for greatest efficiency. The addressing information on the information packet shows the ultimate destination of the packet. The router determines the most efficient path to the ultimate destination by sending the packet through the available networks that have the least activity. Conceptually, this is very similar to driving to a destination using low-traffic secondary roads rather than a busy interstate route. Although the actual mileage may be somewhat higher on the secondary roads, travel time to the destination may be shorter than the more direct route with heavier traffic.

Network Controller/Server

A network controller is used in terminal–host networks consisting of a number of terminals connected to one or more mainframe host computers. The function of this controller is to direct the communications traffic between the host and the terminals and peripheral devices.

LANs do not have a network controller. Rather, communication traffic is directed by a defined protocol that depends on the network topology. The network may have one or more *servers*, which provide network users with a variety of services such as access to files (file servers), help with passing files over the transmission medium (database servers), and a connection to network printers (printer servers).

Network Control Software/Network Operating System

Like a network controller, network control software is also associated with mainframe-based telecommunications networks. The software resides on the host (mainframe), on a small computer (front-end processor) connected to the host and dedicated to communications management, and on other processors in the network. Functions of this software include controlling access to resources, regulating data transmission to and from terminals, improving network efficiency, and detecting and correcting errors.

LANs and WANs employ network operating systems to coordinate and support the operation of the network, such as user access, data traffic, and security. Some network operating systems serve as supplements to the computer's existing operating system. Others, like Windows XP, constitute comprehensive computer operating systems where the networking capabilities have been integrated into the operating system.

The information systems manager, when choosing network software, must consider several factors, such as the number of existing or potential users, the type of network hardware available, the type of applications software programs needed, available resources (human and equipment), and network configuration costs.

Network Topologies

The configuration used to connect the computers and peripheral devices in a LAN is known as the network's *physical topology*. Common alternative configurations available to network designers are bus, ring, and star topologies. These topologies can be used singly or used in combination with one another to form a hybrid network.

Closely related to these physical topologies are *logical topologies*, which "lay out the rules of the road for data transmission" (Hayden 2001, 36). These topologies are largely abstract and not as easily visualized as the physical topologies. This section presents an overview of four physical topologies (bus, ring, star, and hybrid) and four common logical topologies (Ethernet, including fast and switched Ethernet; token ring; fiber-distributed data interface; and asynchronous transfer mode).

Bus Network

In a bus network, a single circuit, or bus, is used to link the computers and other devices composing the network (see Exhibit 6.9). All devices are connected along the bus, or backbone, which may be composed of twisted wire, coaxial cable, or fiber-optic cable. A hardware device known as a *terminator* is used at either end of the bus. Advantages of a bus network are the relative ease of wiring the network and the relatively fast communication rate. Disadvantages are limitations of length of the bus because of signal attenuation, or loss of signal strength, and the fact that if a break in the bus occurs, then all of the devices beyond the break are disconnected from the network. A configuration is called a *line network* if the devices on a single circuit are connected in this manner: Computer A is connected to computer B, computer B is connected to computer C, computer C is connected to computer D, and so on.

A device instructed to send a message listens first to see if the bus is busy. The message is then sent out and received by every other device. Only the intended recipient, however, pays attention to the message. If, by chance,

EXHIBIT 6.9
Bus Network
Topology

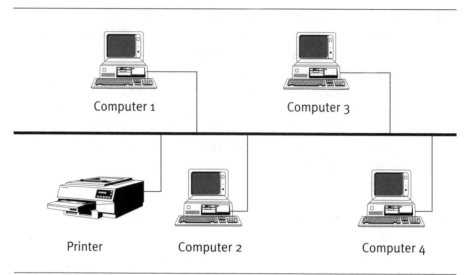

Computer 1   Computer 3

Printer   Computer 2   Computer 4

two devices send out messages at the same time, a collision will occur, which will be detected and the messages will be lost. This problem is resolved by having the two devices involved wait for a random time interval and then resend the message. This protocol is known as *carrier sense multiple access with collision detection* (CSMA/CD), and the trade name for this protocol is *Ethernet*. When a large number of users are attempting to use an Ethernet network, a bottleneck can occur. Fast Ethernet and switched Ethernet represent two possible solutions for this bottleneck. *Fast Ethernet* simply uses a higher-quality line and operates at ten times the speed of traditional Ethernet. *Switched Ethernet* dedicates bandwidth space to segments of users.

Ring Network

A ring network can be conceptualized as a group of devices (nodes) arranged in a circle with a connection between adjacent devices to form a closed loop (see Exhibit 6.10). Data travel in a single direction around the ring, and each device on the network retransmits the signal it receives from the previous device to the next device in the ring. Ring networks offer the advantage of facilitating the construction of high-speed networks that operate over large distances. This is accomplished through the use of a fiber-optic transmission medium for the connection between adjacent nodes along with the use of an amplification device (repeater) at each node. In addition, the operation of the network is not affected by the removal of a node from the ring. Disadvantages include difficulty in troubleshooting the network and adding new nodes to the ring.

A protocol often used with ring networks—the *token-ring* protocol—passes an electronic token (an instruction in computer language) along the

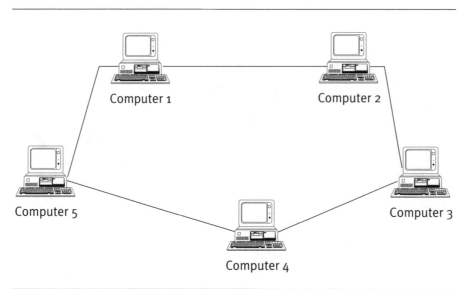

EXHIBIT 6.10
Ring Network
Topology

Computer 1   Computer 2

Computer 5   Computer 3

Computer 4

loop. Only the node computer that holds the token at a given time can place a message on the network. The token is then passed on to the next node. The message passes from node to node until it reaches its destination. Because only one node can access the network at a time, the collisions that are possible with the CSMA/CD protocol (Ethernet) cannot occur here. A fiber-distributed data interface (FDDI) uses a backup token ring that becomes operational in the event that the primary ring fails. If the second ring is not needed for backup and can be used to carry data, the network can operate at rates up to 200 million bps.

Star Network

In a star network, each node has a single point-to-point connection to a center node, called a *hub* or *concentrator* (see Exhibit 6.11). When a given node wants to send a message to a second node, the message must first travel through the central hub. A *passive hub* simply serves as a connector for the wires coming from the various nodes. A message sent from a given node goes to every other node, and the intended recipient node is responsible for claiming its own messages. An *active hub* not only serves as a connector but also regenerates message signals before sending them on to the other nodes. The message signal still goes to all of the nodes, and the appropriate node claims its own messages. Finally, *intelligent hubs* are able to determine the destination address for a particular message and to route the message to that address only.

Advantages of a star network include the ease with which it can be initially wired and repaired and the relative ease with which nodes can be

EXHIBIT 6.11
Star Network
Topology

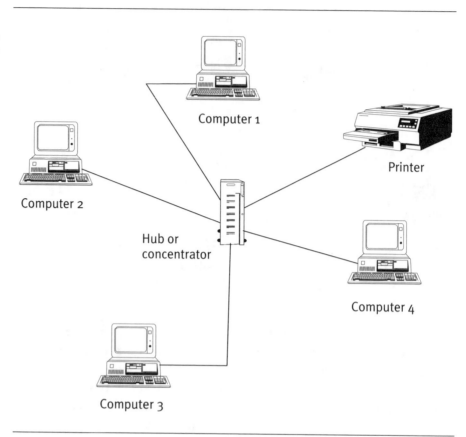

added to an existing network. One disadvantage of a star network is the fact that a malfunctioning hub can bring the entire network down. The use of backup hubs can help to address this difficulty. Additionally, star networks can require more cabling than networks using other topologies. Nevertheless, this topology is in wide use in many network installations.

Hybrid Network

Two or more of these basic network topologies are often combined into a single network known as a *hybrid network*. One example is a WAN formed by linking several LANs that have different topologies. A tree topology connects multiple star networks along a linear bus circuit. Mesh topologies are constructed of multiple connections among network devices, either partially or to the extent that every device is connected to all other devices in the network (full mesh). Possibly the ultimate hybrid network is the Internet, which is a massive interconnection of the full spectrum of network types.

Asynchronous Transfer Mode

Asynchronous transfer mode (ATM) refers to a logical network topology that segments data to be transmitted into small packets of a fixed size, called *cells*. The cells are directed through switches to the appropriate destination node and then reassembled into the original data format. The cells are a fixed size and relatively small; this allows voice, data, and video to be mixed over a network. ATM can run at speeds of up to 1.5 billion bps (Hayden 2001, 40). Understanding the type of data and the speed with which it must be transferred is an important factor when purchasing ATM services. Data may be transferred at a constant or variable bit rate, both of which have guaranteed throughput capacity. Alternatively, transferring at available bit rate allows higher-capacity transfer during nonpeak network time. If time delay is not an issue, ATM service at an unspecified bit rate may be acceptable. These options will differ in price.

Electronic Data Interchange

The networks described in this chapter can serve as the medium for transferring structured information from one computer to another without human intervention. This process, known as *electronic data interchange* (EDI), must incorporate standards and procedures so that the receiving computer will be able to interpret the output of the sending computer. The American National Standards Institute (ANSI) is a primary standard-setting organization for the computer industry. The ANSI X12 standards apply to EDI and are used by HIT product vendors and network communications providers to ensure interoperability across and between networks.

Early applications of EDI in the healthcare field involved the electronic processing of health insurance claims, and claims processing remains an important role for EDI. However, with the connectivity available via the Internet, EDI has become a primary business tool, as data are routinely transferred to various components of the healthcare enterprise and to its strategic partners as well as to fulfill accrediting and regulatory requirements.

Wireless Communication

In each of the computing configurations described earlier, users interact with the information system at a fixed location, often called a *workstation*. However, healthcare professionals deliver their expertise at the site of the patient. While interacting with the patient, they must be able to retrieve needed information and record newly acquired patient data. Mobile computing and wireless communication make this flow of data at the point of care possible.

Mobile Computing Versus Wireless Communication

Mobile computing and wireless communication are in fact two separate concepts. *Mobile computing* refers to the use of a portable computing device such as a laptop, notebook, or palmtop computer. For example, nurses and other caregivers providing healthcare services in patients' homes can download the records of their patients for a given day from a central database into their laptop's hard disk, enter new data and notes into their laptop over the course of the day, and then upload the newly acquired information back to the central system at the end of the day.

Although this procedure is workable, it recreates the very difficulty that led hospitals to adopt networking technology. Because the laptops function as stand-alone computers, the information in the central database is not current until data collected by the portable devices are uploaded back to the central system. If a second provider—say, a physical therapist—calls on the patient later in the day, the nurse's notes, collected earlier but not yet uploaded, will not be available to the therapist.

Even within an inpatient setting, similar problems result when independent mobile computers are used. Until newly acquired information within the hard disk of the mobile computer is transmitted back to the central database or until information from the central computer is sent to the mobile computer, a discrepancy about a given patient remains between two or more databases. This mismatch is not always considered to be a serious problem. For some applications, merely updating the wireless device on a periodic basis is sufficient. For example, physicians may use personal digital assistants (PDAs) at the bedside that contain clinical data, including basic patient data, lab results, and medications prescribed and administered. Updated data are available for download from syncing stations (Briggs 2002, 46). A *syncing station* is a cradle that is wired to a PC. When the PDA is placed in the cradle, data and systems are updated on the PDA and the PC. Mobile devices also need to be recharged from a fixed power source at regular intervals. During the syncing and recharging processes, the mobile device is not accessible for use. Thus, these procedures are usually completed between work shifts or at the end of a workday.

On the other hand, the combination of mobile computing and wireless communication enables portable computers to be connected to an established information systems network without being physically connected. Wireless technology allows computing activities performed on the portable devices in real time, and the central database, as well as the mobile device, always stays current.

Installing a wireless network is considerably less costly than installing additional cabling to create a hardwired system (Sislo 2002), and typically clinicians are supportive of wireless technology (Gillespie 2001, 27).

Despite the obvious benefits of data accessibility, mobile devices are not without drawbacks. Portability, the feature that is a prime benefit, makes the devices physically insecure. Devices may be lost or stolen, creating problems of data security. Due to their size, devices may be easily damaged or need frequent replacement. Special attention must be paid to removing or destroying data on devices that are taken out of service or reissued to new users (Southerton 2007).

Wireless Topologies

Expansion of radio frequency and microwave technologies has enabled broadband wireless options with various ranges, many of which are well suited for use in healthcare facilities. The expectation is that ultimately availability of low-cost, open-standard wireless technology will lead to cable replacement (Ng et al. 2006). With wireless communication networks, even patients and visitors can use their personal communication devices while inside the facility. This capability can reduce some of the frustration associated with patient waiting time in some areas of the enterprise and improve patient satisfaction ratings.

The advent of wireless networks has expanded the traditional classification of networks as LANs or WANs into five classes: (1) wireless global area networks, (2) wireless regional area networks, (3) wireless metropolitan area networks, (4) wireless local area networks, and (5) wireless personal area networks (Siep 2007). As indicated by the labels, the network range may be as extensive as nationwide or limited to a single room.

The conceptual aspect of wired network topologies is applicable in wireless networks in that they can be described in terms of connection structure. Wireless connections may be point-to-point, or linear, which is a direct connection between two clients, such as connecting a personal computing device to a desktop computer to share e-mail and calendar applications. Wireless connections may also be point-to-multipoint, a star configuration. A good example of this structure is a wi-fi hotspot such as you might find in your neighborhood coffee shop where customers can access the Internet and play games or complete work assignments while they enjoy a cup of coffee. When redundancy is important, mesh topologies are useful. Generally speaking, however, wireless networks employ more than one of these configurations.

Three wireless communication topologies are commonly used in networks. Two are typically associated with LANs, while the third is used in a WAN. Each is briefly described in this section.

Spread Spectrum

Spread spectrum is a type of radio frequency technology widely used in healthcare today for wireless communication between devices on a LAN. Benefits of this transmission approach include improved privacy and decreased signal interference. Of the four basic techniques—frequency-hopping spread spectrum (FHSS), direct-sequence spread spectrum (DSSS), time-hopping spread spectrum, and chirp spread spectrum—only FHSS and DSSS are widely used.

Decisions to use this technology in wireless LAN installations should be informed by range of the transmitted signal (to determine network access points), signal frequency (to avoid interference with other systems), and aggregate throughput (data transfer rate).

Infrared Technology

Infrared radiation is a wavelength between visible light and radio waves. Because infrared technology is "line of sight" and cannot pass through walls, it can only be used in a single room. It has found common use in wireless keyboards and mouse devices, remote control units, and cordless modems.

Cellular Digital Packet Data

Cellular digital packet data (CDPD) is a WAN architecture used in cellular networks, like those of cellular telephones, for voice and data transmission. The CDPD transmits and receives packets of data at high speed. An important factor is that using existing cellular data carriers and frequencies offers significant cost savings over capital investment in new cellular media. From a healthcare perspective, CDPD allows remote users to connect to a network without directly connecting to a telephone jack.

Communicating via the Internet

The LANs described in this chapter can be connected to form larger networks, known as *internets* (note the use of a lowercase *i*). For example, each institution's LANs that compose an integrated delivery system can be linked to form an internet known as an *enterprise computer network.*

The largest interconnection of networks in the world today is known as the *Internet* (note the uppercase *I*). The Internet began in 1969 as a US Department of Defense project designed to connect various government laboratories and contractors. However, as the "net" began to be used, it was soon recognized as an indispensable data link between researchers. By the 1990s, the Internet had entered the domain of the general public.

The Internet has become a ubiquitous business and personal tool, bringing instant access to information on almost any topic imaginable, not the least of which is healthcare. According to Internet World Stats (2011), North America boasts 272 million Internet users, about 78 percent of the population. The number of users in North America has increased by about 40 million since 2007. This figure represents more than 151 percent growth in the number of users since 2000. The United States is where 13 percent of all Internet users in the world reside. The continent with the largest percentage of all Internet users is Asia, with an amazing 44 percent.

In 1991 the first web page was launched on the World Wide Web, an environment of multimedia websites and myriad other web pages that are linked electronically and are accessible through the Internet. Individuals have found the Internet and the web to be valuable, and so have businesses, including healthcare organizations; together, they have developed numerous applications to harness these resources. This section provides an overview of the technology issues associated with communication on the Internet, including Internet connection, website hosting, the role of an intranet, and thin client network computer.

Internet Connection

Except for the very few institutions with a staff of in-house engineers, computer specialists, and networking experts who are capable of connecting directly to the Internet, the majority of healthcare organizations obtain their Internet services through an intermediate provider. This provider can be an *online service connection* such as Verizon or AT&T, which provides an array of information services, or an *Internet service provider* (ISP), which provides users with a link to the Internet. A list of ISPs serving a given geographic region can be obtained on www.internetserviceproviders.org. Although Internet connection still can be made using a dial-up or telephone line, most connections are achieved through high-speed cable, fiber optics, or DSL, which are termed *direct network connections*.

A direct network connection uses dedicated digital telephone lines that go directly from the computer to the ISP. They can be fractional T1 lines (about 1 megabit per second) or T3 lines (45 megabits per second). Telephone companies now offer DSL service, which runs over standard telephone wire. It is priced affordably and is found in many home-computing environments. Many cable companies offer direct connections between a computer and the cable television network. The cable company then provides a connection between its cable network and an ISP, or the company might serve as the ISP. A cable modem must be added to the computer to facilitate making a connection into the cable network.

Once a connection has been made between a computer and the Internet, a program is needed to manage the assembly and routing of the messages being transmitted. The *transmission control protocol/Internet protocol*

(TCP/IP) is such a program. According to the Mac OS X Server manual (version 10.4), although the "IP takes care of handling the actual delivery of the data, the TCP takes care of keeping track of the individual units of data (called packets) into which a message is divided for efficient routing through the Internet."

Website Hosting

Most healthcare organizations sponsor a facility website or link to the parent corporation or enterprise website. These websites serve several purposes, including marketing the organization's service lines and providing users with access to an array of e-health applications.

Websites typically consist of multiple "pages" or screen images that a user accesses with the use of software known as a *browser*. The user then interacts with the website using a keyboard and a point-and-click device to input information and navigate through the site's various sections. Common functions of healthcare organization websites include delivering static information such as locations and operating hours, interactive elements such as appointment scheduling, and database capability such as searchable professional staff listings.

Each sponsored website is identified by a unique *Uniform Resource Locator* (URL) or "address." The first part of the URL—www.—indicates a connection to the World Wide Web. The second part of the URL often is an abbreviated version of the organization's name, such as the "ache" in the American College of Healthcare Executives's URL of www.ache.org. The third part of the URL is after the dot (.) and identifies the organization type or domain, such as ".org" (which means the website sponsor is a nonprofit organization). Other common domains include ".gov" for a government entity, ".edu" for an educational institution, and ".com" for a commercial enterprise. This naming convention has become so ubiquitous in our social language that companies with primarily Internet-based transactions are lumped under the term *dot-com industry*.

An organization's website content is stored on a host computer or a server, either in the facility or at a remote location. As websites have become more integrated with business processes, the data storage requirements have increased tremendously. Websites typically function both as an intranet and as a connection to the Internet, thus security issues are extremely important. The need for restricted access to various sections of the website requires assigning and managing multiple access levels as well as monitoring security protocols. Website content must remain current to ensure repeated access by clients, so site maintenance is imperative. A website with incorrect or outdated information creates a negative image for the organization and is quickly ignored by users, which could threaten the organization's market share. In addition, the usual hardware and software updates required by any computer installation must be addressed. For these reasons and others, managing a website is a dynamic process that requires a significant financial investment, close management attention, and skilled technicians.

In today's high-tech social media environment, few organizations design and maintain their own websites. Creating an attractive, highly functional, and dynamic multimedia website requires the talents of skilled graphic designers and programmers who are as efficient in their work as they are artistic. These individuals are mostly employed by companies that offer this specialized technical service to the corporate market on a contractual basis.

The Role of an Intranet

The same Internet infrastructure technology can support communication inside the organization; this structure is referred to as an *intranet* or private network. When an organization shares part of its intranet with customers, strategic partners, and other stakeholders, the intranet becomes an *extranet*. An intranet or extranet uses the same protocols as the Internet and in general looks no different.

A *firewall* is a security protocol to protect the intranet from outside access while permitting organizational access to the Internet. The firewall can also contain software that establishes a *virtual private network* that allows organizations to maintain privacy while sharing public networks for transmission of their data. Data are encrypted before they are sent through the public network and then decrypted at the receiving end. This methodology makes customers feel more comfortable about providing personal information, such as a credit card number, online. Transmission of sensitive patient information can use this same protocol.

As developments in intranet and Internet applications continue, healthcare managers should monitor how their organizations are using this technology. Special attention should be directed toward the security and confidentiality issues created by electronic data access and transmission. Chapter 3 addresses security and confidentiality of healthcare information.

Thin Client Network Computer

Thin client computers are minimally configured PCs that are, as described earlier in the chapter, suitable for a client/server network. Similar machines can also serve as user workstations on the Internet. The healthcare manager will encounter a variety of terminology associated with this type of installation, including *network computer* and *diskless computer*. The Google Chrome OS (operating system) is designed specifically for Internet access and consists of a browser, media player, and file manager (Epipheo Studios n.d.).

Two major advantages result from the use of thin clients or diskless computers rather than fully configured PCs. The first, and most obvious, advantage is cost. Thin clients carry a lower purchase price that can become significant as the number of computers connected to the Internet in typical healthcare settings continues to increase. A second, and somewhat related, advantage relates to the maintenance of these machines. The hard drive of a typical PC contains a number of application packages. As software changes, the information technology department has the formidable task of updating all of the machines. In an environment where thin clients are used, however, the software resides on the web server and thus can be updated relatively easily.

A disadvantage that the manager will face in moving toward the use of thin clients is a cultural one. Users have become accustomed to the power of a fully configured PC on their desk. Making a change to thin clients could face opposition from these users. Another disadvantage, as in all networking situations, is when the server is "down" the user of a thin client is also down.

In this area, as in all decisions concerning information systems acquisition and installation, the healthcare manager is well advised to be aware of all alternatives and select the one best suited for his or her organization.

Summary

The trend toward the creation of integrated health systems and other industry environmental changes has made the information needs of healthcare organizations increasingly complex. Among the strategies necessary to respond to these changes are the development of interoperable computer networks and the use of telecommunications. These technologies are necessary for EDI between and among organizations.

Networks also can be classified according to the manner in which the processing function is distributed among the devices that make up the network: (1) terminal–host system, (2) client/server computing, (3) file/server architecture, and (4) peer network. Each alternative has its own strengths and weaknesses, and the appropriate configuration is dependent on the organization's strategic direction.

A variety of components compose an information network. Transmission media include wired media, fiber-optic media, and radio media. Transmission and receiving components include NICs, modems, multiplexers, bridges, gateways, and routers. Network controllers and protocols associated with the network servers help to direct the communication traffic on the network. Finally, network control software and network operating systems control the accessing and use of network resources and help improve network efficiency.

The configuration with which devices are connected to form a network is known as the network physical topology. Three alternative configurations, each with pros and cons, are bus, ring, and star topologies; two or more topologies can be combined to form a hybrid network. Networks also have logical topologies that guide data transmission. Four logical topologies are Ethernet (including fast and switched), token ring, FDDI, and ATM.

Mobile computing makes information available at the point of care. The addition of wireless communication to the mobile computing device allows the transfer of information between the device and central database to occur in real time. Spread spectrum technology serves as the basis for wireless LANs. CDPD is a WAN architecture that makes data transmission across cellular networks possible.

The Internet is an important resource for healthcare organizations. It provides access to a wide range of information, allows the organization to achieve a presence on a worldwide information network, and provides an infrastructure for communication within the organization and with external entities. Internet technology enables a global network and remote computing as well as novel technology solutions such as cloud computing.

Networking and telecommunications are highly technical and rapidly changing areas. Gaining a basic understanding of these areas, staying abreast of the changes, and knowledgeably interacting with the technical specialists in the field are ongoing challenges for the healthcare manager.

Web Resources

A number of organizations (through their websites) provide more information on the topics discussed in this chapter:

- *Healthcare Informatics* magazine (www.healthcare-informatics.com) publishes a resource guide of information technology companies, products, services, and associations.
- McKesson (www.mckesson.com) provides extensive information about its technology products.
- Microsoft (www.microsoft.com) offers user tips and guides as well as product information.

Discussion Questions

1. Name each of the six components of a computer system and indicate the function of each.
2. Give a brief description of three secondary storage media, including their advantages and disadvantages.
3. Discuss the relative advantage of using a pointing device to enter a patient's vital signs compared with simply typing in the values using a keyboard.
4. Suggest how the use of a patient ID bracelet containing a bar code representation of the patient's ID and a bar code scanner can lead to improved quality of care in a hospital.
5. Explain the difference between devices capable of voice input and voice-recognition technology.
6. Explain what is meant by the resolution of a VDT, and indicate applications where high resolution is important.
7. List the four generations of programming languages, and briefly describe the characteristics of each.
8. Why are users doing so little in-house development of software today?
9. Distinguish between an interfaced system and an integrated system. Provide some examples where one model would provide an advantage over the other.
10. List three specific functions of an operating system.
11. How did the integration of healthcare systems affect the development of computer networks in healthcare organizations?
12. What is the difference between digital and analog waveforms?
13. What are the advantages of fiber-optic media compared with copper media?
14. How do the three physical network topologies differ?
15. Describe some important applications of electronic data interchange in the healthcare field.
16. How does mobile computing differ from wireless communication?
17. Explain the difference between an internet and the Internet.
18. What is the purpose of a firewall?
19. What are the benefits of using a thin client for Internet connection?

HIT SERVICE MANAGEMENT

Learning Objectives

1. Articulate the impact that unplanned work has on the healthcare information technology (HIT) department.
2. Identify a number of different process-improvement frameworks that could be applied to the management of the HIT department and the advantages and disadvantages of each approach.
3. Describe the Information Technology Infrastructure Library (ITIL) service support components and their interrelationships.
4. Articulate why the configuration management database is critical to the service support processes.
5. Describe the ITIL service delivery components and their interrelationships.
6. Describe what service-level agreements are and why they are important to the HIT department.
7. Describe some of the reasons given for HIT service continuity plan failures.

Overview

A consistent area of focus throughout a healthcare manager's career, regardless of responsibility, is the constant effort to achieve efficient, cost-effective operations. While it is certainly true that all healthcare managers will continually be asked to think more strategically, a focus on the strategic aspects of the job at the expense of the operational aspects is a sure recipe for failure as a manager. Debra Walker, former chief information officer (CIO) of Goodyear Tire & Rubber Company, provides a framework for how to think about the effective management of a healthcare information technology (HIT) department for both operational effectiveness and strategic impact. She suggests that the HIT department must master three levels of services. The base level provides a robust and reliable infrastructure for the organization, which is covered in Chapter 6. The second level, which builds on the base level, provides excellent HIT services, which is the focus of this chapter. Walker characterizes the third level by noting that "if [the HIT department] achieves those two things, then [it] gets the credibility that allows [it and the CIO] to play in the third level: partnering with the business to do the very high value-added activities and create competitive advantage" (Field 1998).

Why HIT Service Management Matters

The assertion that the more tactical or operational elements of HIT services are critical to strategic HIT value delivery is consistently reinforced in a number of academic studies (Agarwal and Sambamurthy 2002; Kaplan and Harris-Salamone 2009; Singleton, McLean, and Altman 1988; Smaltz, Sambamurthy, and Agarwal 2006; Watson, Pitt, and Kavan 1998). Much in the same way that Maslow's (1970) hierarchy of needs works in the field of psychology, if lower-level operational HIT needs (e.g., reliable infrastructure, consistent and effective HIT support services) are not being met, the CEO may wonder if the CIO and the organization can be effective in delivering the higher-level strategic HIT needs of the institution.

Ironically, only the most progressive organizations are adopting best practices in HIT service management, while many HIT departments continue to rely on informal, "seat of the pants," error-prone processes (Hoerbst et al. 2011; Schick 2001). This leads to reactive "fire fighting" operating norms within HIT departments, when formal, proactive approaches would be more effective. Recent studies suggest that one of the most accurate indicators of HIT departmental effectiveness in delivering quality services is the percentage of unplanned work in which the department is engaged. *Unplanned work* is any activity in the HIT organization that cannot be mapped to an authorized project, procedure, or change request. While unplanned work can never be entirely eliminated from the HIT department, Kim (2006) suggests that the nature of the unplanned work is very different for high- and low-performing HIT departments. In Kim's study, low-performing HIT departments' unplanned work includes the following:

- *Failed change.* The production environment is used as a test environment, and the customer is the quality assurance team.
- *Unauthorized change.* Engineers do not follow the change management process, making mistakes harder to track and fix.
- *No preventive work.* Failing to conduct preventive work makes repeated failures inevitable. Mean time to repair may be improving, but without root-cause analysis, the organization is doomed to fix the same problems over and over.

- *Configuration inconsistency.* Inconsistencies in user applications, plat-forms, and configurations make appropriate training and configuration mastery difficult.
- *Security-related patching and updating.* Inadequate understanding and inconsistency of configurations make applying security patches extremely dangerous.
- *Too much access.* Too many people have too much access to too many HIT assets, causing preventable issues and incidents.

In contrast, Kim (2006) found that high-performing HIT departments have very different types of unplanned work, which include the following:

- Product failures
- Release failures
- Human/user errors

The key difference between low- and high-performing HIT depart-ments is that high-performing HIT departments put in place holistic controls and processes that cut horizontally across the HIT department, whereas low-performing HIT departments often operate in vertical function-based silos with little to no formal cross-functional controls or processes. Interest-ingly, the Sarbanes-Oxley Act, passed by Congress in 2002, now mandates that holistic and formal controls be established for all for-profit organizations (Library of Congress 2002). However, these controls are not mandated for not-for-profit organizations, which make up the majority of the healthcare delivery field. As such, many HIT departments will continue to have high levels of costly, unplanned work as a result of poor adoption rates of leading organizations' process frameworks that include but are not limited to the HIT process improvement frameworks outlined in Exhibit 7.1.

Sundaresan (2005) notes that "while transforming a typical IT orga-nization into an efficient service delivery organization is difficult, companies that don't make the transition face loss of competitiveness, while the IT organization faces loss of credibility, influence and most importantly impact." Kim (2006) illustrates this sentiment via the following scenario, adapted for our healthcare purpose:

Suppose someone changes an IT asset [such as releasing a seemingly small software patch to a major enterprise application such as an EHR], but the change fails cata-strophically due to lack of preproduction testing and change management authoriza-tion. The failed change results in an "all hands on deck" situation for the IT opera-tional staff; IT drops planned work to remedy the results of the changes. The service

EXHIBIT 7.1
HIT Process
Improvement
Frameworks

Information Technology (IT) Process Improvement Framework	Description
Capability Maturity Model (CMM)	An IT process improvement framework best suited to process improvements surrounding the application development and maintenance domain. The model is based on five levels of maturity (Gartner, Inc. 2001): Level 1: Initial—no repeatable processes Level 2: Repeatable—requirements-identification process in place, policy compliance in place, and basic project management in place Level 3: Defined—application-development processes are well defined, as are applications training and coordination processes Level 4: Quantitatively managed—precise measurement, forecasting, and predictability are added; seeks to reduce special cause–process variation Level 5: Optimizing—continual process improvement efforts at reducing common cause–process variation are added; describes what characterizes an organization at each level but does not describe how to get there
Control Objects for Information Technology (CoBiT)	An IT governance, oversight, and process audit framework recently linked to Sarbanes-Oxley Act of 2002 corporate financial reporting compliance law. CoBiT is made up of four main areas of control objects along with two supporting areas of focus (IT Governance Institute 2005): 1. Planning and organization—assess strategic plan creation, how projects are managed, communications and messaging, and human resources 2. Acquisition and implementation—assess how the organization acquires IT assets, how it implements IT, and how changes are inserted into existing IT assets 3. Delivery and support—assess how end users are supported and served 4. Monitoring—ensure that regular audits of IT controls are accomplished and that reporting is available on internal financial controls 5. Information—assess the degree to which information about the IT operations and internal controls is available for proactive management action 6. IT resources—assess the degree to which adequate IT resources are in place to ensure effective internal controls are in place

(continued)

Information Technology (IT) Process Improvement Framework	Description
CoBiT (continued)	Like the CMM, CoBiT tends to describe what characterizes an organization that has solid internal control mechanisms in place but falls short of how-to descriptions.
International Standards Organization (ISO) 9000	Also from manufacturing, ISO 9000 requires that organizations become accredited or registered, thereby assuring customers that the organization adheres to the ISO quality assurance standards. One criticism of ISO 9000 is that it requires a great deal of administrative overhead to employ ISO 9000 standards and become registered.
Information Technology Infrastructure Library (ITIL®)	An IT process improvement framework centered around seven main IT management domains (itSMF 2004): 1. The business perspective—processes focused on aligning IT investments and activities with business, strategic, and operational needs 2. IT service management (service delivery)—processes focused on ensuring the long-term availability and capacity of IT assets 3. IT service management (service support)—processes focused on holistic approaches to change, release, incident, problem, and configuration management 4. Information communication technology infrastructure management—processes associated with the full lifecycle of IT assets from requests for proposals to acquisition, testing, implementation, and retirement of the IT infrastructure asset 5. Planning to implement service management—planning framework for implementing an IT service management improvement program to include the cultural and organizational change issues associated with it 6. Application management—processes focused on all stages of an application's lifecycle 7. Security management—processes focused on information security to include assessment of information security risks and mitigation strategies

Well suited to organizations whose CIO or IT leader is championing IT process improvements. As opposed to some of the other process improvement models, ITIL provides high-level how-to guidance via its many generic ITIL process flow diagrams and descriptions. |

EXHIBIT 7.1
HIT Process Improvement Frameworks (*continued*)

disruption causes an incident that takes four hours to repair and involves 25 IT staffers from all functional roles: application developers, QA [quality assurance] workers, database administrators, network and systems administrators, and security. Lost IT staff productivity is the first cost of this episode of unplanned work.

Unplanned work also comes at the cost of planned project work. In this case, the application developers and QA staffers are taken from the critical path of an important patient satisfaction project, and the project completion date slips one week. In addition, to address this project delay, IT has to employ a team of contractors longer.

The costs continue to mount. While the IT staff works to restore service, [physicians and nurses] call the service desk to find out why they can't access their [patient's information in the electronic health record (EHR)]. Because of the large [EHR user] base, [hundreds of users] call the service center. The excess calls require the service center to activate the overflow call center, which costs tens of thousands of dollars. Revenue is also disrupted because [the delay in EHR related workflows causes delays in admitting, transfer and discharging patients in a timely manner].

Downtime and IT project resource costs run in the thousands of dollars; service center costs, lost revenue and the delayed IT project costs are in the tens of thousands. . . . Now that this single rogue change affects [the revenue cycle], costs increase almost exponentially. . . . [The impact on the revenue cycle for a large hospital can easily run into the hundreds of thousands of dollars in either lost revenue (workflow disruptions cause a bed to not be available to admit a new patient when needed) or delayed revenue or decreased margins (patient discharged beyond normal length of stay).]

And, there is one more extremely high cost of unplanned work. Any of those late projects, which are getting even further delayed, had some ROI that the [organization] attached to it. So, every moment of unplanned work delaying that project has a quantifiable opportunity cost. . . .

The scenario is all too common in most hospital and healthcare delivery organizations. As such, doing nothing to improve these broken HIT processes will make it increasingly difficult for the CIO and the HIT department to take on the even more challenging strategic HIT issues facing the healthcare field. It is beyond the scope of this text to expand on each of the various HIT process improvement frameworks listed in Exhibit 7.1. While each has its own advantages and disadvantages, the Information Technology Infrastructure Library® (ITIL) is an HIT process improvement framework that is well suited to improvement efforts led by the CIO or HIT leader and department (Young and Mingay 2003). As opposed to some of the other process improvement models, ITIL provides high-level "how to" guidance via its many generic ITIL process flow diagrams and descriptions.

The Information Technology Infrastructure Library
While Control Objects for Information Technology (CobiT) (see Exhibit 7.1) can be thought of as a framework for *what* sorts of things an HIT department

should consider having in place, ITIL can be thought of as a framework of *how* HIT department processes should be interlinked to gain optimum proactive HIT service management. The ITIL was originally created by the Office of Government Commerce (OGC) in the United Kingdom. It is intended to be a holistic framework for providing both the lower-level and higher-level HIT needs of an organization (see Exhibit 7.2). Arguably, current HIT operating budget levels—which typically average 2 percent of operating expenses in community hospitals (Ciotti and Birch 2005) and nearly 4 percent across all health delivery organizations (McGitten et al. 2013)—may make full adoption of the entire ITIL framework challenging. By this we mean that ITIL requires organizations to dedicate some of their resources toward putting in place the more proactive ITIL processes. However, the low-operating HIT budget levels that exist within the healthcare industry mean that most HIT departments do not perceive that they have the excess resources needed to break out of their reactive, fire-fighting mode. By comparison, the financial services industry expends 5 percent to 7 percent on HIT operating budgets (Baschab and Piot 2003; McGitten et al. 2013) and, not coincidentally, is a robust adopter of both the CobiT and ITIL frameworks.

HIT services in most healthcare organizations will, out of necessity, most likely require more proactive approaches with the increasing use of

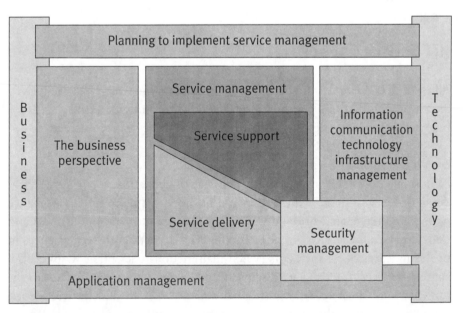

EXHIBIT 7.2
The Information Technology Infrastructure Library

SOURCE: © Crown Copyright material reproduced with the kind permission of the United Kingdom Office of Government Commerce and the Controller of Her Majesty's Stationary Office (HMSO); © Copyright itSMF®, 2001.

mission-critical automation, such as EHR with clinical decision support (CDS) and computerized physician order entry (CPOE). The service management (service support and service delivery) components of the ITIL framework (the middle box in Exhibit 7.2) are particularly well suited to HIT departments that seek to improve their service delivery and support via more proactive, holistic, and integrated HIT service workflows (Grajek and Cunningham 2007).

The IT Service Management Forum (2004) notes that "ITIL . . . provides a framework of 'best practice' guidance for IT service management and is the most widely used and accepted approach to IT service management in the world." HIT service management is composed of two main domains: service support and service delivery (see Exhibit 7.3).

The ITIL processes outlined in Exhibit 7.3, along with project management concepts and practices discussed in Chapter 11, can be thought of as the fundamental HIT services in which every HIT department must excel to be successful, particularly as hospitals and healthcare delivery organizations become even more automated. While informal, seat-of-the-pants HIT service management processes may have been adequate for organizations with largely paper-based records and manual processes, these informal service management processes will no longer be adequate for organizations that increasingly rely on digitally enabled workflows such as EHRs with CDS and CPOE. HIT service support processes are discussed in more detail in the next section.

HIT Service Support

All of the HIT service support processes identified in Exhibit 7.3 are heavily interrelated and should be put in place with forethought. Exhibit 7.4, for example, provides some insight into how these processes are related.

Service Desk

Almost all hospitals or healthcare delivery organizations provide a "help desk" or "service desk," which users call or access online to obtain assistance with computer-related problems. This is likely the most misunderstood and underappreciated service provided by the HIT department. Best practices in providing services for incidents (when malfunctions occur that require HIT support services to repair) are discussed later in the chapter. Here, the healthcare manager must recognize that because the service desk provides such wide exposure into the customer interfacing operations of the HIT department, it becomes—for better or worse—one of the main ways that healthcare executives and managers throughout the organization gauge the effectiveness

IT Service Support	Service desk	The single point of contact for users to report incidents and seek troubleshooting resolution
	Incident management	The process by which trouble calls or incidents are managed to resolution
	Problem management	The process by which recurring incidents are analyzed to determine and provide permanent solutions for root causes
	Change management	The process by which changes are introduced into the computing environment of an organization
	Release management	The process by which major new releases of application or operating system software is implemented
	Configuration management	Closely tied to all of the above IT service support processes, configuration management is the process by which the computing environment is documented—typically in a configuration management database
IT Service Delivery	Service-level management	The process by which service levels are negotiated with end users and tracked for performance adherence
	Availability management	The process focused on ensuring that the IT infrastructure and support services are available to the business functions
	Capacity management	The process focused on ensuring that the IT infrastructure has the processing capacity needed by the business functions
	Financial management	The process of accounting for the complex nature of IT services, understanding cost by unit of service, and assisting management with decisions related to IT services
	Service continuity management	Formerly known as the "disaster recovery" or "business continuity planning" function, this is the process by which organizations identify their most critical applications and design, test, and maintain alternatives for providing IT services in the event of a major service interruption

EXHIBIT 7.3
Elements of HIT Service Management

SOURCE: Adapted from itSMF (2004).

of the HIT services delivered. Therefore, it behooves CIOs and HIT department managers to ensure that the leading customer service practices are in place. The IT Service Management Forum (2001) notes that the service desk is "often a stressful place for staff to work, [and] underestimating its importance, high profile, and the skills required to perform the duties well, can severely hinder an organization's ability to deliver quality IT services."

EXHIBIT 7.4
ITIL Service
Support
Processes

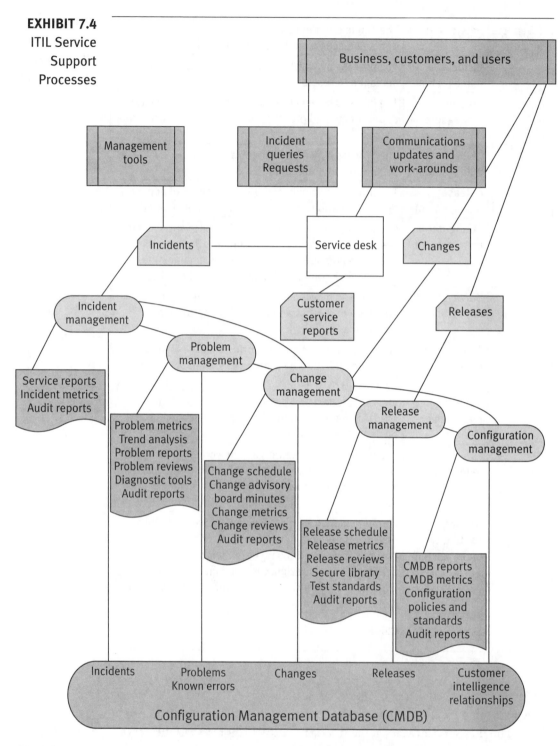

For most of the users of computer resources, the help desk represents the face of the HIT department. While some of the employees of the hospital or healthcare delivery organization have the opportunity to interact with the other service delivery teams within the HIT department, statistically almost *all* employees, at some point in their tenure, will have a need to contact and use the services of the help desk. Gartner Research suggests that, on average, users will place between 1 and 2 calls per month to the help desk (Guevara, Hall, and Stegman 2011). This does not necessarily mean that each and every user will call the help desk at least once a month (e.g., a single user may place six calls in one month and six more the next month to the help desk, while another may not place a call for a year or more). Because many help desks address not only malfunctions or incidents but also how-to questions, over time a user can average 1.1 to 1.6 calls per month. Additionally, as Exhibit 7.4 indicates, a second source of incidents comes from HIT operational management tools that can monitor the HIT infrastructure. When certain thresholds are met (e.g., central processing unit [CPU] capacity on a critical server reaches 75 percent, disk space in the storage area network reaches 85 percent capacity), these management tools will automatically trigger an incident that initially gets sent to the service desk for action.

Hospital or healthcare delivery organizations typically have one of three different types of HIT service desks:

1. *Decentralized.* This is typical of many academic medical centers, where often a central service desk exists, but historically many departments retain their own HIT staff to deal with incidents within their department.
2. *Virtual.* This is a new form of service desk whereby a single contact phone number or website is provided for initiating incidents; however, the actual services may be delivered by a number of different service providers, including internal staff and a third-party provider.
3. *Centralized.* A central pool of resources typically within the HIT department provides centralized service-desk support.

While there are pros and cons for each type of HIT service desk, the key feature that all three must put in place to optimize service support is an integrated view of all incoming incidents. This view not only facilitates a coordinated resolution of the incident but also ensures that trends across the enterprise can be spotted and more proactive approaches can be applied to prevent incidents in the first place (as opposed to simply reacting to them each time they recur).

Incident Management

The goal of incident management is "to restore normal service operation as quickly as possible with minimum disruption to the business [or clinical workflows], thus ensuring that the best achievable levels of availability and service are maintained" (itSMF 2001). In most organizations with a central service desk function, all incidents are channeled through the service desk. Typically, central HIT service desks are organized to provide three levels of support.

1. *First-level support services.* All incidents initially come to the individuals that staff the first-level support services. These individuals typically log the call or request into a "trouble ticket" or "incident management" database so that incidents can be tracked from start to finish. Additionally, the first-level support staff are typically trained to handle most routine, recurring incidents such as resetting a user's password, assisting with routine office-automation software, and answering how-to questions. When HIT service desk technicians are armed with service desk tools that allow remote control of a user's desktop device, organizations can expect 65 percent resolution on the first call into the first-level support technicians. With increased training and access to a knowledge base of symptoms/resolutions, first-call resolution rates above 80 percent can be obtained (Anton 2001).

2. *Second-level support services.* Incidents that cannot be addressed by the first-level support technicians because they require greater expertise and training or require that a technician physically go to the user's location are handed off to dedicated desktop or field-support technicians for resolution.

3. *Third-level support services.* Incidents that are routed to third-level support are typically the most difficult and unique problems and often require deep root-cause analysis and reengineering of the application or system affected.

Exhibit 7.5 depicts a sample workflow diagram showing how incidents may flow through the various levels within a service desk.

In this example of a typical organizational central HIT service desk, the end user can either call in an incident, a request, a problem, or a question (IRPQ) or, for nonurgent IRPQ, simply open an incident report via the service desk's web-based incident portal application. In either case, first-level service desk technicians will initially address the IRPQ and attempt to resolve it on the spot. In this example, the service desk technicians also have access to an ITIL best practice—configuration management database (CMDB), which is covered later in this chapter. In short, this is essentially a knowledge store

EXHIBIT 7.5
Sample IT
Service Desk
Workflow

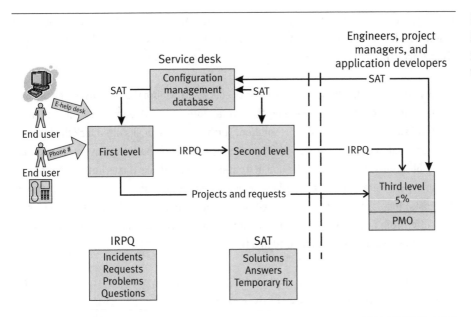

of solutions, answers, and temporary fixes (SATs) as well as a knowledge store for system configuration settings that first-level technicians can use to potentially expedite the resolution of an end user's incident. However, if the first-level service desk technician cannot immediately resolve it, the IRPQ gets escalated to a second-level service desk technician. Finally, for organizations that have implemented a portfolio or program management office (PMO) as outlined in Chapter 11, often the service desk becomes the "front door" for requesting new HIT projects, which, as Exhibit 7.5 suggests, get escalated immediately to the PMO.

Second-level HIT service desk technicians make use of the CMDB and may create new knowledge within it when they discover a permanent solution or find a reliable temporary workaround or fix to a recurring problem. As the exhibit indicates, when second-level service desk technicians cannot resolve the issue, the IRPQ is then moved to the third-level service desk technicians, who typically are members of the organization's HIT network engineering, server administration, or applications development group where root-cause analysis occurs along with efforts to engineer a permanent solution to the IRPQ. Ideally, first- and second-level service desk technicians should be able to find SATs 95 percent of the time, while third-level service desk technicians should be needed for only 5 percent of IRPQs.

Without a disciplined, effective front-door approach to all trouble calls and requests for services, the HIT department can quickly become swamped with requests that circumvent the service desk process. Additionally, without the integration with some of the other ITIL processes (e.g., change management, release management, configuration management, which are discussed later in this chapter) the service desk can be seen as largely ineffective. Ciccolini and McDermott (2005, 1) suggest that

> in many cases, the front-line service desk acts as little more than an answering service, logging incidents and forwarding them to a more senior IT person [second- or third-level support technicians] for resolution. Further, service desks often lack the information needed to address end-user incidents—particularly those that involve proprietary applications. The under-utilization of front-line service desks poses both cost and credibility problems for IT organizations. Incident resolution costs (and indirect opportunity costs) increase as cases are passed on to more senior IT specialists. Business users suffer from productivity declines and perceptions of IT often sour as customers fail to see their issues being addressed in a timely fashion.

Best practices in incident management to overcome these costs and productivity declines include the following:

- Insisting that all users employ the service desk as the front door for submitting all IRPQs
- Using effective automated service desk tools, such as telephony to track phone metrics (e.g., average time a customer is on hold), and service desk management software to log and track all incidents through to resolutions
- Ensuring that service desk technicians have access to an effective CMDB, which serves as an effective knowledge base of system configuration settings, upcoming changes to the infrastructure, upcoming new releases, known problems and errors, resolutions, and workarounds
- Ensuring that service desk technicians have access to service-level management data (covered later in this chapter)

One of the most important functions of the service desk—in addition to quickly finding a resolution to an incident and returning users to productive use—is providing data to spot trends that require a root-cause analysis and a more permanent resolution. For instance, in tracking monthly incident metrics, the HIT manager spots the same incidents recurring each month. As Exhibit 7.4 indicates, these recurring incidents become the input to the next HIT service support process—problem management.

Problem Management

The goal of problem management is "to minimize the adverse effect on the business of incidents and problems caused by errors in (any of the components of) the infrastructure and to proactively prevent the occurrence of incidents, problems, and errors. . . . A problem is the unknown underlying cause of one or more incidents. It will become a known error when the root cause is known and a temporary workaround or a permanent [solution] has been identified" (itSMF 2001).

With incident management, the primary goal is to restore service to end users as quickly as possible. This often results in temporary workarounds or Band-Aid solutions being implemented to allow the end user to use whatever HIT asset is needed to perform his or her job. Problem management, on the other hand, is focused on determining the underlying root cause(s) of incidents. Root-cause analysis should not be a foreign concept, as The Joint Commission (2003) requires root-cause analysis to be conducted to get to the underlying causes of sentinel events that occur in healthcare settings. Furthermore, the National Aeronautics and Space Administration or NASA uses root-cause analysis routinely to determine underlying causes of spacecraft system malfunctions. These same root-cause analysis processes are applied by leading HIT departments as a means of providing world-class HIT support services. Root-cause analysis is composed of the following four elements (Rooney and Vanden Heuvel 2004):

1. *Data collection*. HIT department analysts collect all known information about a particular problem from myriad sources, which include but are not limited to the incident management database, the configuration management database, and change control logs.
2. *Causal factor charting*. Analysts create a flowchart of events, configuration settings, and other known facts that created the problem. This charting process often identifies gaps in knowledge that require more data collection to investigate the problem. Therefore, the data collection and causal factor charting should be viewed as iterative processes that work in tandem. Additionally, it is not uncommon for multiple contributing causes to problems to exist.
3. *Root-cause identification*. After all of the potential contributing causes have been identified in a flowchart, analysts identify the underlying root causes for the problem.
4. *Recommendation generation and implementation*. Based on the particular root causes, people from the HIT department with the relevant skill sets are gathered to generate ideas about resolving the identified root causes, select the "best" recommended solution(s), and develop and implement the plan (this typically involves the change management process discussed next).

Healthcare organizations with formal problem management processes in place can expect to see a reduction in the number of overall incidents that are generated, a decrease in average time to resolve incidents, and an increase in customer satisfaction over time.

Change Management

To effectively administer needed changes to the *HIT infrastructure*—broadly defined as any HIT application or architecture component—organizations generally defer to a change review committee or change advisory committee. This committee is made up primarily of HIT personnel from all of the various teams within the HIT department along with key users from the business and clinical areas. Typical representation of such a group includes but is not limited to the following:

- Network engineer or architect
- Server/hardware engineer or architect
- Key application analyst
- Support center manager
- Nurse manager
- Business office manager
- Physician (as needed for changes that involve physician workflow)
- Vendor representative (as needed when changes affect a vendor-supplied application or hardware device)
- Third-party consultant and other technical expert (as needed)

This group meets as often as necessary to proactively manage upcoming changes. Typically, organizations have a means of dealing with both urgent and routine changes. Urgent changes follow a fast-track approach, such as quickly rolling out the latest virus-protection signature files to all end-user devices after an organization is hit with a new virus. Routine changes include those for which lead times are known and can be planned in a less hurried manner, such as adding disk-encryption software to all end-user devices, which can be planned far in advance and rolled out in a measured way.

As Exhibit 7.4 indicates, requests for changes can come from the business or clinical units (e.g., request to interface two preexisting applications that have not previously been interfaced), can come from incidents, or can stem from a problem management process that has recommended changes to alleviate root causes to identified problems. Additionally, change management process must ensure that ongoing changes are documented in the organization's CMDB.

Release Management

The purpose of release management processes is to ensure that either a new software or a new hardware being added to a live environment has been built and tested in such a way that it is put into service without causing negative effects (described earlier in this chapter). For instance, as part of the health-care organization's testing of a new version of a mission-critical application, an HIT manager discovers that the software will run only on hardware with an upgraded operating system and upgraded hardware memory. In this case, the decision is made to release this new version of software as part of a package that includes an upgrade of its associated hardware. Organizations without rigorous release management practices suffer from disruptions in service due to unplanned work as described by Kim (2006).

The full release management process as outlined by the IT Service Management Forum (2001) includes the following processes, all of which are tied to the CMDB at a minimum (as it is the definitive knowledge source for documenting changes to all HIT resources):

- Release policy (clarify roles and responsibilities within the HIT department, and establish business rules or operating norms associated with how releases will be managed)
- Release planning (develop a succinct but comprehensive plan for each specific release to include a contingency plan to remove the release and return to a preexisting version should the release fail)
- Development or purchase of software/hardware (determine if the release requires the purchase of hardware/software components)
- Building and configuration of the release (include the development of detailed instructions for implementing the release)
- Release testing (conduct a performance test of the release, ideally with the end users of the product, to ensure it operates as expected)
- Release acceptance (the end users and the HIT manager[s] responsible for the release formally accept the release)
- Roll-out planning (essentially extend the release plan that was initially developed at the beginning of the project to add specific details of the exact installation process)
- Communication preparation and training (plan and develop the communications targeted at the end users as well as the training that end users and system administrators may need prior to the release implementation)
- Distribution and installation (distribute the release and install it as appropriate)

In essence, the release management process requires explicit and deliberate coordination and communication mechanisms to be evident within and beyond the HIT department. Release management processes are closely tied to both change management and configuration management. In fact, leading organizations are advised, when putting in place these ITIL processes, to centralize oversight of the change, configuration, and release management processes (Farah 2004; OGC 2005) and to closely tie this centralized oversight into the project management process identified in Chapter 4 (Moreira 2004).

Configuration Management

A common feature of almost all hardware and software is the ability to manipulate its configurations. Examples of configuration settings can be simple (such as the screen saver that can be selected on a personal computer) or complex (such as the fail-over settings for adding CPU capacity to a virtual server environment). Most hospitals and integrated hospital delivery networks use a hundred or more different applications and dozens of different hardware platforms. Thus, maintaining comprehensive knowledge of the configuration settings on each becomes an important task for HIT departments that want to avoid all of the reactive, unplanned work that results when new changes or releases are introduced without knowledge of their impact on preexisting configurations (Kim 2006). Configuration management processes focus on the identification, recording, and reporting of HIT components to include software versions and the interrelationships between the components (itSMF 2000, 2001).

Configuration management includes the following five subprocesses:

1. *Planning.* This entails high-level outline planning and detailed three- to six-month planning that address envisioned additions to the hardware or software environment that likely will have an impact on configuration settings of one or more of the HIT assets within the healthcare organization.
2. *Identification.* This explicitly identifies configurable components of the HIT infrastructure and documents their ownership and the interrelationships between them. Examples include but are not limited to servers, network components, software licenses, desktops, and computer facilities.
3. *Control.* This ensures that no change is enacted within the HIT infrastructure without appropriate documentation validating that the envisioned affected configuration items have been adequately tested prior to implementation.

4. *Status accounting.* This ensures accurate reporting of the configuration setting of all of the items that make up an organization's HIT infrastructure throughout their lifecycle.

5. *Verification and audit.* This involves routinely auditing the documentation that exists on configuration items to ensure accuracy.

One tool that can facilitate the configuration management process is the CMDB. As noted in Exhibit 7.4, all of the HIT service support processes (incident management, problem management, change management, and release management) can have an effect on HIT asset configuration settings. As such, a single CMDB that is used by the entire HIT department can provide a powerful means of dynamically documenting change states in asset configurations as well as serving as an up-to-date tool to plan changes and releases.

HIT Service Delivery

The previous section of key HIT departmental processes was largely focused on establishing a rigorous, interconnected set of operational methodologies. This section, on HIT service delivery, focuses on tactical methodologies that focus on ensuring that services are delivered as expected by the HIT department's customers. Exhibit 7.6 depicts how the HIT service delivery processes work together. (For definitions of HIT service delivery processes, please refer to Exhibit 7.3.)

Service-Level Management

The purpose of service-level management is to proactively review, with the HIT department's customers, the value of the services being delivered. Service-level management is typically operationalized via the establishment of service-level agreements (SLAs) between the HIT department and specific sets of customers. The contents of a typical SLA include the following (itSMF 2004):

- Description of the services to be provided or a particular deliverable (e.g., provide dual power and redundant server hosting services in the hospital's central computer room)
- Agreed-on service hours (e.g., help desk services from 7:00 am to 7:00 pm)
- Description of the response times and resolution times for various scenarios (e.g., resolve within two hours all PC support incidents categorized as urgent)

EXHIBIT 7.6
ITIL Service
Delivery
Processes

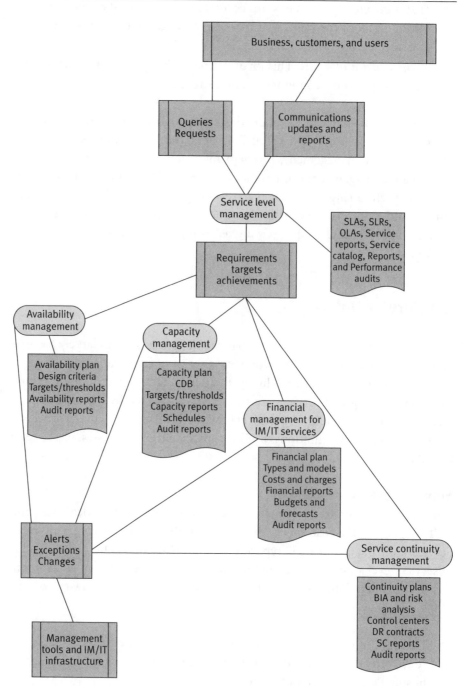

SOURCE: © Crown Copyright material reproduced with the kind permission of the United Kingdom Office of Government Commerce and the Controller of Her Majesty's Stationary Office (HMSO); © Copyright itSMF®, 2001.

- Description of service availability, security, and business continuity expectations (e.g., in the event of catastrophic loss of the hospital's central computer room, inpatient electronic medical record application will be available via the disaster recovery remote site within 72 hours)
- Explicit articulation of customer responsibilities and HIT department responsibilities (e.g., customer is required to initiate all requests for service via the HIT central service desk)
- Explicit articulation of critical business periods (e.g., end-of-year financial closeout may require heightened service levels and responsiveness) and exceptions (e.g., holidays)

Some HIT departments do not enter into SLAs at all; hospital users simply get whatever service the HIT department is able to provide. Others enter into SLAs whereby the HIT department specifies the terms or conditions of the services it is able to provide within specified time periods without any input from its customers. Both of these examples (no SLAs and SLAs dictated by the HIT department) are suboptimal practices that do not align HIT service delivery expectations with the drivers of the hospital's business. High-functioning HIT departments, on the other hand, take the time with all of their major customers to negotiate and agree on specific service-level expectations at a given cost. Typically, HIT departments with more resources can be more responsive. Often, however, hospital budgets limit the amount of dollars available for the delivery of HIT services. For this very reason, it becomes paramount that HIT managers put in place SLAs with their customers. The purpose of these agreements are not only to set realistic expectations (in the case of the budget-constrained hospital) but also to continually work together to assess performance against the SLA and make adjustments (perhaps by increasing the HIT budget to attain higher service levels).

Another important component of service-level management is the development of a service catalog, which describes all of the HIT services that the healthcare organization's customers can expect to receive from the HIT department. These service catalogs can range from simple brochures detailing the services and means of accessing the services to fully web-enabled dynamic service catalogs that link to various applications that serve as entry points to numerous HIT services.

Capacity Management

The Information Systems Audit and Control Association, considered the definitive professional society for certifying and educating information systems audit professionals, defines *capacity management* as "the process of monitoring, analyzing and planning the effective use of computer resources"

(Anderson and Peris 2007). Specifically, first, capacity management is an explicit process to create a better understanding of the business and clinical needs for computer resources (such as the impact that adding a patient portal to a preexisting EHR system will have on existing computer resources). This is largely an outward-looking analysis of the organization's changes in business goals and approaches. Changes in goals and approaches might necessitate changes in the hardware or software environment that supports the business and clinical processes. The second focus of capacity management is more inwardly focused, whereby CPU performance, disk space utilization, growth of applications running on computer resources, growth of users accessing computer resources, and network traffic patterns are constantly monitored so that HIT managers can proactively address potential problems that can be forecasted as a result of rigorous monitoring. As such, the definitive goal of capacity management is to consistently and accurately predict and implement needed changes in the computer resources of an organization to ensure that sufficient capacity exists within the computing resources for unimpeded business and clinical operations. Organizations that do not have capacity management processes in place experience high amounts of unscheduled downtime and high costs associated with mitigating the impact of unforeseen computer resource upgrades needed to restore capacity (Schess 2002).

Availability Management

Availability management is closely related to capacity management in its focus on ensuring that computer resources are available when users need them. Availability management consists of the following five components (itSMF 2001):

1. *Availability*—the percentage of agreed-on service hours that a particular computer resource or service is available for use (e.g., the service center is available for taking trouble calls from 7:00 am to 7:00 pm)
2. *Reliability*—the prevention of malfunctions and the ability to keep services and computer resources operational (e.g., by using backup power distribution units, power-related failures are mitigated)
3. *Maintainability*—the ability to quickly restore services or computer resources back to normal operations (e.g., an effective service center that can quickly resolve incidents and restore computer resources to an operational state)
4. *Serviceability*—the ability of external contractors to augment internal HIT department resources to service parts of the HIT infrastructure (e.g., an effective escalation process whereby vendor specialists can be called in to help resolve vendor-specific hardware or software issues)

5. *Security*—the implementation of appropriate access controls to ensure continued services (e.g., the ability to accurately restore user passwords for bona fide employees when such a need arises)

The availability management process focuses on measuring system downtime, network downtime, average time it takes to resolve an incident, and other metrics that describe when systems and services are not available to users. These metrics then become the internal benchmarks with which HIT managers assess improvements in availability of computer resources.

Financial Management for HIT Services

Many small HIT departments do not set up a distinct function to holistically manage the finances associated with providing HIT services. As healthcare institutions continue to automate an increasing number of their operational processes and as the complexity of managing computer resources increases as a result of this significant growth in automation, the need to effectively manage HIT as a business in and of itself will also continue to grow (Lutchen 2004). In fact, Ferranti (2007) suggests that organizations with more than 100 HIT employees will typically have a senior manager who oversees the HIT department finances and reports directly to the CIO. Typical functions associated with the financial management of HIT services include but are not limited to the following:

- Creation of the annual HIT budget and management of that budget to ensure annual expenditures do not exceed the budgeted amounts
- HIT asset procurement management to ensure purchased items are within the budget and to seek maximum volume discounting on purchases
- Creation of the schedule of costs and oversight of charge-back processes and receipt of funds from customers
- Vendor management to continually seek vendor discounts and manage relations with vendors
- Oversight of anti-fraud policies and procedures, such as Sarbanes-Oxley Act compliance (particularly true for for-profit healthcare organizations)

As noted in Exhibit 7.6, the finances required to provide a given level of HIT services are driven by the clinical and business needs of the healthcare organization. As the need for responsiveness goes up, so does the need for additional finances to support these higher service-level targets. Likewise, organizations' attempt to increase the number of HIT development initiatives they wish to undertake within a budget cycle typically will also drive up the funding levels needed to support increased simultaneous development efforts. Thus, it is critical to negotiate definitive SLAs with all of the customers of the HIT department to ensure that adequate funding needs can be identified that align with the desired service-level needs. Often, cutting back on HIT budgets forces organizations to remove resources that had previously been assigned to providing HIT services. In these situations, it is paramount that HIT leaders renegotiate SLAs to ensure that misunderstandings about service-level expectations can be avoided. The old adage "you get what you pay for" holds particularly true in providing HIT services to healthcare organizations. To avoid a mismatch in customer expectations, fully understanding the service-level constraints of given levels of funding is important to the effective financial management of HIT services.

Service Continuity Management

While service interruptions due to unforeseen downtime of healthcare HIT assets are fairly well understood, expected, and largely routinized, major service interruptions due to natural disasters such as earthquakes, hurricanes, or fires typically require a much different response. HIT *service continuity management* is the process for restoring the healthcare organization's HIT services as quickly as possible after a service interruption (itSMF 2001). Examples of devastating impacts on healthcare operations were plentiful in the New Orleans area following Hurricane Katrina in 2005. Some healthcare operations, such as Charity Hospital, simply ceased to exist as a result (Rowland 2007). As noted earlier, healthcare delivery organizations' poor financial health often makes it difficult to invest adequately in HIT services such as continuity plans. While it is not uncommon for organizations to have continuity plans, in the event of a real disaster or major disruption in service, the executions of these plans often fail. Clarke (2004) refers to these types of plans as "symbolic plans" or "fantasy plans." He notes, "symbolic [continuity] plans are the ones that are charade. They're touted as workable but, in fact, they're not based on actual expertise or experience and, by definition, they over promise. . . . [Furthermore,] symbolic plans can create a dangerous false sense of security" (Clarke 2004, 21–22).

To ensure that the HIT department has workable HIT service continuity plans in place, the United Kingdom's Office of Government Commerce (2005) suggests that the organization undertake a business impact analysis whereby the senior leadership team identifies the business and clinical processes that are absolutely critical to the functioning of the enterprise. For instance, a balanced scorecard–performance reporting application may not be essential, but the admissions, discharges, and transfers and billing applications will likely be considered critical. The business impact analysis also assesses the following for each critical process (OGC 2005):

- Lost revenue or costs associated with a disruption that may accrue
- Likelihood that the degree of damage or loss will escalate after a disruption
- The staffing, skills, facilities, and services necessary to enable critical and essential business processes to continue operating at a minimum acceptable level
- Realistic estimates of the time required to restore minimum service levels
- Realistic estimates of the time required to fully recover service levels

After the business impact analysis is completed, a risk assessment is conducted to assess the extent to which a healthcare organization is vulnerable to different potential threats. For instance, a hospital in Lubbock, Texas, has a higher likelihood of sustaining damage from a tornado than a hospital in Vancouver, British Columbia. After assessing the business impacts as well as the potential risks and their likelihood of occurrence, an HIT service continuity strategy is developed. The key elements of this strategy should describe the following:

- Implementation of the strategy
- Arrangements made for standby recovery locations, either via contracts with third-party vendors specializing in disaster recovery hosting services or via reciprocal support agreements with other organizations
- Risk-reduction measures (While the organization cannot do much about being located in a tornado alley, for example, identifying a need to move the computer room from the basement of the building because it is within the 100-year flood zone to a higher floor is certainly something that can be accomplished to reduce risk.)
- Detailed step-by-step procedural checklists to restore service levels (These should "be action oriented—simple checklists for teams to follow, supported by supplements containing more detailed information on each action required" [Hiles 1992].)
- Timeline for testing the plan in a realistic manner (e.g., periodically simulating a disaster and invoking the standby contracts to bring up one or more of the critical applications at an alternate location. This is an important element of service continuity planning, as it overcomes Clarke's [2004] criticism of symbolic plans and ensures that

the organization has a tried-and-tested approach to restore critical HIT-dependent business processes.)

The Continued Evolution of the ITIL Service Management Practices

As a framework of information technology service management practices, ITIL continues to evolve and be refined. The ITIL framework was reconceptualized as the ITIL Service Management Lifecycle (TSO 2007). The individual information technology operational service support management processes (i.e., incident management, problem management, release management, change management, and configuration management) continue to be recognized as important best practices in managing HIT departments. In addition, they remain core to current conceptualizations of ITIL (Whittleston 2012). These individual information technology service support management practices are now part of a lifecycle framework that emphasizes the need to view information technology services as a continual service improvement process. Exhibit 7.7 provides an overview of the ITIL service management lifecycle and shows how the individual ITIL processes discussed in this chapter are related to the latest evolution of service management.

This new conceptualization of ITIL suggests that the delivery of services should begin with a strategy for how those services might be provided to the various businesses, customers, and users of the services. Most important, it highlights the importance of establishing policies and standards that will help in effectively delivering information technology services. The financial management for information technology services, discussed in this chapter, falls into this ITIL service management lifecycle category.

The output of the service strategy lifecycle element becomes the input for the service design element, where plans to create and modify services as well as tactical service delivery management processes (i.e., service-level management, capacity management, availability management, financial management, and service continuity management) are addressed. In turn, the output of the service design element becomes the input to the service transition element, in which the proactive management of the transition of a new or changed service and/or service management process is placed into production. The output of the service transition element becomes the input for the service operation element, which involves the day-to-day operations of services and service management processes.

Finally, the latest evolution of the ITIL service management practices is the conceptualization of a continual service improvement element, which is to be embedded throughout all of the ITIL practices, creating feedback loops

EXHIBIT 7.7
Service
Management
Lifecycle

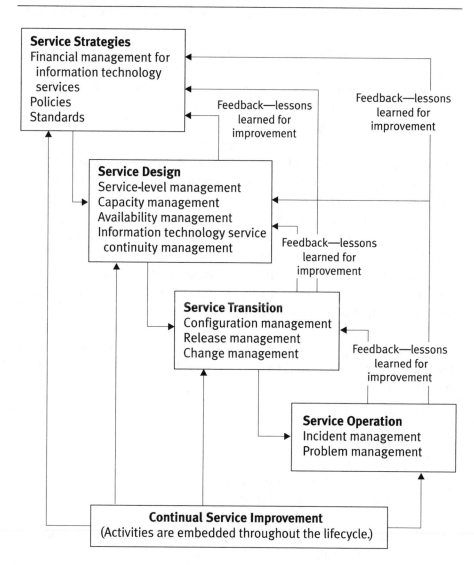

SOURCE: Adapted from TSO (2007).

of lessons learned throughout the lifecycle that should be used to continually improve services.

Summary

Healthcare administrators have long recognized the need for efficient and effective operations throughout the healthcare enterprises that they lead. However, because few senior executives have come from HIT backgrounds, the internal workings of the HIT department have often been a "black box" to senior leadership. In this chapter, we open the HIT department black box and present ten operational and tactical key processes that, when managed in a loose, informal manner, will create costly unplanned work that limits the resources available for new strategic initiatives. To maximize efficiencies and effectiveness, many healthcare enterprises are adopting frameworks to enhance their internal operations.

A number of frameworks are presented here, including the ITIL framework, which Young and Mingay (2003) suggest is the framework best suited for HIT department-led process improvement efforts. ITIL categorizes the ten key HIT department processes into two: (1) service support management, which includes incident management, problem management, change management, release management, and configuration management, and (2) service delivery management, which includes service-level management, capacity management, availability management, financial management, and services continuity management. As more and more healthcare enterprises are becoming automated, demands on professional HIT department services will continue to increase. HIT departments that have implemented, or are implementing, formal process improvement frameworks like ITIL will create greater efficiencies and thereby leverage HIT resources toward more strategic initiatives.

Web Resources

A number of organizations (through their websites) provide more information on the topics discussed in this chapter:

- Information Technology Infrastructure Library (ITIL; www.itil-official site.com). This is the official ITIL website.
- ITIL Open Guide (www.itlibrary.org/index.php?page=ITIL). This website is maintained by the ITIL practitioner community for sharing information about ITIL.
- IT Service Management Forum International (www.itsmfi.org). This is an international forum that promotes best practices in information technology service management.
- IT Service Management Forum US (www.itsmfusa.org). This is the US chapter of the IT Service Management Forum International.

Discussion Questions

1. Why does unplanned HIT work increase costs?
2. Identify some process improvement frameworks that are applicable to an HIT department. What are the advantages and disadvantages of each?
3. Describe the five HIT service support processes and how they are interrelated.
4. What is a CMDB, and why is it an important component of HIT service support?
5. Describe the five HIT service delivery processes and how they are interrelated.
6. What is an SLA, and why is it an important component of HIT service delivery?
7. List some of the reasons given for HIT service continuity plan failures.

SYSTEMS SELECTION
AND CONTRACT MANAGEMENT

Learning Objectives

1. Describe the steps in the healthcare information technology (HIT) system selection process.
2. Articulate why it is important to clarify objectives prior to engaging in system selection.
3. Describe vital features that an organization should include when negotiating and crafting contract terms and conditions.
4. Articulate the purpose of an HIT total-cost-of-ownership analysis.
5. Articulate the purpose of a benefits realization assessment.

Overview

When he saw a large wooden horse at the gates of Troy, presumably left as a peace offering by the Greek army, the Trojan priest Laocoön gave birth to the now famous phrase, "beware of Greeks bearing gifts." As the mythology tells us, the Trojans ignored Laocoön's warning and accepted the gift horse, which resulted in the fall of Troy (Phrase Finder 2011). Clearly, this Trojan Horse analogy is entirely too strong for healthcare information technology (HIT) vendors; however, it is nevertheless prudent for healthcare managers to play modern-day Laocoön when working with any outsider whose interests and risk profile may not be aligned with those of the organization. To be sure, failed IT implementations can sometimes be attributed to poor execution on the part of the hospital or health system project team. Although this chapter is not about failure to execute scenarios, it does focus attention on how to establish productive relationships with potential HIT vendors.

Mike Murphy, president and CEO of Sharp Healthcare in San Diego, once commented, "I have been disappointed that many of the products are not really ready for prime time when they are sold" (Smaltz et al. 2005b). Similarly, David Hoidal, while CEO of the University of Alabama at Birmingham Health System, noted that "it's disappointing that the lack of functionality that cuts across multiple applications leaves healthcare system like ours to bear the cost and the burden of making everything work together" (Smaltz et al. 2005b). These anecdotal insights from leading CEOs suggest that having a sound system selection process with contract management is instrumental in making informed HIT investment decisions. This chapter[1] focuses on the crucial system selection process and contract management function.

The System Selection Process

For many healthcare providers, selecting and implementing a new enterprise information system can be one of the most costly and high-risk investments they will make over the course of many years. Especially in the case of an enterprise electronic health record (EHR), revenue cycle, or enterprise resource planning (ERP) solution, the capital and ongoing operational investment can run into hundreds of millions of dollars, and the system itself will have a direct impact on the daily lives of staff, clinicians, administrators, and (most important) patients and their families. These core systems are long-term investments, so a lot of fear and uncertainty are associated with the selection process because it is an activity that occurs infrequently but has far-reaching consequences.

The good news is that system selection is relatively straightforward, and the guidelines and principles of a well-managed system selection process apply equally well to the process of selecting a departmental solution (such as a pharmacy information system) and an enterprise EHR.

The primary activities in a system selection process are as follows:

- Clarification of the objectives
- Formation of the system selection governance structure and processes
- Establishment of a system selection plan
- Education: Understanding the marketplace
- Down selection: Narrowing the field
- Documentation of the requirements: Developing the request for proposal
- Conducting detailed product demonstrations
- Completion of other due diligence activities
- Final selection
- Contract negotiations
- Benefits realization

Clarification of the Objectives

As with any organizational management decision, the first step is to document the problems that the organization is trying to solve with the new system or define the opportunities that the organization will be able to pursue because of the investment in a new system. This step addresses what the great philosopher and baseball legend Yogi Berra once said, "If you don't know where you are going, you will wind up somewhere else" (Things People Said 2011).

For instance, the organization can develop a set of requirements that address known problem areas with current applications or processes. Even more important, once the organization has created this initial list of needs, it must vet these requirements to understand which ones truly are must-have capabilities and which ones are less important. Too often, the organization becomes enamored by a new technology or popular product without knowing the clear purpose for that system. Technology should always be implemented to support the achievement of a desired process or outcome. Key questions for which an organization should have clear answers include the following:

- Is the system required to meet a regulatory mandate?
- What aspects of the organization's strategic business plan will it support?
- Will it help to drive business growth or support service-line development?
- Will it enhance patient safety and quality outcomes?
- Will it improve the flow of clinical, financial, or operational information across the enterprise?

Ideally, the objectives for the system must be clearly identified and agreed on before any products are reviewed. A project charter that lists these objectives, the expected benefits, the main project participants, the participants' roles and responsibilities, and the process for monitoring project progress is an excellent tool to support communication and buy-in. The project charter's objectives can be the basis for a return-on-investment analysis, which is required for the approval of capital investment in many organizations.

Formation of the System Selection Governance Structure and Functions

One of the most difficult tasks in systems implementation is achieving the desired level of adoption in the organization. An excellent way to lay the foundation for enthusiastic adoption is to bring all the stakeholders to the table as early as possible, obtain their endorsement of the objectives, and then ensure their active participation in the selection process. This leads to a shared sense of ownership in the result as well as a better-educated and better-prepared user population. Note here that the HIT department should almost never be seen as the main driver of the system selection. Having executive-level sponsorship for the project and highly visible leadership by members of the intended user population (be they physicians, nurses, pharmacists, or others), with the information technology (IT) department providing support to the process in the background, is ideal. Also important is to establish a project organizational governance structure that ensures strong and ongoing sponsorship, effective management and oversight, and sufficient involvement of operational staff so that all requirements are properly defined and evaluated. A hierarchical structure works well, where operational work groups perform the bulk of the analysis, feeding the information up to a selection committee for decision making. In some cases, it may be appropriate to seek the assistance of an external consultant with expertise in the specific technology and vendor marketplace to help guide the process and provide subject matter expertise on the marketplace. An example organizational governance structure is provided in Exhibit 8.1.

Most organizations have a preexisting executive committee that can serve in the executive oversight role. Under that committee, typically a system selection committee composed of representative stakeholders is formed. For instance, if the technology is a pharmacy system, the committee membership could comprise the pharmacy director/vice president (VP), the finance director/VP, the chief nurse, the chief medical information officer, one or two representatives from the medical staff, the IT applications director, and other key stakeholders of the potentially affected workflow areas. On the other hand, if the system is an enterprise EHR, then the system selection committee must have much broader stakeholder representation. For efficiency, establishing functional work groups for focused activities is often useful. For example, the system selection committee may form an ancillary services work group to develop requirements for the ancillary modules of the EHR, while a decision support work group might work on developing requirements and evaluating vendor responses for order set development, alerts and reminders, and so on. Finally, external consultants sometimes augment the process in organizations that prefer to have a consultant that has broad experience in running a system selection process.

Establishment of a System Selection Plan

Another best practice is to develop a system selection plan and timeline that are not only efficient but also realistic. If the process is rushed to meet an

EXHIBIT 8.1

Sample HIT Project Organization: Roles and Responsibilities

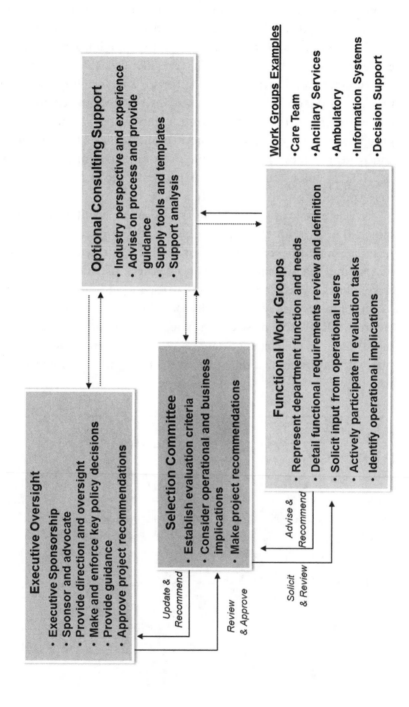

Executive Oversight
- Executive Sponsorship
- Sponsor and advocate
- Provide direction and oversight
- Make and enforce key policy decisions
- Provide guidance
- Approve project recommendations

Selection Committee
- Establish evaluation criteria
- Consider operational and business implications
- Make project recommendations

Optional Consulting Support
- Industry perspective and experience
- Advise on process and provide guidance
- Supply tools and templates
- Support analysis

Functional Work Groups
- Represent department function and needs
- Detail functional requirements review and definition
- Solicit input from operational users
- Actively participate in evaluation tasks
- Identify operational implications

Work Groups Examples
- Care Team
- Ancillary Services
- Ambulatory
- Information Systems
- Decision Support

Update & Recommend

Review & Approve

Solicit & Review

Advise & Recommend

SOURCE: Reprinted from material in "The Vendor Selection Process" by Paul Murphy, 2011, Encore Health Resources White Paper, Houston, Texas, pp. 1–12. Used with permission.

aggressive deadline, decisions may need to be made too quickly—and this can result in errors or omissions and in members of the selection team feeling left out of the process or forced into a solution they were not ready to accept. Some tasks in the selection process can be very time intensive, so it is important to ensure that selection team members understand or are conscious of the time commitment required of them, the time impact of competing projects and responsibilities, and specific calendar events (such as public holidays and summer vacations). Equally important is to match the selection project timeline to the complexity of the systems being evaluated and the committed availability of the selection team members, both at the functional work group level and the system selection committee level. Organizations should anticipate activities that will require extra time to coordinate and plan (such as product demonstrations), and prepare early. An example of a system selection work plan is provided in Exhibit 8.2.

The system selection plan depicted in the exhibit outlines a 17-week intended process for the steps leading up to, but not including, the contract negotiation and beyond. This assumes that the organization has no delays in forming the system selection governance structure and functions, the stakeholders are available and can participate on schedule, and so forth. In large, complex organizations with many stakeholders undertaking a complex enterprise EHR system selection, selecting a vendor of choice could easily take twice as long. The important point is to have an explicit system selection plan with a timeline that the organization thoughtfully develops and attempts to follow.

EXHIBIT 8.2

Sample System Selection Work Plan

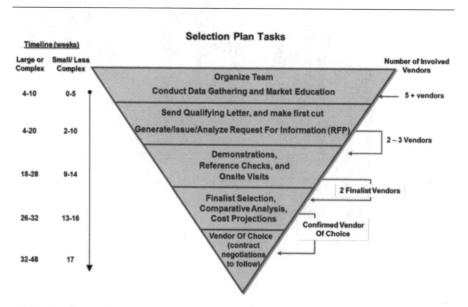

SOURCE: Adapted from material in "The Vendor Selection Process," by Paul Murphy, 2011, Encore Health Resources White Paper, Houston, Texas, pp. 1–12. Used with permission.

Education: Understanding the Marketplace

In highly competitive markets with many quality products, the vendors' reputation and services may represent the biggest differentiator between one system and another. System selection committee members typically conduct some initial data gathering on the leading vendors in the marketplace to find out details such as the following:

- How long has the vendor been in business?
- What is the vendor's reputation for providing customer support during implementation and ongoing maintenance?
- How much effort will the vendor put into product development and enhancement?
- What is the vendor's business plan?
- How has the vendor performed financially over the past several years?

If the vendor is financially or organizationally unstable, it may not be able to adequately support an organization or continue to invest in the quality of the product. In the HIT marketplace, vendor acquisitions are common, and the new owner may not provide the same level of service as given by the original vendor.

A number of subscription-based sources are available for assessing HIT functionality and the extent of a vendor's installed base for its products. The first is Gartner (www.gartner.com), a consulting firm that specializes in providing market research in the IT industry. Many healthcare organizations' IT departments maintain subscription services to Gartner, which also tracks the HIT industry specifically. For instance, for EHR applications, Gartner tracks by vendor the level of sophistication of various EHR capabilities such as the following:

- Clinical data repository
- Privacy
- Interoperability
- Controlled medical vocabulary
- Workflow
- Clinical decision support
- Clinical documentation
- Display
- Order management (computerized physician order entry)
- Knowledge management
- Continuum of care

Furthermore, Gartner tracks the number of implementations of various vendors' EHR components (Handler 2004, 2005, 2006).

Another source for assessing the extent of installed base of various vendors' EHR offerings is the HIMSS Analytics database (www.himssanalytics.com). This information is generally free to healthcare organizations that are willing to submit their own data regarding their particular installed base of various products. Furthermore, because the HIMSS Analytics database tracks organizational demographic information (e.g., number of beds, adjusted patient days), it can create peer-comparison reports that can be used to benchmark peers running similar financial or clinical application suites.

Finally, KLAS Enterprises (www.klasresearch.com) provides another source for doing research on HIT products. Regardless of a healthcare manager's tolerance for risk, the acquisition of most HIT is an expensive endeavor—one that requires particular due diligence with respect to narrowing the field, negotiation, and contracting.

Down Selection: Narrowing the Field

Down selection is the term for taking an initial set of vendors that are in the marketplace and narrowing down the field to just a few finalists. Often, there are many potential suppliers of a product; some may be industry veterans with tried-and-tested solutions, while others may be newcomers with exciting new technologies but a short track record. It is usually not possible or even desirable to do a full and detailed evaluation of every potential vendor and product. To use time and resources efficiently, it is best to narrow the field of vendors as quickly as possible to the top two or three candidates before engaging in very detailed, time-consuming analysis. Think of this initially as a process of elimination rather than a process of selection. Weed out the obvious misfits so that the system selection committee can focus on the leaders. An effective way to narrow the field is to establish a list of selection criteria that match closely the organization's objectives. Following are some criteria that are often used:

- Essential product functionality
- Existing client base for the system
- Ability to integrate with other systems
- Technology platform
- Vendor reputation and financial health
- Cost to acquire and implement
- System usability

The selection team may apply a percentage weighting to each of the selection criteria so that everyone understands the relative importance of functionality versus cost versus technology and so on. This weighting will prove highly valuable in the final selection as it provides an objective way to score the finalist vendors.

If a very large number of vendors exist in the marketplace, what can be useful sometimes is to write a short *qualifying letter* that requires each vendor to indicate its ability to comply with basic, objective selection criteria, such as the vendor must have existing clients that are similar to the organization or the vendor must hold desired certifications such as the Centers for Medicare & Medicaid Services' Meaningful Use certification for EHRs. This qualifying letter helps to quickly eliminate outliers with the minimum of effort.

Documentation of the Requirements: Developing the Request for Proposal

During the initial stages of the system selection process, high-level objectives and knowledge gained by the system selection committee members during the marketplace education stage are used to down select to a few key vendors. Some organizations spend a great deal of time developing lists with hundreds or even thousands of functional requirements for the system to which the vendors are then required to respond. This is very time-consuming for both the selection team and the vendors and can provide limited value (the vendor responses also take a lot of work to review). Often, it is better to think "bigger picture" and then create a request for proposal (RFP) or alternatively a request for information (RFI) that contains fewer than 100 questions addressing the primary functions and features desired by the organization. The RFP or RFI is a formal notice—often issued by an organization's purchasing department—that the organization is interested in purchasing a particular type of HIT product. If the selection team is unsure of the features available in the current market, the team may invite one or two vendors to provide a high-level demonstration of their products as a form of education before creating the RFP.

The RFP should be divided into sections addressing different aspects of the system and vendor. It should begin with a few paragraphs that inform the vendors about the organization and its objectives for the system selection, followed by a series of questions about the vendor, the product it is proposing, the functionality offered, underlying technology, associated services, comprehensive costs, and any other relevant information that will help the selection team in decision making. The work groups should participate in drafting questions in their area of expertise. The RFP questions should require the vendor to explain key aspects of the proposed solution rather than merely give a simple yes/no response. For example, instead of "Does your system include medication ordering?", the question should be "Describe medication orders functionality, including related decision support and any features designed to enhance patient safety." Typical RFP sections include the following (see also Exhibit 8.3).

According to mThink (2003), system selection committee members should ensure "vendors account for all costs, such as implementation and maintenance, and don't overlook hidden costs for items such as training and infrastructure costs (wireless, mobile devices, etc.). Here is a list of common expenses:

- Hardware
- System software (e.g., operating system, database licensing, etc.)
- Vendor software
- Interfaces
- Conversions
- Ongoing licensing [and] maintenance
- Increased staff needs
- Networking

EXHIBIT 8.3
Sections in a
Typical Request
for Proposal

Information Category	Details Sought
Corporate overview	Vendor corporate history, size, organization, financials
Client base	Current client base using relevant products, geographic spread, clients similar to the organization
Healthcare reform and regulatory compliance	Meaningful use compliance plan, support of quality measures reporting, interoperability support for medical home, etc.
Product availability	Products matching required functions (e.g., inpatient, ambulatory, clinical, administrative, technical, reporting), date released, Office of the National Coordinator for Health Information Technology certification status, delivery and support models
Interface availability	Interfacing approach, relevant experience
Technology platform	Use of current, industry-standard technologies
Preliminary and ongoing costs	One-time and ongoing costs, including hardware, software licensing, implementation, training, support, and subscriptions
Implementation and support approach	Phasing, resource requirements (vendor and organization), ongoing support services
Development direction, unique attributes	Future product and technology plans, alignment with organizational vision, market differentiators

- Peripherals (printers, PCs, bar-code readers, handheld devices)
- Training
- Facility renovation to accommodate hardware and training."

Some organizations provide a separate spreadsheet form in which the vendors are required to list costs by category. This helps to ensure that all the costs are identified and can be compared across the vendors' price quotes. Comparing vendor costs should be "apples to apples," carefully separating one-time costs (e.g., licenses, implementation services, training services) from ongoing costs (e.g., annual maintenance, subscriptions) and ensuring that the functionality being included matches across the quotes.

In addition, the RFP should include detailed instructions for vendor responses, including the format for response, dates of submission, and rules for communication. It is important to limit vendor communications to a small number of people on the selection team so that the process can be properly managed and to ensure that all vendors receive the same information. It is a best practice in the selection process to inform the responding vendors that the responses documented in their RFP and quotes will be attached to the final contract as a commitment. This helps to set the vendors' expectations that they will be held accountable to their RFP promises and prevents rework during the negotiation. Analysis of the RFP responses and how well they match the system selection criteria helps to determine which vendors are asked to continue to the next step—conducting detailed product demonstrations.

Conducting Detailed Product Demonstrations

Detailed product demonstrations are usually one of the most time-consuming steps in the selection process. Demonstrations for an enterprise EHR can take more than a full day per vendor and require the attendance of many key personnel. For this reason, it is best to use the information from the qualifying letter and RFP to eliminate all but the top two or three vendors before inviting them for demonstrations. A formal agenda for the product demonstrations is helpful as it sets the expectation that all vendors follow the same approximate sequence and show equivalent functions and features. Paul Murphy of Encore Health Resources, a firm that specializes in assisting hospitals with system selection processes, suggests that organizations should avoid very detailed scripts as these may force the vendor into a workflow that does not match the design of their system and will confuse the audience. Scripted demonstrations tend to take much longer to prepare for and conduct. A simple evaluation document that outlines the major requirements outlined in the RFP will allow system selection committee members to easily record their observations. This is vital to performing an objective comparative analysis.

Completion of Other Due Diligence Activities

The term *due diligence* in the context of this chapter means the effort to educate oneself when evaluating options available for purchase. To round out the selection process, talking to existing users of the finalist vendors' products is always valuable to hear about their experience with the system and the vendor. Using an evaluation form for these reference calls is also recommended. If the organization can afford it, it should conduct site visits with a select group of representatives from the selection team. Many selection committees create a clear agenda for the site visit and share it with the host before traveling to the site. Site visits are also an opportunity to forge relationships with other organizations that can become great sources of advice and assistance during the implementation process and beyond.

Finally, ensure that any questions left unanswered from the RFP, demonstrations, and reference checks are addressed through additional meetings with the finalist vendors. Often valuable is for the technical team at the provider organization to meet directly with technical representatives from the vendors to more fully understand the details of the system infrastructure and technical support requirements.

If the vendors were asked to supply cost quotes during the RFP, the selection team should review these proposed prices again and ask the vendor to confirm the total quoted costs. Frequently, new costs are introduced during due diligence. As a result, creating a total-cost-of-ownership (TCO) analysis prior to final system selection is often helpful in understanding the total costs an organization is likely to incur. A sample TCO for an EHR project appears in Exhibit 8.4.

The intent of the TCO analysis is to uncover not only the fees payable to the HIT vendor but also any additional third-party software fees. Equally important is that a TCO analysis allows the organization to gain an understanding of its own staff costs, as knowledgeable subject matter experts (SMEs) from the current staff often are assigned full-time to the project and will need to be back-filled with new hires or temporary hires; these are often significant costs that are historically underestimated in large HIT projects. Many organizations build in a budgetary reserve of 5 to 15 percent of the anticipated TCO to cover any unforeseen costs (e.g., a hospital acquisition midway through HIT implementation, which would increase licensing and implementation costs).

Final Selection

It is helpful to return to the original selection criteria and rate each of the finalist vendors against each of these weighted criteria based on all the findings from the activities performed by the selection committee. Much of the scoring is subjective, but the selection criteria help the selection team to make decisions regarding the pros and cons of each solution and weigh those decisions in an objective way. Once the final vendors are ranked (e.g., first preference, second preference), identify the top-ranked vendor as "Vendor of Choice," pending contract negotiations. In this way, the first-place vendor is aware that the organization has a second option, and thus the vendor may be more willing to negotiate the terms more favorably to close the deal.

Contract Negotiations

A well-conducted selection process should set the stage for a streamlined negotiation. By clearly identifying the expectations for the products being purchased or licensed and working through the pricing and implementation support elements of the RFP response, the selection team will already have laid out many of the terms that are of highest priority in the contract negotiations prior to the actual formal discussions.

As a general guideline, the most productive contract negotiations are those in which all parties are committed to developing an agreement that is fair, clearly sets out expectations for the implementation project and subsequent support relationship, provides legal and financial protection to the purchaser, and establishes a relationship based on mutual respect and collaboration. Organizations that take a combative stance or adopt an aggressive, no-compromise attitude during the negotiations must recognize that contract negotiations are the first step in a new business relationship that may continue for many years and thus will find this negative approach unproductive in the long term.

The first step in negotiations is to identify the members of the negotiations team, which include senior executives who have the authority to make financial commitments on behalf of the organization, management-level members of the selection committee who understand the product and its intended functionality, a representative from the organization's purchasing department, and the organization's legal counsel.

Contract negotiations should be treated as a project in itself, with designated negotiation committee members, documented goals and objectives, and a timeline and meeting schedule that includes internal review sessions in between the negotiating meetings. In most cases, including legal counsel, who will take the lead in managing the legal aspects of the contract negotiation, is necessary. Because legal counsel can be expensive, especially for an organization that is not large enough to have an internal legal professional, the legal discussion may be put on hold until all or most of the business terms have been resolved.

Before the first negotiation session with the vendor, the internal negotiating committee should meet to agree on the negotiating strategy, which includes the issues that are most important (e.g., better pricing on software

EXHIBIT 8.4

Sample Ten-Year Total Cost of Ownership for a Typical EHR

Products	FY06	FY07	FY08	FY09	FY10	FY11	FY12	FY13	FY14	FY15	Total
Volume Based Software Licenses					Capital Based License fees						
Chunk 1 (350K Visits)											
25 % at Signing	$$$,$$$										$$$,$$$
20 % at Delivery	$$$,$$$										$$$,$$$
5 % on final workflow walkthru		$$,$$$									$$,$$$
5 % on integrated testing kickoff		$$,$$$									$$,$$$
25 % on First Live Use (FLU)		$$$,$$$									$$$,$$$
10% FLU + 90 Days			$$$,$$$								$$$,$$$
10% FLU + 12 months			$$$,$$$								$$$,$$$
Chunk 2 (up to 500K Visits)			$$$,$$$								$$$,$$$
Chunk 3 (up to 750K Visits)			$$$,$$$								$$$,$$$
Chunk 4 (up to 850K Visits)					$$$,$$$						$$$,$$$
Oncology Module		$$$,$$$	$$,$$$	$$$,$$$	$$$,$$$						$$$,$$$
Third Party Database		$$,$$$	$$,$$$								$$,$$$
Add'l Vendor One Time Products		$$,$$$	$$,$$$								$$,$$$
Third Party One Time Products			$$,$$$								$$,$$$
Interfaces (Live)											
25% at Signing		$$,$$$	$$,$$$								$$,$$$
25% at Delivery			$$,$$$								$$,$$$
25 % at FLU			$$,$$$								$$,$$$
25% at FLU + 90			$$,$$$								$$,$$$
Medication Interfaces (Phase II)				$$,$$$							$$,$$$
					Capital Based Implementation Fees						
Implementation (Base)		$$$,$$$	$$$,$$$								$$$,$$$
Implementation (Oncology)		$$,$$$	$$$,$$$								$$$,$$$
Implementation (Interfaces)		$$$,$$$									$$$,$$$
Post-Live Activities		$$,$$$									$$,$$$
Project Team Training		$$$,$$$									$$$,$$$
Estimated Travel		$$$,$$$									$$$,$$$
Rollout			$$$,$$$								$$$,$$$
					Capital Based Hardware Fees						
Hardware Environment											
AIX Servers		$$$,$$$				$$$,$$$					$,$$$,$$$
SAN		$$$,$$$		$$,$$$		$$$,$$$			$$,$$$		$$$,$$$
Test/Training Server	$$,$$$				$$,$$$		$$$,$$$				$$,$$$
Clairty RDBMS Server	$,$$$				$,$$$						$,$$$
Crystal Enterprise Server		$$,$$$					$$,$$$				$$,$$$
Print Server		$,$$$					$,$$$				$$,$$$
Patient Portal Server		$$,$$$					$$,$$$				$$,$$$
Citrix Servers		$$$,$$$		$$$,$$$			$$$,$$$				$$$,$$$
Citrix Server Optional				$$$,$$$					$$$,$$$		$$$,$$$
Blade Enclosure		$$,$$$		$$,$$$					$$$,$$$		$$$,$$$
Citrix Licenses		$$,$$$		$$,$$$					$$$,$$$		$$$,$$$
Training/Implementation for AIX		$$,$$$				$$,$$$		$$,$$$			$$,$$$
SQL Enterprise Licenses	$$,$$$						$$,$$$				$$,$$$
Citrix Administrator		$$$,$$$					$$$,$$$				$$,$$$
Citrix Technical Training	$$,$$$										$$,$$$
Network Infrastructure Upgrades	$$,$$$		$$$,$$$					$$$,$$$			$,$$$,$$$

	Operating Based Software Fees (Maintenance and Subscription Fees)								
Volume Based PP Chunk 1 (350)	$$,$$$	$$,$$$		$$$,$$$	$$$,$$$	$$$,$$$	$$$,$$$	$$$,$$$	$,$$$,$$$
Yearly Support - Optional		$$,$$$	$$$,$$$	$$$,$$$	$$$,$$$	$$$,$$$	$$$,$$$	$$$,$$$	$,$$$,$$$
Oncology		$$,$$$	$$$,$$$	$$$,$$$	$$$,$$$	$$$,$$$	$$$,$$$	$$$,$$$	$$$,$$$
Third Party dB - Required	$,$$$	$$,$$$	$$,$$$	$$$,$$$	$$$,$$$	$$,$$$	$$$,$$$	$$$,$$$	$$$,$$$
Third Party dB - Optional		$$,$$$	$$,$$$	$$$,$$$	$$$,$$$	$$,$$$	$$,$$$	$$$,$$$	$$$,$$$
Third Party Maintenance Fees	$$,$$$	$$,$$$	$$$,$$$	$$$,$$$	$$$,$$$	$$$,$$$	$$$,$$$	$$,$$$	$$$,$$$
Vendor Consulting On Hand	$$,$$$	$$,$$$	$$$,$$$	$$$,$$$	$$$,$$$	$$$,$$$	$$$,$$$	$$$,$$$	$$$,$$$
Patient Portal Software	$,$$$	$$,$$$	$$,$$$	$$$,$$$	$$,$$$	$$,$$$	$$,$$$	$$,$$$	$$,$$$
Interface Maintenance	$$,$$$	$$,$$$	$$,$$$	$$$,$$$	$$,$$$	$$,$$$	$$,$$$	$$,$$$	$$,$$$
Subscription Applications	$0	$$,$$$	$$,$$$	$$$,$$$	$$,$$$	$$,$$$	$$$,$$$	$$$,$$$	$$$,$$$
	Operating Based Additional EMR Staffing								
Clinical Applications IS Team	$$$,$$$	$$$,$$$	$$$,$$$	$$$,$$$	$$$,$$$	$$$,$$$	$$$,$$$	$$$,$$$	$$$,$$$
Oncology Specific IS Team	$$$,$$$	$$$,$$$	$$$,$$$	$$$,$$$	$$$,$$$	$$$,$$$	$$$,$$$	$$$,$$$	$$$,$$$
Other IS Staff	$$$,$$$	$$$,$$$	$$$,$$$	$$$,$$$	$$$,$$$	$$$,$$$	$$$,$$$	$$$,$$$	$$$,$$$
Core Trainers	$,$$$	$$$,$$$	$$$,$$$	$$$,$$$	$$$,$$$	$$$,$$$	$$$,$$$	$$$,$$$	$$$,$$$
End User Trainers - Initial		$$$,$$$	$$$,$$$	$$$,$$$	$$$,$$$	$$$,$$$			$$$,$$$
End User Trainers - Addtl.		$$$,$$$							$$$,$$$
Onsite Support Personnel - Initial	$$$,$$$	$$$,$$$	$$$,$$$	$$$,$$$	$$$,$$$		$$$,$$$	$$$,$$$	$$$,$$$
Onsite Support Personnel - Addtl.		$$$,$$$	$$$,$$$	$$$,$$$	$$$,$$$	$$$,$$$	$$$,$$$	$$$,$$$	$$$,$$$
Total Spend	**$,$$$,$$$**	**$,$$$,$$$**	**$,$$$,$$$**	**$,$$$,$$$**	**$,$$$,$$$**	**$,$$$,$$$**	**$,$$$,$$$**	**$$,$$$,$$$**	**$$,$$$,$$$**
	Required and Optional Split of Costs								
Total Required	$,$$$,$$$	$,$$$,$$$	$,$$$,$$$	$,$$$,$$$	$,$$$,$$$	$$$,$$$	$$$,$$$	$$$,$$$	$$,$$$,$$$
Total Optional	$0	$0	$$$,$$$	$$$,$$$	$$$,$$$	$$$,$$$	$$$,$$$	$$$,$$$	$$$,$$$
	Capital and Operational Split of Costs								
Total Capital	$,$$$,$$$	$,$$$,$$$	$,$$$,$$$	$$$,$$$	$$$,$$$	$$$,$$$	$$$,$$$	$$$,$$$	$$,$$$,$$$
Total Operational	$$$,$$$	$$$,$$$	$,$$$,$$$	$$$,$$$	$$$,$$$	$$$,$$$	$$$,$$$	$$$,$$$	$$$,$$$

Legend:
$,$$$ Thousands
$$,$$$ Tens of Thousands
$$$,$$$ Hundreds of Thousands
$,$$$,$$$ Millions
$$,$$$,$$$ Tens of Millions

Notes:
1. For confidentiality reasons, real dollar figures could not be used
2. This 10-year total cost of ownership model is from a 5-Hospital, 1000+ bed academic medical center with 700+ physicians
3. The total estimated operational spend over the 10-year period is 75% of the total spend, while the capital spend is only 25% of the total spend

licenses, additional implementation resources, better support services). Naming a primary spokesperson during the negotiating meetings as well as an individual to be responsible for handling communications between meetings creates clarity, prevents confusion about the most current status of issues, and helps prevent conflicts. Another efficient practice is to have the negotiating team prospectively vet and gain agreement on which items are of the highest priority, which items the organization will be unwilling to compromise, and which items are open for compromise and can therefore be used as "bargaining chips." Some items that an organization should pay particular attention to when negotiating and crafting terms and conditions include but are not limited to the following (Chesney 2005; O'Connor 2005):

- *Project scope*, such as levels of effort, resource requirements, timing, costs, and deliverables. Areas that vendors are keenly sensitive to include endless customizations that the organization wants to make to their product. Recognize that vendors will want to minimize their risk as well and will want to limit customizations. Seek to strike a mutually agreeable balance.

- *Consequences of nonperformance*, which might include options to require the vendor to provide additional resources at no additional cost to mitigate the nonperformance, give the organization the right to a set sum of money for liquidated damages, or give the organization the right to withhold payments. Because much of an EHR or ERP implementation, for instance, requires large-scale workflow reengineering, recognize that vendors will not want to take on the risk that the organization cannot make decisions regarding changes in the workflow.

- *Personnel commitments.* Clearly specify the personnel by name, and retain the right to be involved in personnel selection should changes be required during the project. Establish also the expectations regarding on-site work versus off-site work; redesigning workflows using an automated tool typically requires vendor expertise on site for a large portion of the effort.

- *Project management methodology.* This identifies, among other things, governance and decision rights, change processes, escalation processes for problem resolution, testing and acceptance criteria, expectations regarding standard meetings, and regular project-performance reporting expectations.

- *Payment terms.* Most vendors will want to link payment terms to measured time intervals. The healthcare organization should link payment terms to explicit deliverables that involve demonstrated, stable functional use of the product. It should also specify limits in increases in ongoing maintenance and support costs and ensure that those ongoing costs are indexed to the negotiated price and *not* a "book" price—list price of the application, which averages in the range of 18 to 22 percent of the negotiated price.

- *Site of litigation.* This site should be the organization's state. While litigation is clearly something to be avoided, should it become necessary specifying the site up front when the organization's legal counsel is better positioned to address it is ideal.

- *Vendor's accounting cycles.* Attempt to negotiate on price at the end of an accounting quarter—or, even better, an accounting year. Sometimes, particularly for publicly traded vendor organizations, substantial discounts may be offered during these windows of opportunity.

To start the process of contract negotiations, it is customary for the negotiating team to obtain a copy of the vendor's standard contract for the products and services being proposed and to identify any issues in the contract that are important to address, such as some of the items noted in the preceding list. These issues may be entered into an *issues matrix*, which may be sent to the vendor in advance of the first meeting so that the vendor is prepared to discuss alternatives at the outset. Examples of typical categories and items found in an issues matrix include the following:

Scope Definition
- Software, hardware
- Interfaces and conversions
- Professional services
- Custom development items
- Service support levels

Business Terms
- License term, renewal, termination
- Upgrades and enhancements
- Future products and services
- Risk-sharing terms
- Pricing and discounts, payment terms
- Implementation work plan

Legal Terms and Conditions
- Acceptance terms
- System performance and response times
- Regulatory compliance
- Governing law

- Indemnity, warranties, and remedies
- Assignment
- Intellectual property and confidentiality
- Liability

Include space to record negotiating positions, relevant dates, contract identifiers, and status. An example of a one-page negotiations issues matrix is provided in Exhibit 8.5.

Using the issues matrix as the primary tool to track progress, the negotiating team can conduct several rounds of meetings to work through the issues on the list and agree on the terms. During meetings, stay focused and adopt a tone of collaborative problem solving. It is always appropriate to call a short time out to discuss an item in private (e.g., if a new issue is raised and the team needs to agree on the organization's position). It is normal to compromise on certain items in order to "win" on priority issues; this is where the advance discussion and planning will help to keep the selection process moving forward. In negotiating the terms of a system implementation, a best practice is to seek payment terms that tie payments to achievement of milestones (rather than regular calendar payments) as this encourages the vendor to activate the product in the desired timeframe and reduces risk for the purchasing organization. Many organizations seek to establish risk-sharing arrangements, where the vendor may receive higher payments if it accomplishes certain tasks or outcomes ahead of schedule and, conversely, may be penalized financially if it falls behind schedule. Risk-sharing arrangements like this ensure that each party has "skin in the game"; however, note that this also places a burden on the purchasing organization to hold up its end of the agreement to provide resources and make decisions as required to accomplish the desired results.

Because the contract with the vendor will include costs and services to support implementation of the new system, it is usually best to draft a preliminary implementation plan to make sure that both parties have a shared understanding of the resources and timeline, including the achievement of major milestones.

At the conclusion of contract negotiations, the team can create an internal communication document for senior leadership that summarizes the business deal, key terms and conditions, concessions received, and other risk-mitigation agreements.

Monitor Contract Performance

Remember the importance of clearly defining the project scope up front, such as levels of effort, resource requirements, timing, costs, and deliverables.

EXHIBIT 8.5

Sample Negotiations Issues Matrix

Discussion Topic	Our Position	Vendor Response	Cross-Reference to Contract Section	Date Discussed	Current Status (Open, In process, Resolved)
License	The license to use the software should be perpetual.				
Term	Customer will consider entering into a 7–10 year term for support.				
Scope of use	The agreement would include the entire enterprise, as well as future sites. The list of sites is: • [insert list]				
Products	The following products are included in the base deal: *Clinical* • [insert product names] *Revenue cycle* • [insert product names] *Departmental* • [insert product names] The following products should be considered options to be purchased in the future: • [insert product names]				
Pricing	Provide best and final pricing by: • Application				

If the organization has a professional project management office, the HIT project will have built in performance measurements and updates. However, if the organization has not yet made an investment in comprehensive project management methodologies, it should at the very least ensure that someone in the organization (not someone from the vendor's firm) is tracking progress on full-time equivalent resource consumption, project timelines and milestones, and other costs and deliverables. To fully gain the contracting benefit of having specified these items in the terms and conditions of the contract, the organization must demand regular project-performance updates with the members of the vendor team.

Benefits Realization

An often overlooked but incredibly important part of the system selection process is that, at some point after the new HIT goes into productive use, the organization must conduct a formal benefits realization assessment to see if the desired benefits envisioned for the particular HIT investment were actually achieved. The best approach for accomplishing this is to collect baseline *before* performance indicators (e.g., length of stay, readmission rates by diagnosis-related group, overtime hours by staff type) in the areas of performance the organization hoped to improve with HIT; then, about 12 months after the new HIT goes into production, the organization can collect the *after* measures of those same indicators and compare the two sets of data. This is a powerful, "close the loop" step that can provide valuable lessons and validation to the board of directors or senior leadership team—that the HIT investment made is actually reaping the benefits envisioned.

Summary

The selection of information systems by an organization, particularly those systems that affect a large portion of operational functions, is a process that requires rigorous due diligence and systematic, participative decision making. In this chapter, we provide a framework for conducting a system selection process that includes the following activities:

- Clarification of the objectives
- Formation of the system selection governance structure and process
- Establishment of a system selection plan
- Education: Understanding the marketplace
- Down selection: Narrowing the field
- Documentation of the requirements: Developing the request for proposal

- Conducting detailed product demonstrations
- Completion of other due diligence activities
- Final selection
- Contract negotiations
- Benefits realization

The key to increasing the chances of having a successful outcome to a system selection process is to resource it like any other formal process and to include the key stakeholders throughout the organization who will be affected by the system selection decision. The organization must ensure that these stakeholders are active participants in both the due diligence and the decision to move forward with a vendor of choice.

Note

1. Portions of this chapter have been reprinted and/or adapted from *The Executive's Guide to Electronic Health Records* by Detlev H. Smaltz and Eta Berner (Chicago: Health Administration Press, 2007) and from the 2011 unpublished work by Paul Murphy, strategy advisory service leader at Encore Health Resources. Material from Paul Murphy's work—"The Vendor Selection Process" (July 2011) and "Selection Process Exhibits" (July 2011)—is used with permission of Encore Health Resources.

Web Resources

A number of organizations (through their websites) provide more information on the topics discussed in this chapter:

- Gartner (www.gartner.com/technology/research.jsp). Gartner provides subscription-based research notes on information technology that covers a full spectrum—from technical to IT-based business processes.
- HIMSS Analytics (www.himssanalytics.org). HIMSS Analytics provides data and analytic expertise.
- KLAS (www.klasresearch.com). KLAS provides ratings of healthcare technology that help organizations make informed decisions.

Discussion Questions

1. What are the major activities that make up the system selection process?
2. What are some examples of functional work groups and the types of work that they might accomplish in support of a system selection project?
3. Why is it important to create a system selection plan at the outset of a system selection endeavor?
4. What is the down selection activity, and why is it an important step in the system selection process?
5. What is a request for proposal (RFP), and what is its purpose?
6. What are some of the typical sections that make up an RFP?
7. What is a total cost of ownership, and why is it important to estimate prior to making a system selection?
8. What are some of the important items that an organization should consider when going into contract negotiations with a vendor?
9. What is a benefits realization assessment?

APPLICATIONS: ELECTRONIC HEALTH RECORDS

Learning Objectives

1. Define the term *electronic health record* (EHR).
2. Understand the key capabilities of a robust EHR.
3. Articulate the benefits of a robust EHR.
4. Articulate some of the key cost categories associated with the purchase and implementation of an EHR.
5. Describe the EHR Adoption Model.
6. Understand the concept of meaningful use of an EHR, and describe some of the criteria that both individual providers and hospitals need to achieve to earn incentives for meaningfully using an EHR.

Overview

There has been an evolution of the terms used to describe a digital version of a medical record. Currently, *electronic health record* (EHR) is the most commonly used term to describe "a longitudinal electronic record of patient health information generated by one or more encounters in any care delivery setting. Included in this information are patient demographics, progress notes, problems, medications, vital signs, past medical history, immunizations, laboratory data and radiology reports. The EHR automates and (with appropriate operations management) can streamline the clinician's workflow. The EHR has the ability to generate a complete record of a clinical patient encounter—as well as supporting other care-related activities directly or indirectly via an interface—including evidence-based decision support, quality management, and outcomes reporting" (HIMSS 2012b). A key component of this definition from the Healthcare Information and Management Systems Society (HIMSS) is the ability to record patient information that is generated in *any* care delivery setting. In other words, the EHR should provide caregivers with the ability to communicate patient information collected from across organizational boundaries. Regardless of where care was delivered, the EHR is designed to gather that information for a full, longitudinal detailed view of a patient's medical history. In the past, terms like the computer-based patient record (CBPR or CPR) or an electronic medical record (EMR) were used and should be viewed as less robust versions of what today has evolved into the EHR.

Components of an EHR

Dick, Steen, and Detmer (1997) published an Institute of Medicine (IOM) report titled *The Computer-Based Patient Record*, which originally articulated the key features of the contemporary EHR. Later, HIMSS Analytics expanded on the original key components/features of an EHR that Dick and his colleagues suggested (Garets and Davis 2006) and developed the seven-stages EMR Adoption Model (EMRAM), depicted in Exhibit 9.1. These seven stages not only have become the de facto standard description of the key components of a complete EHR but also, with the addition of the stages of adoption of these key components/features, have provided a means of tracking the degree of EHR adoption throughout the industry.

We cover the EHR adoption stages in more detail later in this chapter. The rest of this section provides a brief overview of each of the seven key components of an EHR—primarily in the context of the EMRAM.

Stage 1: Ancillary Systems

The ancillary systems component of an EHR includes automated information systems to support workflow in the laboratory, radiology, and pharmacy departments. In the laboratory department, for instance, this includes captur-

EXHIBIT 9.1
US EMR Adoption Model[SM]

Stage	Cumulative Capabilities
Stage 7	Complete EMR; CCD transactions to share data; Data warehousing; Data continuity with ED, ambulatory, OP
Stage 6	Physician documentation (structured templates), full CDSS (variance & compliance), full R-PACS
Stage 5	Closed loop medication administration
Stage 4	CPOE, Clinical Decision Support (clinical protocols)
Stage 3	Nursing/clinical documentation (flow sheets), CDSS (error checking), PACS available outside Radiology
Stage 2	CDR, Controlled Medical Vocabulary, CDS, may have Document Imaging; HIE capable
Stage 1	Ancillaries—Lab, Rad, Pharmacy—All Installed
Stage 0	All Three Ancillaries Not Installed

SOURCE: Reprinted from "U.S. EMR Adoption Model[SM] Trends." www.himssanalytics .org/docs/HA_EMRAM_Overview_Eng%20011812.pdf. Used with permission from HIMSS Analytics.

ing test results from various laboratory test devices and automatically pulling that into an automated stand-alone laboratory information system or an integrated laboratory EHR module that physicians and other caregivers can access to obtain their patients' test results. Similarly, in the radiology department, this includes providing results of radiological exams to the physicians that ordered them. In the pharmacy department, it provides an automated means of managing the process of dispensing and delivering drugs to patients.

Stage 2: Clinical Data Repository (CDR)

The CDR collects data from a variety of information systems and makes the data available to physicians and other caregivers in a unified view of each of their respective patients. While CDRs from different EHR vendors may differ slightly, they typically aggregate data from ancillary systems such as lab results, pathology reports, and radiology reports as well as pharmacy data and other data relating to the patient (e.g., demographics; admission dates; transfer dates, if applicable; discharge dates; diagnosis codes). The CDR often also uses a controlled medical vocabulary.

Stage 2: Controlled Medical Vocabulary (CMV)

CMV is "a tool used to standardize information for purposes of capturing, storing, exchanging, searching and analyzing data" (*Health Informatics* 2012). The purpose of a CMV is to address the many needs and limitations of healthcare's information infrastructure; examples are as follows (*Health Informatics* 2012):

- Reducing ambiguity that is inherent in normal human languages (for example, how "heart attack," "myocardial infarction," and "MI" may mean the same thing when describing a patient condition but represent different conditions to a computer coding that information)
- Making the exchange of information consistent between different providers, care settings, researchers, and others even at different points in time
- Overcoming differences in medical information recording from one place to another
- Summarizing medical information (in a consistent manner)
- Allowing symbolic manipulation of data (searches for specific analysis)
- Providing automated reasoning (clinical decision support)

Some common CMVs include the following:

- *Systematized Nomenclature of Medicine-Clinical Terms (SNOMED-CT).* "SNOMED CT provides the core general terminology for the electronic health record . . . and [as of 2012] contains more than 311,000 active concepts with unique meanings and formal logic-based definitions organized into hierarchies. When implemented in software applications, SNOMED CT can be used to represent clinically relevant information consistently, reliably and comprehensively as an integral part of producing electronic health records" (IHTSDO 2012).

- *Logical Observation Identifiers Names and Codes (LOINC).* LOINC is a universal code system for identifying laboratory and clinical observations (Regenstrief Institute 2012).
- *Unified Medical Language System (UMLS).* "The UMLS integrates and distributes key terminology, classification and coding standards, and associated resources to promote creation of more effective and interoperable biomedical information systems and services, including electronic health records" (NLM 2012).

In short, the main value of a CMV is in providing a means for health-related information systems—particularly, EHRs and EHR component modules—to become semantically interoperable.

Stage 2: Document Imaging

Many healthcare providers make copies of paper records that are either generated within their own setting or that patients bring with them from another care setting (e.g., clinic, hospital). Making these images of paper records available through the EHR is another capability that helps ensure providers have as much information available as possible as they assess and care for patients.

Stage 2: Health Information Exchange (HIE) Capability

The US Department of Health & Human Services's Office of the National Coordinator for Health Information Technology (ONCHIT) believes that HIE capability (exchange of health information electronically) is essential to both providing the best possible care for patients and driving down the overall cost of that kind of high-quality care at a national level (Williams et al. 2012). Contemporary EHRs should have the basic ability to securely and electronically send and receive data about relevant patients to aid patient assessment and care decisions. ONCHIT is working to establish standards for accomplishing this in a more unified, consistent manner. Note that data about a patient should be able to be securely and appropriately exchanged not only intra-organizationally (i.e., across all inpatient, outpatient, ancillary, and complementary care settings within the organization) but also inter-organizationally (i.e., across distinct, legal, organizational entity boundaries).

Stage 3: Clinical Decision Support (CDS) and Clinical Decision Support System (CDSS)

CDSS has been defined in a variety of ways. Garg and colleagues (2005), in a review of CDSS and its effects on practitioner performance and patient outcomes, says, "CDSS are information systems designed to improve clinician decision making. Characteristics of individual patients are matched to a computerized knowledge base, and software algorithms generate patient-specific recommendations."

Most major EHR system vendors have CDSS capabilities; that is, they can generate a variety of alerts and reminders, such as error checking for drug–drug and drug–food adverse effects as well as conflict checking for drug–lab orders. A more advanced CDSS also has the ability to supply evidence-based medicine protocols (e.g., order sets that have been shown in the medical body of literature to have the best statistical outcomes for patients with specific diagnoses or conditions). These advanced CDS capabilities provide easy access to any local and/or remote subscription-based knowledge sources, such as MD Consult, OVID, the Medline medical literature database, and national or local clinical guidelines. The most advanced CDSS also can provide guidance—in the form of variance and compliance alerts—for all clinical activities related to clinical protocols and outcomes (HIMSS Analytics 2012b; Middleton et al. 2004).

Key CDSS implementation considerations that in the past were determined locally with input from the clinical staff include

- the choice of which alerts/reminders to include,
- how alerts/reminders are delivered to the clinician, and
- the circumstances under which clinicians are allowed to override the alerts/reminders.

Too-frequent alerts with only minimal justification result in what has been termed *alert fatigue*, which not only generates complaints from clinicians but also results in frequent overrides and ignoring of even the most important alerts. For instance, many medication knowledge bases that can be purchased to be integrated with the EHR to provide alerts for drug–allergy interactions, for example, produce an alert for the specific drug as well as for any drugs in that class—even if patients have already taken the related drugs with no ill effects. Furthermore, alerts are triggered by elements in the EHR; that is, if the clinician had originally included, for instance, an allergy to aspirin when the patient said the aspirin upset her stomach but the clinician never changed the entry when he realized this was not a "real" allergy, then the alert will be triggered anyway. Conversely, if the system is set up so that a blank allergy field suggests that the patient is *not* allergic to anything, when in fact the empty field only means that allergies have not yet been assessed or the documentation is incomplete, then unsafe medication orders may not generate an alert. For these reasons, determination of how to implement the CDSS functions of the EHR is definitely too important to leave to the health information technology (HIT) staff. There should be significant involvement by providers during the design phase of the CDSS implementation.

ONCHIT has emphasized CDSS, especially in regard to *e-prescribing* —the transmission of prescriptions electronically from clinician to pharmacy. As part of the national effort, the American Medical Informatics Association (AMIA) developed what has been called a "road map" for CDS. This road-map suggests that while CDS tools are promising, much has yet to be done to realize their full potential—particularly in the following three areas (Ford, Menachemi, and Phillips 2006):

1. Applying the best clinical knowledge available at the point when it is needed
2. Achieving high adoption of CDS and effective use
3. Continuous improvement of clinical knowledge and CDS methods

Osherhoff and his colleagues (2005) suggest a phased implementation of CDS with physician thought-leader input as the plans are developed as well as a responsive feedback and modification process as the CDS capabilities of the EHR are implemented. Training and support for physicians are considered essential, and including training on what the alerts mean and how to respond to them is also very important.

Stage 3: Nursing/Clinical Documentation

Contemporary EHRs have the ability to document vital signs, flow sheets (time-based trending of particularly relevant clinical data to assess a patient's condition over time), nursing notes, and care plans. They also can keep a comprehensive record of all medications that have been administered to the patient.

Stage 3: Picture Archiving and Communication Systems (PACS)

PACS capture and store medical images such as x-ray images, CT (computerized tomography) scans, MRI (magnetic resonance imaging) scans, and other medical diagnostic images. They also have the ability to allow caregivers from across the organization to electronically access those images. Contemporary EHRs provide a means to make PACS images available to caregivers outside of the radiology department.

Stage 4: Computerized Physician Order Entry (CPOE)

HIMSS (2012c) defines CPOE as "the portion of a clinical information system [or EHR] that enables a patient's care provider to enter an order for a medication, clinical laboratory or radiology test, or procedure directly into the computer. The system then transmits the order to the appropriate department, or individuals, so it can be carried out. The most advanced implementations of such systems also provide real-time clinical decision support such as dosage and alternative medication suggestions, duplicate therapy warnings, and drug-drug and drug-allergy interaction checking." Both the Health Information Technology for Economic and Clinical Health (HITECH) Act of 2009 and employer advocacy groups, such as the Leapfrog Group (www.leapfroggroup.org), share the goals to improve quality of care and reduce the cost of care via providing incentives to healthcare practitioners who adopt CPOE. The Leapfrog Group is a continually growing coalition of *Fortune* 500 companies that promotes CPOE, which research data have shown to have the ability to reduce the possibility of adverse drug events (Reckmann et al. 2009). Hospitals that have CPOE are promoted to the employees of Leapfrog Group companies and advocate for higher reimbursement levels for care. This push from Leapfrog and federal legislation such as the HITECH Act for healthcare delivery organizations and systems to increase patient safety has prompted the growing interest in CPOE adoption. Remember, however, that CPOE alone is unlikely to realize the proposed benefits—unless the technology is coupled with an EHR with the foundational features discussed in this chapter and unless it is linked to at least minimal CDS that provides advice on appropriate drug ordering, such as alerts for drug–drug or drug–allergy interactions.

Stage 5: Closed-Loop Medication Administration

Closed-loop medication administration, also called *end-to-end medication administration*, includes CPOE with CDS for error checks, bar code or other automated methods for checks during medication administration, and an electronic medication administration record (e-MAR) linked to the pharmacy and the CPOE. Closed-loop medication administration obviously requires that the component parts (CPOE, CDSS, e-MAR) be in place and integrated; thus, the process is clearly a later stage in the EMRAM but is vital for achieving much-higher levels of patient safety (Smaltz and Berner 2007).

Stage 6: Physician Documentation

Physician documentation that was produced and managed as a paper record—such as progress notes, consult notes, discharge summaries, problem lists, and diagnosis list maintenance—can now be entered and maintained electronically within the EHR. Not only should the EHR support direct entry of data by physicians, but it also should support structured data entry, which necessitates a defined vocabulary (as noted previously). This does not mean that physicians need to be taught a new language to use the system, but the database that underlies the record should be structured. There have been some attempts to use mechanisms to process actual spoken or written natural language, but these have not been as successful in gaining full EHR benefits in the way that structured data have. What is needed if unstructured input is going to be allowed is a mechanism to link from the dictated language to the structured language—that is, *natural language processing* (NLP), which continues to make progress as a technology that captures and transcribes physician dictation into text; at this writing, NLP is not yet a fully fail-safe means of leveraging practitioner input for direct patient care decisions, although it is an excellent means of conducting medical research such as the ability to identify, extract, and categorize information found within clinical narrative text such as in dictated physician notes (Al-Haddad et al. 2010; Terry 2012). However, templates for recording patient information have been used with some success. Indeed, using structured templates for routine types of care (e.g., a template for adult-acquired pneumonia) provides the added benefit of being able to do real-time evaluation and management (E&M) coding, which can have a huge impact on expediting billing and consequently reducing accounts receivable days.

Stage 7: Analytics and Reporting

EHRs should have the ability to provide advanced reporting to analyze patterns of clinical data to improve quality of care and patient safety as well as care efficiencies.

Security and Access

In addition to the elements of the seven stages is one of IOM's original recommendations for EHRs that has become absolutely required: protect the confidentiality and integrity of the patient's information. The system must be able to track, in a rigorous way, who has accessed the record. This essential function aligns the evolution of the EHR with the original HIPAA (Health Insurance Portability and Accountability Act) legislation and the HITECH Act extensions to HIPAA (e.g., more rigorous requirements related to protecting personally identifiable patient information). While timely access, both onsite and remotely, by a wide range of providers needs to be unequivocally guaranteed, unauthorized access must be prevented.

Benefits and Goals

An EHR can increase the efficiency of the clinical care processes not only by getting rid of inefficient paper-based documentation but also by reducing the need to search for lost charts, lab data, or other pieces of patient information. An EHR can potentially increase the efficiency of claims processing by using the actual clinical data to provide documentation for claims. Having the data on care processes in electronic form can also help in monitoring what is happening in the patient care settings at the individual level and in using analytical techniques for identifying patterns in that care process. The monitoring can involve both cost-effectiveness and quality.

Many parts of the clinical processes, the claims processes, and monitoring the patient care setting were accomplished primarily with paper medical records. While bills were generated, risk assessments were conducted, and quality assurance and quality improvement activities were performed, they all relied primarily on painstaking *chart abstraction*—the manual process of reviewing paper-based medical records and extracting the pieces of information needed for the particular task at hand. The use of an EHR can introduce possible improvements in both the processes and outcomes of care. These are improvements that are difficult to accomplish with a paper chart. We discuss those aspects in this section, but first let's look at four benefits of an EHR related to improving efficiency and monitoring.

Benefit 1: Access to Information
One of the most obvious benefits of an EHR is access to information—that is, getting the clinical information when and where it is needed. Goals such as 24-hours-a-day, 7-days-a-week accessibility are common expectations for an EHR. Access and communication go hand in hand, because easy access not only makes it convenient for individual clinicians to get the information they need but also improves communication among providers.

Benefit 2: Better Organization of Data
This benefit includes having basic patient data located in a central place so that the data have to be entered only one time. Other efficiency goals include improving the quality of the data in the record by avoiding illegible handwriting and getting an assurance that the data are complete and accurate.

Benefit 3: Claims Processing Efficiency
Even though the record is a clinical record, the clinical data can improve claims processing efficiency if this information drove the billing process. Data that are accessible in electronic form can ease the process of gathering and

providing documentation for claims purposes. In addition, linking the clinical indications to laboratory test orders can improve the accuracy and efficiency of that process.

Benefit 4: Improved Monitoring of Performance

An EHR allows for individual provider profiles of performance as well as aggregate profiles of all providers, something most of the insurance carriers and managed care organizations are already doing. These data can be used within the organization to target quality improvement initiatives. As noted, manual chart audits are difficult and labor intensive. One important point to emphasize, however, is that while microfiche, optical scanning, and other document imaging procedures may provide a better means of storage and may make accessing information easier than was possible with the paper-based medical record system, they will not make the profiling and auditing any easier. To do that, the clinical information must be stored in such a computer-readable/searchable manner that the information can be easily retrieved in multiple different ways.

With an EHR, clinical and financial outcomes can be more easily monitored and linked to quality improvement processes; this is extremely difficult to do with traditional paper records. Individual caregivers can also develop their own profiles of behavior so that they can monitor and modify that behavior. Furthermore, individual profiles of behavior can provide insight into needed, targeted continuing education. Educational activities can be more easily targeted to real clinical needs, not just the practitioner's interests. Finally, a robust EHR's ability to aggregate data across patients provides a means for population-based monitoring and specific disease management.

Stages of EHR Adoption

While it is true that some healthcare facilities have focused on CPOE (Stage 4) even before getting the back-end ancillary systems automated and integrated, it is generally recommended that other systems (stages under 4) be in place and working well before the workflow changes needed for CPOE are undertaken. Exhibit 9.2 shows the stages of adoption of EHR capabilities across the United States as of early 2012.

Most hospitals have moved beyond having just automated departmental systems such as pharmacy, radiology, and laboratory (HIMSS Analytics 2012b). In fact, the majority of hospitals are at Stage 3 capabilities or below—at 44.9 percent in 4th quarter 2011 and 43.9 percent in 1st quarter 2012 (see Exhibit 9.2). This degree of integration can provide very useful, accessible information for clinicians and can promote more direct clinician interaction with the computer, which potentially pave the way for easier adoption and attainment of CPOE *meaningful use* (a new federal incentive

Stage	Cumulative Capabilities	2011 Q4	2012 Q1
Stage 7	Complete EMR; CCD transactions to share data; Data warehousing; Data continuity with ED, ambulatory, OP	1.2%	1.2%
Stage 6	Physician documentation (structured templates), full CDSS (variance & compliance), full R-PACS	5.2%	6.2%
Stage 5	Closed loop medication administration	8.4%	9.4%
Stage 4	CPOE, Clinical Decision Support (clinical protocols)	13.2%	13.2%
Stage 3	Nursing/clinical documentation (flow sheets), CDSS (error checking), PACS available outside Radiology	44.9%	43.9%
Stage 2	CDR, Controlled Medical Vocabulary, CDS, may have Document Imaging; HIE capable	12.4%	12.1%
Stage 1	Ancillaries—Lab, Rad, Pharmacy—All Installed	5.7%	5.5%
Stage 0	All Three Ancillaries Not Installed	9.0%	8.4%
		N=5337	N=5318

EXHIBIT 9.2
US EMR Adoption Model[SM]: Levels of Adoption, 2012

SOURCE: Reprinted from "U.S. EMR Adoption Model[SM] Trends." www.himssanalytics .org/docs/HA_EMRAM_Overview_Eng%20011812.pdf. Used with permission from HIMSS Analytics.

program discussed later in this chapter). In addition, most research studies have shown that automation of nursing processes (a Stage 3 capability) actually saves time for nurses, which provides a motivation for accepting these automated systems. In contrast, although it is likely to bring other benefits, CPOE may take more of a physician's time at the front end than do current manual ordering processes. This impact on physician time just from CPOE would be compounded if the automated clinical systems offered no other value. This is why most consultants recommend getting to Stage 3 capabilities before tackling the Stage 4 CPOE.

Adoption of CPOE is still seen as a problem today, as many practicing physicians still have a number of objections to it—such as impact on time, the view that the data-entry component is low-level work, and alert fatigue from overly aggressive systems, just to name a few. Despite the fact that EMRs with CPOE have been around for more than 30 years, a study by HIMSS Analytics (2012b) involving more than 5,300 US hospitals found that at the beginning of 2012 only 1.2 percent of the participating organizations had implemented a complete EHR—what HIMSS Analytics refers to as a Stage 7 Hospital (see Exhibit 9.2). To gain the full benefits of meaningfully using an EHR with CPOE, federal legislation has been enacted to enforce EHR adoption throughout the United States. These mandates reward the meaningful use of an EHR and penalize practitioners and organizations that continue to avoid meaningful use.

Federal Initiatives to Promote the Meaningful Use of an EHR

The 1999 landmark report *To Err Is Human*, published by the IOM, suggested that in the United States between 44,000 to 98,000 deaths a year were due to medical errors. This report heightened the concerns about patient safety by many groups, including healthcare executives, clinicians, health policymakers, and the general public; more important, it captured the attention of the legislative and executive branches of the US government. The report advocated for the increased use of EHR, CPOE, and CDSS as means of preventing errors, leading President George W. Bush, in his 2004 State of the Union address, to emphasize the need to computerize patient health records (*Washington Post* 2004).

While it is difficult to make predictions in any fast-changing arena, the momentum for change in HIT has certainly increased. For one thing, a federal-level office (ONCHIT) now exists, headed by an HIT "czar" who is charged with overseeing a variety of government HIT initiatives, including the deployment of national interoperable EHRs (the term *interoperability* refers to the ability of systems to talk to each other within and between facilities and organizations). Congress had initially appropriated funding for ONCHIT and for grants through the Agency for Healthcare Research and Quality (AHRQ 2004), focusing on the development of standards, prototype data networks, review of privacy and security practices at a statewide level, and demonstration projects in urban and rural settings of model systems.

In addition to appropriations to AHRQ for targeted HIT projects, an increasing amount of federal legislation is geared toward reducing medical errors, increasing the use of information technology in healthcare, and changing the way healthcare organizations are trying to improve quality. In 2005, the Patient Safety and Quality Improvement Act was signed into law, establishing a voluntary error-reporting database. The Joint Commission (2011) now publishes an annual report called *Improving America's Hospitals*, which publicizes myriad quality and safety measures stratified by US hospitals. Furthermore, the Centers for Medicare & Medicaid Services (CMS n.d.[c]) has several online sources of quality data on hospitals and home health care, such as the Medicare Inpatient Hospital Dashboard, which provides comparative quality and cost data. Websites like Healthgrades (www.healthgrades.com) already provide various quality performance indicators for a growing number of hospitals (Healthgrades 2009).

Other legislation provides grants to hospitals for implementing systems for electronic transmission of prescription orders (e-prescribing) and a variety of proposals to differentially reward high-quality care (pay for performance). The latter will almost certainly require electronic tracking and transmission of outcome data. In addition to these carrots (or sticks, depending on one's perspective), a bill has been proposed to modify the antikickback provisions of the Stark antitrust laws to provide a "safe harbor" for hospitals that work with their referring physicians to develop integrated information systems (Gottlieb 2010).

Finally, the HITECH Act, which is part of the American Recovery and Reinvestment Act (ARRA) of 2009, gives significant incentives both to hospitals and independent physicians that meaningfully use a certified EHR and imposes penalties to providers for not using a certified EHR by 2015 (ONCHIT 2012a). The intent of these incentives goes beyond rewarding the act of implementing an EHR; they are meant to motivate the use of an EHR that results in significant measurable improvements in the quality and affordability of care (Blumenthal and Tavenner 2010).

While these national laws and developments are encouraging the widespread adoption of HIT, several factors have made healthcare executives (and private clinicians) cautious about embracing new technologies. First, executives are confronted by a rich assortment of products, options, and vendors, so making a choice is difficult in an area as rapidly changing and as expensive as HIT. While it may not be too painful (financially and otherwise) to replace a $2,000 laptop for the CEO every few years as technology changes, the same cannot be said for a $30 million system for her hospital. Second, because of the many different EHR vendors, many hospitals have adopted the *best of breed* approach to purchasing departmental systems—that is, buy the locally perceived top-of-the-line radiology system from one vendor, the best billing system from another vendor, and the preferred system of the chief of pathology from a third vendor. This approach, while satisfying the individual department's needs, can make interoperability between these departmental applications a challenge within a hospital, much less between institutions. A related purchasing approach is known as *best of suite,* wherein hospitals adopt the best financial suite of applications from one vendor and the best clinical suite of applications from a different vendor that has similar cross-suite interoperability challenges. A third purchasing approach is buying all or most applications from a single vendor; this may solve the problem of communication within a hospital but does not make it easy to electronically send data to a different hospital with a different proprietary system. In addition, because the healthcare organization has invested so much in a single vendor's product, it becomes difficult to change vendors (Ford et al. 2010).

ONCHIT (2012b), working closely with CMS, oversees the development of the requirements to certify vendor EHR products. Both the standards of meaningful use and an objective certification process are intended to help buyers of EHRs make more informed decisions and essentially assure buyers that the systems they purchase meet established standards and can work seamlessly with other vendors' systems. In fact, ONCHIT maintains a list of the current certified HIT products for both ambulatory practices and hospitals (see www.healthit.gov/policy-researchers-implementers /certified-health-it-product-list-chpl).

The Meaningful Use Standards

The HITECH Act specifies the three key elements of meaningful use as follows (CMS n.d.[c]):

1. The use of certified EHR technology in a meaningful manner, such as e-prescribing (using an automated system to submit prescriptions directly to a retail pharmacy rather than writing a prescription on paper)
2. The use of certified EHR technology for electronic exchange of health information to improve quality of healthcare
3. The use of certified EHR technology to submit clinical quality and other measures to CMS

These high-level criteria for meaningfully using an EHR are broken into three stages, as envisioned to be implemented between 2011 and 2015 and beyond:

- Stage 1 sets the baseline for electronic data capture and basic information sharing and had a 2011–2012 expected implementation goal. As of February 2013, CMS reports that more than 234,000 healthcare providers have received incentive payments for achieving Stage 1 meaningful use (CMS 2013).
- Stage 2 begins in fiscal year 2014 for hospitals and in calendar year 2014 for eligible hospitals with an expectation to demonstrate meaningful use of an EHR across an even larger portion of their respective patient populations. The latest criteria can be found on the ONCHIT website at www.healthit.gov/policy-researchers-implementers/mean ingful-use-stage-2.
- Stage 3 continues to expand on the baselines established in Stage 1 and Stage 2.

Both the actual granular criteria that were adopted to represent the final Stage 1 criteria and the criteria that will be finalized over time to represent the detailed Stage 2 and Stage 3 criteria are accomplished through a public process of rulemaking administered by ONCHIT and CMS. For instance, the Stage 1 meaningful use criteria include specific items for eligible individual physicians and a separate set for hospitals (outlined in Exhibit 9.3). For eligible professionals (physicians), there are a total of 25 objectives of which they must meet 15 core objectives and select 5 additional objectives

Stage 1 Meaningful Use Core Objectives Criteria	
Eligible Professionals	*Hospitals and Critical Access Hospitals*
15 Core Objectives	14 Core Objectives
1. Use CPOE for medication orders directly entered by any licensed healthcare professional who can enter orders into the medical record per state, local, and professional guidelines. 2. Implement drug–drug and drug–allergy interaction checks. 3. Maintain an up-to-date problem list of current and active diagnoses. 4. Generate and transmit permissible prescriptions electronically (e-prescribing). 5. Maintain active medication list. 6. Maintain active medication allergy list.	
7. Record all of the following demographic information: (a) preferred language, (b) gender, (c) race, (d) ethnicity, and (e) date of birth	7. Record all of the following demographic information: (a) preferred language, (b) gender, (c) race, (d) ethnicity, (e) date of birth, and (f) date and preliminary cause of death in the event of mortality in the eligible hospital
8. Record and chart changes in the following vital signs: (a) height, (b) weight, (c) blood pressure; (d) calculate and display body mass index (BMI); (e) plot and display growth charts for children 2–20 years, including BMI. 9. Record smoking status for patients 13 years old or older.	
10. Report ambulatory clinical quality measures to CMS or state Medicaid programs.	N/A
11. Implement one CDS rule relevant to specialty or high clinical priority along with the ability to track compliance with that rule. 12. Provide patients with an electronic copy of their health information (including diagnostics test results, problem list, medication lists, medication allergies) upon request. 13. Provide clinical summaries for patients for each office visit. 14. Have the capability to electronically exchange key clinical information (for example, problem list, medication list, allergies, and diagnostic test results) among providers of care and patient-authorized entities. 15. Protect electronic health information created or maintained by certified EHR technology through the implementation of appropriate technical capabilities.	

EXHIBIT 9.3
Stage 1 Meaningful Use Criteria

(continued)

EXHIBIT 9.3
Stage 1
Meaningful Use
Criteria
(*continued*)

Stage 1 Meaningful Use Menu Options Criteria	
Eligible Professionals	*Hospitals and Critical Access Hospitals*
5 Menu Options (*Note:* 5 of the following list of 10 objectives must also be met in Stage 1 to qualify for incentives.)	
1. Implement drug formulary checks. 2. Incorporate clinical lab-test results into EHR as structured data. 3. Generate list of patients by specific condition to use for quality improvement, reduction of disparities, research, or outreach. 4. Use certified EHR technology to identify patient-specific education resources, and provide those resources to the patient if appropriate. 5. The provider, hospital, or critical access hospital that receives a patient from another setting of care or provider of care or that believes an encounter is relevant should perform medication reconciliation. 6. The provider, hospital, or critical access hospital that transitions its patient to another setting of care or provider of care or that refers its patient to another provider of care should provide a summary-of-care record for each transition of care or referral. 7. Have the capability to submit electronic data to immunization registries or immunization information systems and actual submission according to applicable law and practice. 8. Have the capability to submit electronic syndromic surveillance data to public health agencies and actual submission according to applicable law and practice.	
9. Send patient reminders per patient preference for preventive/follow-up care.	9. Record advance directives for patient 65 years old or older.
10. Provide patients with timely electronic access to their health information (including lab results, problem list, medication list, and allergies) within 4 business days of the information being available to the provider.	10. Have the capability to submit electronic data on reportable (as required by state or local law) lab results to public health agencies and actual submission according to applicable law and practice.

SOURCE: Adapted from CMS (n.d.[c]).

from a menu list of 10 as outlined in the exhibit (20 of the 25). For eligible hospitals and critical access hospitals, there are 24 objectives of which they must meet 14 core objectives and select 5 additional objectives from a menu list of 10 as outlined in the exhibit (19 of the 24). Many of the objectives for physicians and hospitals are similar, with some appropriate differences relevant to each group's use of an EHR. These objectives are then quantified for Stage 1.

Take, for instance, the first objective—use of CPOE. It requires a provider to use CPOE to directly enter at least one medication order for more than 30 percent of all the provider's unique patients who have at least one medication on their medication list. To meet Stage 1 incentives, the provider must show that more than 80 percent of all unique patients he sees have at least one medication entry (or an indication that the patient is not currently prescribed any medication) recorded as structured data. To meet Stage 2 incentives, the provider must enter more than 60 percent of medication orders, more than 30 percent of laboratory orders, and more than 30 percent of radiology orders. For eligible hospitals, the objective to maintain a problem list requires that more than 80 percent of all unique patients admitted to the inpatient or emergency department have at least one problem entry (or an indication that no problems are known for the patient) recorded as structured data. For Stage 2, this objective has been merged into the summary-of-care document at transitions of care and referrals. For a complete list of the EHR incentive measures for eligible professionals and hospitals, see the CMS website (www.cms.gov/EHRIncentivePrograms).

For eligible professionals who achieve meaningful use objectives, incentives are available through either Medicare or Medicaid (but not both; a provider may take advantage of whichever is most advantageous to her assuming she meets minimum patient volume criteria) depending on the first calendar year that they began to meaningfully use certified EHR technology (CMS 2010b). See Exhibit 9.4 for the EHR incentive table. For eligible hospitals and critical access hospitals that achieve meaningful use objectives, the incentives are calculated differently (following a formula that begins with a $2 million base incentive, increased principally on the basis of Medicare and/or Medicaid patient volumes) and can range from $2 million to more than $10 million.

Beyond the incentives, physicians and hospitals that do not successfully demonstrated meaningful use of an EHR by 2015 or later are subject to a negative payment adjustment on their Medicare and/or Medicaid claims. This makes clear that CMS has both incentives and penalties in place to drive meaningful use of EHRs.

Declining Physician Resistance

A lingering obstacle to the use of clinical systems, in particular EHRs with CPOE, has been physician reluctance. Physicians clearly want to do what is in the best interests of their patients' care, but studies have shown that EHRs—particularly CPOE—change work patterns for physicians in significant ways (Morrison and Smith 2000). In addition, while the costs are obviously less for smaller practices, they may still be substantial. Prior to the development of the HITECH Act's meaningful use incentives, some suggested that the financial benefits of the EHR should largely accrue to payers,

EXHIBIT 9.4
EHR Incentive Payment Schedule for Providers

Maximum EHR Incentive Payments by Program Based on the First Calendar Year (CY) for Which the Eligible Professional Receives Payment

CY	CY 2011		CY 2012		CY 2013		CY 2014		CY 2015		CY 2016	
	Medicare	Medicaid	Medicare	Medicaid	Medicare	Medicaid	Medicare	Medicaid	Medicare	Medicaid	Medicare	Medicaid
2011	$18,000	$21,250										
2012	$12,000	$8,500	$18,000	$21,250								
2013	$8,000	$8,500	$12,000	$8,500	$15,000	$21,250						
2014	$4,000	$8,500	$8,000	$8,500	$12,000	$8,500	$12,000	$21,250				
2015	$2,000	$8,500	$4,000	$8,500	$8,000	$8,500	$8,000	$8,500		$21,250		
2016		$8,500	$2,000	$8,500	$4,000	$8,500	$4,000	$8,500		$8,500		$21,250
2017				$8,500		$8,500		$8,500		$8,500		$8,500
2018						$8,500		$8,500		$8,500		$8,500
2019								$8,500		$8,500		$8,500
2020										$8,500		$8,500
2021												$8,500
Total (if EP does not switch programs)	$44,000	$63,750	$44,000	$63,750	$39,000	$63,750	$24,000	$63,750	$0	$63,750	$0	$63,750

NOTE: Medicare Eligible Professionals may not receive EHR incentive payments under both Medicare and Medicaid.
NOTE: The amount of the annual EHR incentive payment limit for each payment year will be increased by 10 percent for EPs who predominantly furnish services in an area that is designated as a Health Professional Shortage Area.
SOURCE: Reprinted from CMS (2010b).

the hospital/health system, and the patients themselves—as opposed to the individual physician (Berner et al. 2006; Doolan and Bates 2002).

Physician adoption was seen as a problem, but the meaningful use incentives (and penalties by 2015); the growing body of young caregivers and professionals who were raised with computers and have now entered healthcare; and the rise of instant messaging, texting, email, social networking, and other mobile computing and communication technologies all suggest that clinician anxiety about using computers is likely to be replaced by excitement and demand for them. The *Journal of the American Medical Informatics Association* published an estimate of the adoption rates for EHRs among physicians (see Ford, Menachemi, and Phillips 2006, 2009) that has largely been corroborated by the National Center for Health Statistics' annual survey of EHR adoption in physician office settings (see Hsaio et al. 2011; Simborg, Detmer, and Berner 2013). Between 2011 and 2015 as physician practice adoption moves above the 50 percent mark (Hsaio et al. 2011), hospitals and healthcare organizations that do not have an EHR in place may begin to see a decline in their ability to attract physicians and inpatient referral patterns, as physicians and empowered patients may begin to favor a transparently safer and more information-integrated environments that EHRs are envisioned to provide. To further track EHR adoption in the ambulatory setting, HIMSS Analytics has created a new Ambulatory EMR Adoption Model, which can be found at www.himssanalytics.org/emram/AEMRAM.aspx.

Costs and Benefits of an EHR

Federal legislation and programs clearly have created monetary incentives to adopt EHRs, but it is important to understand both the scope of the effort to implement a robust EHR and the other benefits that the IOM and HITECH Act advocate. A study by the Rand Corporation published in *Health Affairs* suggested that $81 billion in aggregate could be saved annually as a result of EHR adoption, but some CEOs wondered how much of that actually could accrue to their respective organizations (Hillestad et al. 2005). They certainly were aware of the legislative incentives and penalties associated with adoption of EHRs and were cognizant of consumer and employer empowerment that may increasingly demand healthcare providers to use EHRs, but at the same time they were leery of a number of unknowns, including (but not limited to) the following (Hillestad et al. 2005):

- Will their organization be able to successfully undergo the significant cultural and workflow process changes needed to achieve benefits?
- Are the vendor's product capabilities real or marketing hype?

- What hidden costs are associated with an EHR project?
- Will the physicians adopt the new EHR-enabled processes and workflows?

In this section we address the costs questions of these CEOs along with the envisioned benefits of the EHR.

Costs

Costs for small physician practice EHRs have declined significantly, but hospital-based EHRs continue to be relatively expensive. While we applaud the efforts to release to the public government-developed EHR software, such as the US Department of Veterans Affairs's VistA system, we issue a caution that the actual cost of that software's license is only the tip of the proverbial iceberg. An EHR project, because it affects so many workflows and individuals, is really a large-scale organizational and cultural transformation project. The bulk of the costs of an EHR is spent on workflow-reengineering efforts and ongoing support and maintenance. A particularly useful way to assess the long-term costs of an EHR is to develop a ten-year total cost of ownership (TCO) model for the project. All hospitals and healthcare organizations consider the purchase price of the hardware and software licenses and even the ongoing software maintenance costs and additional staff needed to be added to the HIT department, but few of them accomplish a comprehensive assessment of the total costs of the project (Smaltz and Berner 2007).

Total Cost of Ownership

Exhibit 9.5 provides the one-time and the recurring cost components for assessing the TCO of an EHR project. Most of these cost items likely resonate with CEOs, COOs, CFOs, and CIOs, but we advocate taking the time to cost out each component over a ten-year period to reduce "blind spots" and thus assist the organization in making a well-informed decision about its total investment package over time. Exhibit 9.5 also provides a nice outline of some of the elements that an EHR planning team should take into consideration when estimating the total ten-year spending on the project. These include not only the obvious one-time charges (such as the purchase of the software licenses for the EHR and/or the purchase of the hardware on which the EHR software resides) but also the recurring charges (such as the ongoing operational personnel needed for the care and feeding of the EHR system, the personnel needed to provide ongoing training, and the personnel needed to provide integration with future applications that might need to integrate with the EHR).

Exhibit 9.6 is a sample ten-year TCO of an outpatient EHR with CDS and CPOE capabilities at a 5-hospital, 1,000-plus bed academic medical center with more than 700 physicians. For confidentiality reasons, the exhibit does not include actual dollar figures but uses appropriate orders of

Scope Element	One-Time	Recurring
Software and intellectual property	Perpetual software license Content licensing	Term, ASP (application service provider) license; support fees
Timing	Project management Post-live/cutover management	Ongoing support Subsequent improvement phases
People	Implementation • Application • Functional • Infrastructural • Integration • Project management • Sponsorship • Education • Backfill • Vendor and third-party support	Support • Application • Functional • Infrastructural • Integration • Project management • Sponsorship • Education
Process/redesign (logical scope)	People and organizational change needs Third-party support Infrastructure changes	Ongoing support
Infrastructure— technology, facilities	Computing/servers/ storage Network Third-party system interfaces End-user devices Space-fit-out, moves	Maintenance Refreshment at end of life

EXHIBIT 9.5
Components of Total Cost of Ownership of an EHR

magnitude to give you an itemized perspective of the TCO of an EHR for such an organization.

The real value of developing a ten-year TCO of an EHR or any major project is to explicitly and deliberately force an analysis and articulation of all the expenses the organization will incur, not just the initial purchase costs. While not obvious from the example in Exhibit 9.6, given that the actual dollars are masked, do note that in most EHR projects the capital expenditure over the ten-year period is only about 25 percent or less of the total spending. The vast majority—about 75 percent or more—of the expense of an EHR accrues on the operating side of the balance sheet (Smaltz and Berner 2007). For healthcare organizations that are looking to plan beyond the next budget cycle, accomplishing ten-year TCOs for any major investment, let alone an EHR, provides a systematic means of both making an informed decision at the time of purchase and being more able to proactively reduce the project-execution risks of such a complex project.

EXHIBIT 9.6

Sample 10-Year Total Cost of Ownership for an Outpatient EHR

Products	FY06	FY07	FY08	FY09	FY10	FY11	FY12	FY13	FY14	FY15	Total
Capital Based License Fees											
Volume Based Software Licenses											
Chunk 1 (350K Visits)											
25% at Signing	$$$,$$$										$$$,$$$
20% at Delivery	$$$,$$$										$$$,$$$
5 % on final workflow walkthru		$$,$$$									$$,$$$
5 % on integrated testing kickoff		$$,$$$									$$,$$$
25 % on First Live Use (FLU)		$$$,$$$									$$$,$$$
10% FLU + 90 Days			$$$,$$$								$$$,$$$
10% FLU + 12 months			$$$,$$$								$$$,$$$
Chunk 2 (up to 500K Visits)			$$$,$$$								$$$,$$$
Chunk 3 (up to 750K Visits)				$$$,$$$							$$$,$$$
Chunk 4 (up to 850K Visits)					$$,$$$	$$$,$$$					$$$,$$$
Oncology Module	$$$,$$$				$$$,$$$						$$$,$$$
Third Party Database	$$,$$$	$$,$$$			$$$,$$$						$,$$$,$$$
Add'l Vendor One Time Products	$$,$$$	$$,$$$									$$,$$$
Third Party One Time Products		$$,$$$									
Interfaces (Live)											
25% at Signing	$$,$$$	$$,$$$									$$,$$$
25% at Delivery		$$,$$$									$$,$$$
25 % at FLU		$$,$$$									$$,$$$
25% at FLU + 90		$$,$$$									$$,$$$
Medication Interfaces (Phase II)				$$,$$$							$$,$$$
Capital Based Implementation Fees											
Implementation (Base)		$$$,$$$	$$$,$$$								$$$,$$$
Implementation (Oncology)		$$$,$$$	$$$,$$$								$$$,$$$
Implementation (Interfaces)		$$,$$$	$$,$$$								$$$,$$$
Post-Live Activities		$$,$$$	$$,$$$								$$$,$$$
Project Team Training		$$$,$$$	$$,$$$								$$$,$$$
Estimated Travel		$$$,$$$	$$$,$$$								$$$,$$$
Rollout			$$$,$$$	$$$,$$$							$$$,$$$
Capital Based Hardware Fees											
Hardware Environment											
AIX Servers		$$$,$$$					$,$$$,$$$				$,$$$,$$$
SAN		$$$,$$$		$$,$$$			$$$,$$$		$$,$$$		$$$,$$$
Test/Training Server	$$,$$$					$$,$$$	$$$,$$$				$$,$$$
Clairty RDBMS Server	$,$$$					$,$$$	$,$$$				$,$$$
Crystal Enterprise Server		$$,$$$					$$,$$$				$$,$$$
Print Server		$,$$$					$,$$$				$,$$$
Patient Portal Server		$$,$$$					$$,$$$				$$,$$$
Citrix Servers		$$$,$$$		$$$,$$$			$$$,$$$				$$$,$$$
Citrix Server Optional				$$$,$$$					$$$,$$$		$$$,$$$
Blade Enclosure	$$,$$$			$$,$$$			$$,$$$		$$,$$$		$$,$$$
Citrix Licenses	$,$$$			$,$$$			$$,$$$		$$,$$$		$$$,$$$
Training/Implementation for AIX		$$,$$$					$$,$$$				$$$,$$$
SQL Enterprise Licenses	$$,$$$					$$,$$$					$$,$$$
Citrix Administrator		$$$,$$$						$$$,$$$			$$$,$$$
Citrix Technical Training		$$,$$$									$$,$$$

	Operating Based Software Fees (Maintenance and Subscription Fees)									
Volume Based PP Chunk 1 (350)	$$,$$$		$$$,$$$	$$$,$$$	$$$,$$$	$$$,$$$	$$$,$$$	$$$,$$$	$$$,$$$	$,$$$,$$$
Yearly Support - Optional			$$,$$$	$$,$$$	$$,$$$	$$,$$$	$$,$$$	$$,$$$	$$$,$$$	$$$,$$$
Oncology		$,$$$	$$,$$$	$$,$$$	$$,$$$	$$,$$$	$$,$$$	$$,$$$	$$,$$$	$$$,$$$
Third Party dB - Required	$,$$$		$$,$$$	$$,$$$	$$,$$$	$$,$$$	$$,$$$	$$,$$$	$$,$$$	$$,$$$
Third Party dB - Optional		$$,$$$	$$,$$$	$$$,$$$	$$$,$$$	$$$,$$$	$$$,$$$	$$$,$$$	$$$,$$$	$$$,$$$
Third Party Maintenance Fees		$$,$$$	$$,$$$	$$,$$$	$$,$$$	$$,$$$	$$,$$$	$$,$$$	$$,$$$	$,$$$,$$$
Vendor Consulting On Hand		$$,$$$	$$$,$$$	$$,$$$	$$,$$$	$$,$$$	$$,$$$	$$,$$$	$$,$$$	$$$,$$$
Patient Portal Software		$,$$$	$$,$$$	$$,$$$	$$,$$$	$$,$$$	$$,$$$	$$,$$$	$$,$$$	$$,$$$
Interface Maintenance		$$,$$$	$$,$$$	$$,$$$	$$,$$$	$$,$$$	$$,$$$	$$,$$$	$$,$$$	$$$,$$$
Subscription Applications	$0	$$,$$$	$$,$$$	$$,$$$	$$,$$$	$$,$$$	$$,$$$	$$,$$$	$$,$$$	$$,$$$
Operating Based Additional EMR Staffing										
Clinical Applications IS Team	$$$,$$$	$$$,$$$	$$$,$$$	$$$,$$$	$$$,$$$	$$$,$$$	$$$,$$$	$$$,$$$	$$$,$$$	$$$,$$$
Oncology Specific IS Team		$$$,$$$	$$$,$$$	$$$,$$$	$$$,$$$	$$$,$$$	$$$,$$$	$$$,$$$	$$$,$$$	$$$,$$$
Other IS Staff		$$$,$$$	$$$,$$$	$$$,$$$	$$$,$$$	$$$,$$$	$$$,$$$	$$$,$$$	$$$,$$$	$$$,$$$
Core Trainers	$$,$$$	$$$,$$$	$$$,$$$	$$,$$$						
End User Trainers - Initial		$$$,$$$	$$$,$$$						$$$,$$$	
End User Trainers - Addtl.		$$$,$$$			$$$,$$$	$$$,$$$	$$$,$$$	$$$,$$$	$$$,$$$	$$$,$$$
Onsite Support Personnel - Initial	$$$,$$$		$$$,$$$	$$$,$$$						
Onsite Support Personnel - Addtl.		$$$,$$$	$$$,$$$							
Total Spend	$,$$$,$$$	$,$$$,$$$	$,$$$,$$$	$,$$$,$$$	$,$$$,$$$	$,$$$,$$$	$,$$$,$$$	$,$$$,$$$	$,$$$,$$$	$,$$$,$$$
Required and Optional Split of Costs										
Total Required	$,$$$,$$$	$,$$$,$$$	$,$$$,$$$	$,$$$,$$$	$$$,$$$	$$$,$$$	$$$,$$$	$$$,$$$	$$$,$$$	$$$,$$$
Total Optional	$0	$$$,$$$	$$$,$$$	$$$,$$$	$$$,$$$	$$$,$$$	$$,$$$	$$$,$$$	$$$,$$$	$$$,$$$
Capital and Operational Split of Costs										
Total Capital	$,$$$,$$$	$,$$$,$$$	$$$,$$$	$$$,$$$	$$$,$$$	$$$,$$$	$$$,$$$	$$$,$$$	$$$,$$$	$$$,$$$
Total Operational	$$$,$$$	$,$$$,$$$	$,$$$,$$$	$,$$$,$$$	$,$$$,$$$	$,$$$,$$$	$,$$$,$$$	$,$$$,$$$	$,$$$,$$$	$,$$$,$$$

Legend:
$,$$$ Thousands
$$,$$$ Tens of Thousands
$$$,$$$ Hundreds of Thousands
$,$$$,$$$ Millions
$$,$$$,$$$ Tens of Millions

Notes:
1. For confidentiality reasons, real dollar figures could not be used
2. This 10-year total cost of ownership model is from a 5-Hospital, 1000+ bed academic medical center with 700+ physicians
3. The total estimated operational spend over the 10-year period is 75% of the total spend, while the capital spend is only 25% of the total spend

Benefits

A common reaction by most CEO, COO, and CFOs when they become aware of the costs of implementing an EHR is to immediately ask, "Where's the return on investment (ROI)?" Our colleague Dr. John Glaser has a nice analogy that he uses when someone confronts him with that question. He replies with, "What's the ROI of a chainsaw?" After letting his questioner ramble on a bit about the inherent efficiencies of chainsaws over axes or the lower number of full-time equivalents needed when employing a chainsaw versus an ax, he comes to their rescue with an obvious, thought-provoking insight: "What if you are making a dress? You'd be hard pressed to find an ROI for chainsaws if the task at hand were to efficiently make dresses. An equally important question follows that, 'What if the chainsaw is in the hands of a 10-year old child?'" Again, in the hands of a user without the requisite skills or ability to effectively use a chainsaw, the ROI is equally dubious. Glaser's message is clear: Depending on what you want to do with an EHR and who will be using it, the ROI is variable (Glaser and Garets 2005).

First and foremost, EHRs should not be treated as a proverbial silver-bullet technology that one throws at the problem of inefficient patient care processes. Rather, an EHR project is an organizational, cultural transformation that just happens to have a technological component. The benefits of the project will depend on (1) which processes an organization is willing to reengineer to take on the associated long-standing or ingrained status quos; (2) to what extent an organization is willing to invest in ensuring that the process owners and users are fully engaged and committed to reengineering the EHR-enabled processes; and (3) whether users are being fully trained in using the new EHR tools. In other words, as mentioned earlier as well, proper project execution is paramount to achieving the promise and value of the EHR. Assuming the healthcare organization has the leadership and buy-in as well as the project management prowess to effectively implement an EHR, an organization can expect to accrue a number of benefits from an EHR (see exhibits 9.7 and 9.8) beyond the meaningful use incentives.

The financial benefits in Exhibit 9.7 are fairly self-explanatory and are those that organizations generally consider when comparing costs with benefits. Not all benefits are strictly financial, although they can be framed in financial terms. The product line benefits in Exhibit 9.8 are often overlooked when assessing the positive impact of an EHR. As legislation and payer models begin to reward health maintenance activities, as opposed to health intervention activities, an EHR can, with pinpoint precision, identify patients that need, for instance, A1C screenings, immunizations, mammograms, prostrate screenings, and other proactive or preventive services. EHRs (especially those integrated with CPOE and CDS) have been touted as a key approach to reducing medical errors (Bates et al. 1998; IOM 1999). A number of

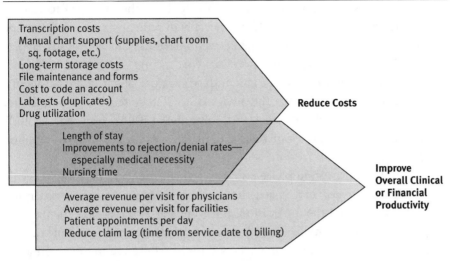

EXHIBIT 9.7
Typical Financial Benefits of EHRs

SOURCE: Smaltz and Berner (2007). Reprinted with permission from Health Administration Press, Chicago.

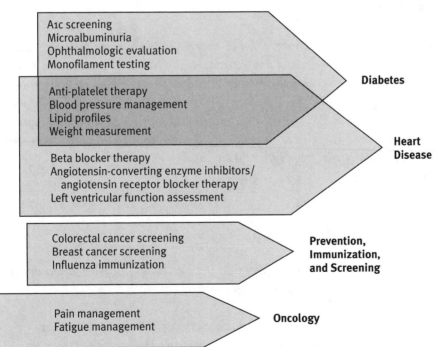

EXHIBIT 9.8
Typical Product Line Benefits of EHRs

SOURCE: Smaltz and Berner (2007). Reprinted with permission from Health Administration Press, Chicago.

research studies have documented that EHRs have the potential to lead to substantial benefits in patient safety, especially in reducing medication errors. Given that the costs of adverse drug events (ADEs) are enormous, avoidance of ADEs can translate into potential cost savings. Evans and colleagues (1998) found significant savings in length of stay, use of anti-infective agents, and total hospital costs when the advice of a CDS system for antibiotic use was followed. Similarly, Kaushal and colleagues (2006) analyzed the ROI on a CPOE system and estimated a cumulative net savings of $16.7 million dollars.

While EHRs can improve efficiency, the efficiencies may not be evenly distributed. An EHR may speed the time between a medication order and the patient receiving the medication, but some parts of that process may take longer than without the EHR. An analysis of multiple studies of time savings with electronic documentation systems showed a decrease in documentation time for nurses, but physician time was more variable; in some cases, the time for electronic documentation meant an increase in physician time at the front end (Poissant et al. 2005), but reduced search time for patient records may compensate for time lost in documentation.

Summary

With federal laws and incentives to meaningfully use an EHR in place for both individual physicians and hospitals, the stage is set for EHR adoption to continue to rise. Both the federal government as well as employer advocacy groups like the Leapfrog Group hope that the meaningful use of an EHR achieves the objectives, originally identified in the IOM report *To Err Is Human,* to prevent unnecessary deaths from healthcare errors, make healthcare demonstrably higher quality, and reduce the overall cost of providing healthcare.

Web Resources

A number of organizations (through their websites) provide more information on the topics discussed in this chapter:

- Centers for Medicare & Medicaid Services (CMS; www.cms.gov /Regulations-and-Guidance/Legislation/EHRIncentivePrograms /index.html?redirect=/EHRIncentivePrograms/). This website provides official guidance on CMS EHR incentive programs.

- Healthcare Information and Management Systems Society (HIMSS; www.himss.org/asp/topics_ehr.asp). HIMSS is the largest HIT professional association, and its website provides overview information on EHRs.
- International Health Terminology Standards Development Organisation (IHTSDO; www.ihtsdo.org/snomed-ct/snomed-ct0). IHTSDO's website presents information on standard medical nomenclature.
- Office of the National Coordinator for Healthcare IT (ONCHIT; www.healthit.gov/providers-professionals/ehr-implementation-steps /step-5-achieve-meaningful-use). ONCHIT's website provides guidance on both EHR implementations as well as incentives for meaningful use of an EHR.

Discussion Questions

1. What are some of the key capabilities of a robust EHR?
2. What is CPOE, and why is it seen as vital to achieving the nation's patient safety and healthcare quality goals?
3. What are some of the benefits of a robust EHR?
4. What are some of the main categories of cost associated with purchasing and implementing an EHR?
5. Why did the federal government in the HITECH Act of 2009 create a meaningful use standard for EHRs?

APPLICATIONS: MANAGEMENT/ ADMINISTRATIVE AND FINANCIAL SYSTEMS

Learning Objectives

1. Describe the components typically included in an enterprise resources planning system.
2. Provide examples of transaction processing applications, and discuss how they support financial management.
3. Discuss desirable features of an automated enterprise scheduling system.
4. Distinguish between clinical decision support software and executive information systems.
5. Understand the use of computer applications as tools for research and medical education.

Overview

For many years, the healthcare field lagged other businesses in the design and implementation of robust information systems. Problems have included undercapitalization of the system development process and management failure to oversee system implementation effectively. However, the situation has changed substantially due to heightened competition, increased regulation, and changing payment mechanisms affecting the entire industry. Changes in the delivery and financing of healthcare since the late 1980s have been pivotal to establishing information management as a key strategic resource in most healthcare organizations. Healthcare managers have come to rely on information systems as essential tools for robust growth, effective competition and, in some cases, survival.

Most healthcare organizations began their automated information processing activities with computer systems that supported administrative operations—in particular, financial and accounting systems. While a significant number of current healthcare applications still serve financial purposes, the drive for robust clinical information systems has become a top priority for most healthcare organizations. Note, however, that clinical information systems not only provide direct support to patient care processes but also populate the data repositories essential for performance measurement, external reporting, cost management, and other organizational accountability activities. Thus, the "ideal" clinical and administrative applications integrate into a comprehensive system that supports the continuum of information needs in an enterprise.

Most early information system applications in healthcare organizations were designed as stand-alone systems, and purchase decisions were based on maximizing desired specific functionality at acceptable costs. In the current environment, however, clinical and administrative applications are expected to integrate, sharing functionality and transferring data across various elements of the enterprise information system as well as exchanging information with systems external to the enterprise. Purchase decision criteria now include interoperability, compliance with data transmission standards, and many other complex factors.

Migrating these stand-alone *legacy* systems into an integrated environment proved to be one of the most difficult challenges that healthcare information technology (HIT) teams encountered in building systems to meet the expanding information needs of healthcare enterprises (Gilchrist et al. 2008; Hicken, Thornton, and Rocha 2004; Kraatz, Lyons, and Thompkinson 2010). In fact, some teams concluded that "starting from scratch" would be easier than retrofitting various systems from multiple vintages. As technologies and system configurations continue to evolve, however, repeated "start-overs" usually are not a realistic option for several reasons. Purchase and implementation costs of full-scale systems can be prohibitive, although purchase price has become almost the least important criterion in system selection. Operations and planning are dependent on data and information stored in existing systems, and migrating data archives may be difficult or even impossible. In light of the extent of technology dependence in healthcare organizations, the disruption in service delivery and business operations during a full-system transition could be tremendous. Thus, managers must select system components with forethought for the capability to transition to next-generation products for better interconnectivity and interoperability in both clinical and administrative applications.

Enterprise resources planning (ERP) systems are bundled applications, or "single vendor solutions" (Raths 2006), that integrate operational information derived from financial, human resources, materials management, and other function-based areas into a robust database used to achieve business management objectives (Legnick-Hall and Legnick-Hall 2006). These systems connect inventory and facilities management, resource scheduling, accounting and financial management, and other business events in a real-time environment. As with clinical systems, the market for ERP applications emerged from the need to update legacy software. However, a large number of vendors continue to develop and market applications that will operate as stand-alones or that can be integrated or interfaced with other applications. The administrative applications typically incorporated in an ERP include the following:

- Financial information systems
- Human resources information systems
- Resource utilization and scheduling systems
- Materials management systems
- Facilities and project management systems
- Office automation systems

Each of these system components is described in this chapter with illustrative examples. Special features of these types of applications designed to meet the needs of nonhospital healthcare organizations, such as physician practices and home health care, are addressed. Additional uses of information systems in healthcare, such as medical research, education, and decision support, are discussed briefly.

Financial Information Systems

The highly competitive and regulated environments in which healthcare organizations operate require timely and accurate financial information that enables managers to monitor and guide operational performance. In the face of answering demands for accountability and cost containment while still providing high-quality services, managers are acutely aware of the importance of sound financial management in guiding operational performance. Financial information systems support operational activities such as general accounting, patient accounting, payroll, contract management, and investment management. Financial systems also provide information to management for controlling and evaluating organizational performance. Analysis of current and historical information helps in projecting future financial needs of the organization.

Financial information systems require input from transaction-processing systems, external sources, and strategic organizational plans (see Exhibit 10.1). Transaction-processing systems record the organization's routine activities, collecting information from other administrative subsystems, including payroll, accounts payable, accounts receivable, general ledger, and inventory control. These transactions are the basis for many financial reports required by management. To support effective financial decisions, financial

EXHIBIT 10.1
Financial
Information
System

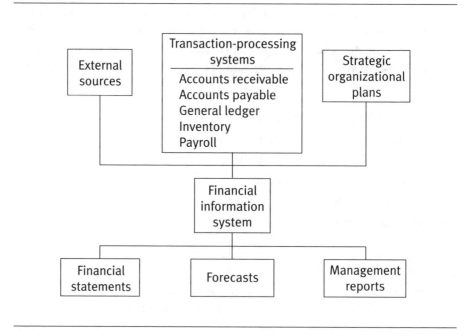

systems also need external data such as government statistics, inflation rates, and information about the marketplace. An organization's strategic plan should contain financial goals and objectives that help provide the framework for preparation of financial reports.

A fully integrated financial information system brings related information together for planning, monitoring, and control. Individual financial subsystems include the following:

- Payroll preparation and accounting, linked to a human resources information system
- Processing of accounts payable, linked to purchasing and inventory control systems
- Patient accounting, patient and third-party billing, and accounts receivable processing
- Cost accounting and cost allocation of non-revenue-generating activities and general overhead expense
- General ledger accounting
- Budgeting and budget control
- Internal auditing
- Financial forecasting
- Investment monitoring and analysis
- Financial statement preparation

- Financial reporting for operating supervisors, executive management, board members, external regulators, and third-party financing agencies

The development of a financial information system depends on the existence of a good accounting system. Sophisticated cost accounting, essential in a negotiated pricing environment, enables the financial information system to generate accurate information on personnel and other physical resources used to deliver services. For services provided under managed care contracts, providers, managed care organizations, and employers need cost information to help negotiate rates and monitor contract performance. Integrated financial reporting based on a solid cost accounting system provides information for product costing, analysis of labor productivity, inventory control, and examination of the productivity return on capital investments.

Significant proportions of total payments for healthcare services provided are based on either a fixed payment per case (e.g., diagnosis-related groups) or a fixed payment per person per month (i.e., capitation payment systems). For effective management in this environment, a financial information system must have the capability to convert or link cost and net revenue information to multiple units of payment.

A market analysis prepared by the Dorenfest Institute for HIT Research and Education (2006) for the HIMSS Foundation reported that ten suppliers dominate in sales of financial applications software, suggesting a highly concentrated market. This concentration is due in part to two high-profile mergers that produced two powerhouses in the HIT industry: McKesson, which acquired HBOC, Inc., and Siemens, which merged with Shared Medical Systems. These two companies hold significant market share in every type of financial application.

Human Resources Information Systems

Employees of a healthcare organization constitute its most important resource. Most organizations spend more than 60 percent of their operating budget on employee salaries and benefits. Thus, a good human resources information system (HRIS) is a very important tool to assist managers in personnel planning, staffing, and productivity analysis. The common functions of an HRIS include, but certainly are not limited to, the following:

- Maintaining, updating, and retrieving information from a database of employee personnel records
- Providing automatic position control linked to the budget
- Producing labor analysis reports for each operating unit or cost center

- Producing reports used for assessing personnel problems, such as turnover and absenteeism
- Maintaining an inventory of special skills and required certifications of employees
- Producing labor cost allocations with linkage to the payroll system
- Providing information on employee productivity and quality control, assuming that appropriate labor standards have been developed
- Managing employee sick leave, vacation, and other earned time off
- Comparing the organization's compensation and benefit packages with industry norms

Large amounts of data are required to provide these types of reports and others that may be needed. The HRIS information processing and reporting functions are supported by information drawn from various databases that contain individual employee data, wage and salary data, the organization's job-classification structure, benefit packages, employment contracts, and many other related data elements. Actual ownership of the various databases may be distributed among multiple departments. Thus, the structure of the databases is an important factor in data transfer from one element of the system to another.

Although essential for efficient business practices, the availability of computerized employee-record files creates a security issue. Because protecting the employee's right to privacy is essential, organizations need to establish software and hardware security systems and set policies for accessing and updating electronic files containing personnel data and information. (See Chapter 5 for discussion on data security policies.)

In addition to supporting operational work in the human resources department, a well-designed HRIS will produce reports for management planning and control (see Exhibit 10.2). For example, HRIS management reports can be used to monitor turnover rates, unfilled positions, labor costs, employee productivity, and utilization of benefits. Attitudes of employees and physicians can be monitored through periodic satisfaction surveys. This survey data used in conjunction with activity and utilization data can be an important component of planning changes to benefits provided to employees.

Software applications are used to maintain records related to verifying physician credentials and defining practice privileges in the organization as well as for ongoing evaluation of physician clinical performance. Credentials and privileging systems are important for monitoring quality standards and for maintaining documentation required by accrediting and regulatory bodies. The task of verifying academic and training credentials and malpractice exposure is frequently outsourced to a certified *credentials verification organization* (CVO), such as Healthplex (www.Healthplexcvo.com) and Professional

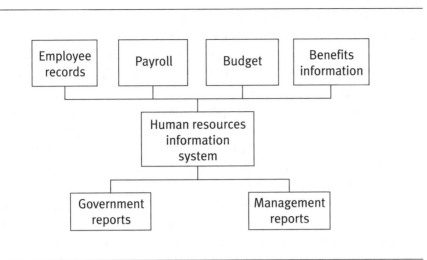

EXHIBIT 10.2
Human
Resources
Information
System

Credentials Verification Service, Inc. (www.pcvs.net). Data transmitted by the CVO must be connected to relevant data from the organization's clinical and administrative systems to develop practice profiles for monitoring physician productivity and conformance to quality standards. Often, there is a need to integrate external benchmark and industry standards for comparison with actual performance data. Because of the sensitive nature of the data in this system and the specificity of facility accreditation requirements for this function, a stand-alone system often is used to achieve the desired functionality and system security. Example applications include MD-Staff (www.mdstaff.com), a cloud-based network that includes background screening, credentialing, and provider management options. In early 2012, MD-Staff reported more than 600 installations.

Resource Utilization and Scheduling Systems

Under fixed-price and capitation payment systems, cost containment and efficient resource utilization are pivotal to success. External mandates for utilization review by regulatory agencies and insurance companies are more than balanced by internal drivers for ensuring that resource utilization is optimized. Managers must ensure that services are available when needed and that personnel and technology are efficiently allocated and scheduled. These efficiency needs are met through computerized monitoring and scheduling systems.

Information systems monitor inpatient occupancy rates, clinic and emergency department activity, and utilization of individual service facilities such as the operating suite or diagnostic units. Patient scheduling systems are used for advance booking and scheduling of facilities—both for patient and physician convenience and for efficient allocation of resources, particularly staffing. Comprehensive and timely data are essential to monitor use of expensive diagnostic and treatment technologies to achieve optimal revenue returns on capital investments.

Advance bed-booking and preadmission systems are particularly useful in situations where most of the admissions are elective (e.g., a specialized surgical facility). Advance booking also provides time for necessary precertification for managed care patients and others covered by insurance plans that require review and certification of medical necessity for procedures and inpatient admission. Preadmission information systems can be linked to individual physicians' offices as well. Computer programs can project the average length of stay for each elective admission once historical data (including diagnosis, surgical procedure, age of patient, and gender of patient) have been accumulated. After admissions are scheduled and the data are entered into the computer's master files, the system keeps track of projected occupancy levels for each day.

Admissions monitoring and scheduling systems improve staffing and workflow in healthcare organizations. These systems can reduce daily fluctuations in a hospital's census and improve the effectiveness of flexible staffing systems. Acute care general hospitals must maintain an accurate accounting of bed census and occupancy if they are to survive. Census information helps administrators compare projected income against projected budgets. Administrators can also track demands for specific services and adjust staffing levels and scheduling of facilities as demand patterns change.

Computer programs are also available for scheduling operating rooms in hospitals and ambulatory surgery centers. These systems are designed to improve operating room utilization, contain costs, facilitate planning, and aid in the scheduling of specific surgical procedures. Outpatient clinic appointment and scheduling systems are common in organizations with a large volume of outpatient activity.

Resource utilization and scheduling systems may be designed for use at the department level or for a small entity such as a physician practice, but enterprisewide scheduling systems that meet multiple objectives are becoming common. These robust integrated systems support fiscal objectives such as balanced schedules, optimum staffing, and management of resources across the enterprise. From a patient perspective, the ability to schedule multiple diagnostic procedures in one session, and perhaps schedule all procedures in a single day, contributes to satisfaction with the encounter experience.

The scheduling system can include modules that capture patient insurance and billing information during the registration process, which can be matched against stored contract data to produce appropriate charge records. Most systems can produce automated appointment reminders in a variety of formats, including computer-generated telephone calls, e-mails, or text messages, in addition to mailed documents.

Scheduling systems can be linked with materials management systems to ensure that equipment and supplies are available for scheduled procedures, including initiating the process to transport the supplies to the treatment area. As items are removed from inventory, ordering and restocking procedures are triggered.

Materials Management Systems

Computer systems are invaluable in effective management of supplies and materials, including data exchange with suppliers, automated purchase orders, inventory control, use of bar-code devices for encoding supplies and materials, and computerized menu planning and food service management.

In a typical materials management system, requisitions for supplies and materials are electronically generated and matched against budgetary authorization for financial control. Reports of overdrafts on supply accounts are transmitted to the appropriate supervisor for follow-up action. Once requisitions are cleared, often using an automated workflow process for sequential authorizations, the system generates purchase orders. Purchase orders can be transmitted electronically to suppliers via established data-exchange protocols. As materials are received, bar-coded products can be scanned and matched against an open order file. Many automated purchasing systems also include direct linkage to the accounts payable system if system integration has been planned. Some systems also provide the capability for automatic reordering of selected items as inventory is depleted (see Exhibit 10.3). Supply chain applications reduce processing costs and obtain materials on a just-in-time basis to minimize the need to carry a large inventory.

Detroit Medical Center divides its materials resource management department into several functional areas: linen services, clinical engineering, contract administration, logistics management, procurement, supplier diversity, and systems development (www.dmc.org/vendor). The department communicates with current and potential business associates via a website, providing information about open requests for proposals, standard contracts and policies, and status on open purchase orders. Some areas of the website are open access, which may generate interest from potential vendors, but areas that store proprietary or contract-related information are protected with a secure login and are accessible only to current business partners.

Coding standards are an important element of automated purchasing and materials management systems. Bar codes for all types of medical supplies and pharmaceuticals have become standard and are essential to efficient purchaser–vendor relationships in healthcare.

EXHIBIT 10.3
Materials
Management
System

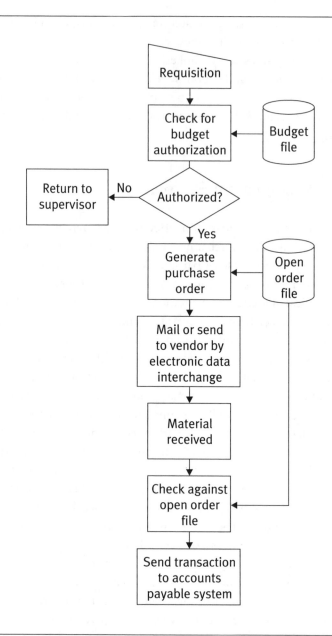

Computerized menu-planning systems store and analyze data on patients' nutritional and dietary requirements, food items in inventory and their costs, and decision rules for selecting from among alternative menus. Decision criteria might include patient preferences or visual appearance of food in addition to nutritional adequacy and cost. (See the sidebar on the next page for an example.)

Healing the Body by Stimulating the Appetite

UAB Hospital in Birmingham, Alabama, has implemented a novel alternative to routine menu plans for inpatients who want more choice in their meal selections. Patients can order "room service" for delivery to their rooms between 6:30 am and 7:00 pm. Meal choices include breakfast foods, soups, salads, hot and cold sandwiches, pizza, meat-based entrees, and desserts. For the adventurous, a seasonal meal planned by a renowned local restaurateur is available.

Patients with dietary restrictions are flagged in the information system to be automatically connected with a dietary representative who will address their meal requests appropriately. Online menus include designations to aid patients in selecting "heart healthy" foods or those allowed on a diabetic diet.

This meal option is supplemented by nutritional education available on the patient education television channel and with telephone access to a registered dietitian.

More information is available at www.uabmedicine.org/patient-and-visitor-guide/patient-information-room-service.

Facilities and Project Management Systems

Computerized systems can help organizations plan, manage, and maintain physical facilities. Examples include preventive maintenance systems, energy management systems, and project scheduling and control systems (particularly useful in new construction and remodeling projects).

Preventive maintenance systems help extend the life of equipment and facilities and reduce costly failures. Routine maintenance can help organizations achieve significant cost savings by preventing repair and replacement costs. Additional benefits accrue, including preventing nonproductive downtime, improving the safety of the workplace, and decreasing the risk of patient or employee injury due to equipment malfunction. Exhibit 10.3 shows the framework for a materials management system.

Energy conservation is an important cost-saving strategy for healthcare organizations as it is in all major industries. Computer applications assist in monitoring routine and peak energy use, providing information to tactics for reducing consumption. Actual utilization figures can be compared against calculated requirements, and a computer model can be developed to find economies and efficiencies. The energy management system also can be employed to implement the selected tactics, such as automatically lowering or raising room temperatures in areas that are unused at night or on the weekend.

Healthcare organizations frequently are involved in capital construction and major remodeling projects, and computer systems are an extremely useful aid in project management. These project scheduling and control systems typically employ a combination of integrated tools to manage personnel and activity scheduling, labor and materials costs, required resources, and periodic progress reporting. As a key component, these tools are used to document (1) all activities required to complete the project; (2) the relationships of these activities to one another, including those that can be carried out simultaneously and those that must follow a time sequence; and (3) time estimates for completing each activity. These data are used to generate a diagram of activities that shows the critical path (longest time required) for project completion and any opportunities for concurrent or fast-tracked activities. As activities are completed, actual completion times can be entered back into the calculation, and more accurate schedules can be prepared for the remaining work. These systems are excellent tools for dynamic scheduling and control of major projects. More detailed coverage of project management related to HIT is provided in Chapter 11.

Office Automation Systems

Office automation helps to coordinate and manage people and workflow, link organizational units and projects, and coordinate work in the organization across levels and functions. Healthcare organizations use a variety of computing tools to carry out general office functions, such as word processing, e-mail, project management, meeting scheduling, and maintenance of personnel calendars for work-related activities. These functions may be conducted using desktop workstations; laptop computers; or a variety of handheld devices, including personal mobile telephones or smart phones. Use of systems for integrated word and graphic processing, scheduling, electronic filing of documents, and message/document transmission can dramatically improve administrative efficiency and reduce the costs of office operations.

Office systems can link parts of the organization together by scheduling meetings using electronic calendars and e-mail or text communication. E-mail systems link offices and individuals, allowing electronic files to be forwarded to others or to be archived in a shared storage area for access by members of a workgroup. Mobile computing using laptops and handheld devices, wireless technology, and the Internet have changed the way people work alone or together. Workgroups and teams can meet and collaborate from anywhere—in the same conference room or in geographically separated offices—with full access to necessary software programs and organizational files.

This work environment is supported by *groupware*—collaborative software that enables sharing of information via an interactive network (e.g., a virtual workspace). This software–hardware combination not only facilitates real-time interaction among members of the group to improve problem solving and project management but also supports independent work tasks.

Audio- and videoconferencing allow real-time interaction among team members. Group members may work asynchronously on project activities while maintaining the integrity of a shared work product. When used effectively, and provided employees are trained to use the electronic tools, the virtual office can be as productive as the traditional office. Typical groupware activities include the following:

- E-mail and discussion forums
- Teleconferencing
- Interactive videoconferencing
- Relational databases (used to search for data and information)
- Document editing and management, including archiving and version tracking
- Group calendars and scheduling

SharePoint, a Microsoft product, is an example of groupware. A description of SharePoint functionality is available at www.sharepoint/microsoft.com. SharePoint can be deployed as an on-premises system or in a hybrid environment that employs cloud computing (Robinson 2011).

Information Systems for Nonhospital Healthcare Organizations

As changes to payment models in the 1980s led to changes in delivery models during the 1990s, nonhospital healthcare organizations began implementing information systems to manage clinical services and business operations. Vendors quickly began designing and marketing software products to meet the special information needs of these organizations. Organization types that fall under the nonhospital category include ambulatory clinics; long-term care (LTC) facilities; home health agencies; physician practices; and many others, including retail clinics. Software applications used in these settings typically include multiple modules that meet the organizations' needs for clinical documentation, operations management, and financial management.

Ambulatory Care Information Systems

Significant components of the healthcare continuum are delivered in outpatient and ambulatory care settings. Information systems that support ambulatory care and assist primary care providers in their practices have become a niche market. The availability of powerful and inexpensive microcomputers and practice management software packages has brought this technology within the reach of even small medical groups and solo practitioners.

A typical practice management system (Slovensky et al. 2006) includes modules to support such business functions as the following:

- Operations management (e.g., scheduling, reminders, billing, authorizations)
- Services (e-mail, groupware)
- Claims processing
- Document processing, spreadsheets, and databases
- Transcription
- Personnel management
- Inventory management
- Waste management
- Energy management

Clinical applications in medical practices and freestanding clinics include electronic health records (EHRs), prescription management, and disease management resources. Patient applications—an emerging software market—include electronic communication, monitoring, educational resources, and telehealth applications. Various vendor products offer full-service suites or selected modules based on the practice's needs.

Automating practice functions increases operational efficiency and reduces errors in information processing, both of which contribute to patient satisfaction and reduced risk and liability exposure. Automating or using web-based patient communication for services—such as callbacks, prescription renewals, and similar activities—can be helpful as well.

Office practice computers can be linked to local hospitals in addition to serving the management needs of the practice. Many hospitals or integrated delivery systems have developed computer linkages with physician offices to enable clinicians to pre-admit patients; order diagnostic tests; and query the patient information system for lab results, progress notes, and other current clinical information. Healthcare organizations use such linkages as incentives to attract physicians to use their facilities in a highly competitive environment. Under some conditions, hospitals may be able to offer financial support to physician practices for the purpose of implementing an EHR that links with the hospital system (Babitch 2009).

An alternative to linking with a hospital system is for two or more clinics or health centers to partner and purchase a shared system. This approach may be an excellent option for a multisite group practice or for affiliated professional groups. One example of this approach is provided by the Metropolitan Collaborative of Health Information Technology (METCHIT), a health center network of four organizations in New York City (Egleson et al. 2010). This initiative was clinician-led, which contributed to the successful deployment of the system components across the network. An important factor in the success of this EHR application was the ability to modify system templates to accommodate mandatory reporting requirements.

Long-Term Care Information Systems

The LTC industry has been a late adopter in implementing computer systems, in part because software vendors have been slow to develop products tailored to the needs of nursing homes and continuing care communities. This situation is changing as the scope and volume of healthcare delivered in subacute-care and postacute-care facilities increase. Typical requirements for LTC systems include census management, initial and periodic resident assessments, documentation of care services provided, documentation of physician orders, nutritional assessments and menu planning in the dietary department, and pharmacy applications.

The ability to communicate clinical information between caregivers and the admitting physician is especially important, as the physician usually is not physically present on a daily basis. Remote access to clinical documentation facilitates timely intervention in an acute episode and contributes to better health outcomes. As with other HIT applications, remote access can be achieved using various computing devices or telephone systems. System security and controlled system access are extremely important.

As LTC facilities become components of larger integrated delivery systems, electronic sharing of clinical and administrative information with hospitals, clinics, ambulatory care facilities, and other system components becomes a business essential. Once again, data sharing among the enterprise units and IT strategic partners is a key driver in system design. However, insufficiency of data standards and security concerns remain as significant barriers to achieving the desired level of connectivity, along with issues related to proprietary systems (Edwards et al. 2010).

Home Health Care Information Systems

Home health care services have expanded rapidly in recent years as an alternative to more costly institutional care. As service volume has increased and the scope of services expanded, information systems have been developed specifically to meet the needs of home care provider organizations.

Many home health agencies use laptop computers and other remote access devices for on-site documentation of patient care and for access to treatment plans and previous encounter documentation. Home health nurses and other caregivers enter information directly at the treatment sites for uploading to the centralized data repository. Relevant data can be accessed during a service visit by any provider. These systems reduce the amount of administrative work needed to document care, allowing nurses and home health aides to spend more time providing patients the care and services they need to achieve desired clinical outcomes.

Electronic devices also can transmit clinical information via telephone lines or the Internet for the purpose of routine health monitoring between visits. Patients and family members follow the documented treatment plan, take and record measurements as indicated, and submit data for evaluation by the clinical personnel overseeing their care.

Other Information System Applications in Healthcare

Information systems support most processes in healthcare. While many applications can be categorized by their use for a defined function, many serve the needs of multiple providers and managers in disparate service areas. Clinical information may be combined with administrative information or used for an administrative purpose exclusively. Alternatively, administrative information may be applied in the delivery of clinical care.

Clinical Decision-Support Systems

Clinical decision-support (CDS) systems are designed to assist physicians and other providers in diagnosis and treatment planning. CDS systems fall into two categories: (1) passive CDS systems and (2) active CDS systems.

Passive CDS systems use the computer to collect, organize, and communicate clinical data for interpretation and analysis by the physician. They make clinical information, including medical history, physical examinations, and diagnostic tests, more readily available and usable but do not process the information for further analysis. Clinical information systems—such as laboratory, pharmacy, radiology, and other clinical services applications—are examples of passive CDS systems in that they capture clinical data and make them available to caregivers. These applications become more useful to clinicians for decision support when they are fully integrated and can provide complete medical information (both current data and historical information on the patient) through simple, user-friendly access. For example, caregivers could view temperature, heart rate, and blood pressure readings over time to see patterns in relation to medication administration, physical activity, or food ingestion.

Active CDS systems provide direct assistance to the physician in diagnosis and treatment planning. They combine patient-specific data with generalized medical knowledge to reach a conclusion or make a recommendation to the caregiver. These systems may use a branching logic or rule-based structure, or a statistical probability algorithm, to suggest an appropriate diagnostic or treatment response to a clinical condition described by the physician.

These systems incorporate validated clinical guidelines and treatment protocols that represent current best practices in clinical medicine. The National Guideline Clearinghouse (www.guideline.gov) is an excellent resource to learn more about this type of resource available to clinicians.

Types of active CDS systems are as follows:

1. *Expert systems* contain three major components—knowledge base, patient-specific information, and inference engine. A general knowledge base of medical information, obtained from a panel of experts in a given medical specialty, has been rigorously validated through scholarly research, clinical practice, and consensus support from the medical community. This knowledge base is matched against patient-specific information retrieved from the healthcare organization's clinical database and may include subjective information as well as objective clinical findings. A rule-based inference engine generates conclusions for consideration by the physician. The system is dependent on the quality of the expert knowledge base and the "reasoning power" of the rules used by the inference engine.

2. *Probabilistic algorithms* employ statistical probabilities, which include a calculated element of randomness, rather than rely solely on knowledge collected from expert human beings. Expert knowledge is based on a combination of academic preparation and experiential learning, and variation may occur in either component of an expert's knowledge base. Extrapolations outside an expert's existing knowledge contribute to experiential learning. While a consensus viewpoint among experts incorporates nonquantifiable variability, a statistical probability allows the decision maker to control the degree of uncertainty tolerated in the system's output.

3. *Clinical reminders and alerts,* incorporated into clinical computer applications, suggest potential medical conditions or other problems that should be given attention in setting treatment plans. Examples include pharmacy information systems that alert the physician to potentially negative interactions between two drugs prescribed for the same patient as well as systems that suggest certain drugs or treatments should not be employed when specific laboratory results contraindicate their use. This function can also be used to suggest less expensive (but equally effective) alternatives when a high-cost drug has been ordered. Alternative drugs may also be suggested when the prescribed drug has significant risks for certain types of patients.

Computers can aid decision making by simplifying access to data needed to make decisions, providing reminders and prompts, assisting in order entry, assisting in diagnosis, and reviewing new clinical data to issue alerts when important patterns are recognized. Systems are more likely to be successful when they give patient-specific suggestions, save time, and are incorporated into the regular workflow of the organization. Researchers at the University of Alabama at Birmingham found that physicians using a decision-support rule accessed via a handheld device (e.g., personal digital assistant [PDA]) made better prescribing decisions than those who did not have the PDA for CDS access (Berner et al. 2006). The study, a randomized controlled trial, examined ordering practices for nonsteroidal anti-inflammatory drugs (NSAIDs). Physicians accessing the rule were more likely to order NSAIDs that were considered "safer" when considering gastrointestinal risk factors.

CDS systems that are well integrated with the enterprise EHR offer great promise for personalized medicine (Downing et al. 2009). Responding to variability among individual patients and applying the ever-increasing body of medical knowledge require information processing on a scale that cannot be achieved by human means. Well-designed systems can process large volumes of knowledge-based data filtered by personal clinical data and even by personal preferences for options among treatment modalities. Patients can be evaluated for risk factors for specific conditions, be advised about prevention and early detection strategies, and be assessed for probable effectiveness of various treatment options should the condition occur.

Executive Information Systems

The business corollary to CDS systems is the executive information system (EIS). Sometimes referred to collectively as *business intelligence*, EIS includes systems designed to access and merge internal and external data into meaningful information reports. Executives identify critical environmental trends and facility performance indicators related to strategic objectives to guide their information capture and analysis. Data to support the EIS may be extracted from clinical and administrative databases serving the healthcare enterprise as well as from public and proprietary data repositories. The information needed from an EIS for decision support generally is not met through standard reports. Users must be able to select the variables and data sources needed to answer specific questions, so ad hoc reporting capability is essential. In many analysis scenarios, it is important to begin with general data aggregations and then reduce subsets of the data to increasingly greater detail, a process referred to as *drilling down*. The EIS must support this type of processing through an easily managed user interface.

Evidence-Based Medicine and Disease-Management Systems

Evidence-based clinical practice guidelines, also referred to in application as *evidence-based medicine* (EBM), are intended to assist clinicians and healthcare organizations in standardizing decisions about the care of individual patients to achieve cost and quality benefits. Accumulated evidence from clinical research is used to formulate statements of the "right" things to do for patients with a given diagnosis or condition. Ideally, guidelines ensure that patients receive appropriate diagnostic tests and treatments in an efficient and cost-effective manner. Guidelines are assumed to lower treatment costs by avoiding unnecessary tests. Hundreds of guidelines have been developed and are archived in the National Guideline Clearinghouse sponsored by the Agency for Healthcare Research and Quality (www.ahrq.gov). Although managed care organizations and health insurers employ such guidelines to make decisions about treatment options, covered services, and other aspects of patient care, practice guidelines are not without significant limitations. Among these limitations are differences in local standards of care, access to recommended technologies, and unique patient characteristics.

While linkages to EBM resources are commonly incorporated in clinical systems for large inpatient facilities or integrated healthcare delivery systems, small clinics or medical practices may rely on independent access to EBM resources via the Internet. In these types of primary care settings, the clinician typically is using some component of the office automation system—desktop computer, laptop, or handheld mobile device—for Internet access. In this type of environment, convenience is an important factor in determining whether the clinician will seek external information. Recent research has shown that primary care providers who report using HIT resources as part of their patient encounter routines are likely to conform to evidence-based standards of care (Davis and Pavur 2011). An important caveat to this finding, however, is that providers who used PDAs as their primary computing device did not have the same level of compliance with these standards. As noted in Chapter 6, the size of the display screen relative to the output being displayed is an important system design characteristic. The small screens on handheld devices and the difficulty of entering precise input data using an ultra-compact keyboard make PDAs a poor choice for this purpose.

Disease management information systems and software products are designed to assist healthcare organizations in designing processes to provide quality care at the most reasonable cost possible. For the most part, they are disease specific and focus on high-volume, high-cost chronic conditions such as asthma, diabetes, and congestive heart failure. The typical approach is to involve patients in self-management of their condition and to create monitoring and feedback processes that encourage compliance with treatment plans. The information system may include capturing blood or urine test data, blood pressure readings, and other clinical information in the patient's home and transmitting it to the healthcare organization via digital telephony or other remote monitoring devices. Communication between patients and providers may be via telephone or the Internet. While routine patient monitoring assists in daily decision making, analyzing aggregated data can guide case managers and physicians in modifying treatment plans for better long-term clinical outcomes.

Computer-Assisted Medical Instrumentation

Virtually every piece of medical equipment used for diagnostic testing and treatment now contains a microprocessor. The processors are used for instrument control, image enhancement, or processing medical data and interpreting the results of the testing or treatment process. Common examples include electrocardiograms, electroencephalograms, and pulmonary function testing. Computer systems interface directly with patient-monitoring devices for continuous surveillance of a patient's vital signs and periodic display of physiological data. These systems are particularly useful in critical care and postsurgical units.

The first step in the process is acquiring data from monitoring equipment attached to the patient and then converting that data for computer processing and display. Data are stored and made available for periodic display or display on demand. Computer programs enhance the measured data through structured analysis of clinical data in accordance with programmed decision rules. Trend data are followed to monitor changes in patient vital signs over time. Patient-monitoring systems can operate at the individual patient bedside, at a central station designed to monitor a small number of intensive care beds, or at a remote location linked back to the critical care unit by telecommunication equipment. For example, output from cardiac monitors may be monitored remotely by trained monitoring personnel, who in turn alert caregivers about aberrant readings. Many of these systems also have electronic linkages for transmission of clinical data to the central EHR.

Coupling automated patient identification with electronic biomedical devices can produce significant efficiency gains in many routine tasks. UAB Hospital in Birmingham, Alabama, for example, uses a bar-code scanner to read codes on the patient's electronic monitor and armband, and then the device transmits recorded vital signs to the EHR. This approach has resulted in a 92 percent efficiency gain in recording vital signs and has decreased the number of errors in documentation significantly (Hicks 2009).

Telemedicine

Telemedicine—now sometimes referred to as telehealth or e-health systems—is the application of computer and communications technologies to support healthcare provided to patients at locations remote from the provider. Telemedicine often involves telephone and online communication between a primary care physician, nurse practitioner, or physician's assistant who is treating patients in a rural area and specialty physicians located at a distant medical center. Audio communications and videoconferencing equipment are used in conjunction with computer access to patient records to establish primary diagnoses or provide expert consultation and second opinions. The systems often employ teleradiology for transmission of medical images for review by specialty physicians. Telemedicine systems can save patients travel time and costs as well as deliver healthcare cost savings.

The University of Texas Medical Branch's Electronic Health Network, self-described as "the largest telemedicine system in the world" (UTMB 2007), provides medical services to indigent populations and correctional facilities across Texas, in addition to corporate and school programs. One of UTMB's more interesting programs is providing telemedicine services to the National Science Foundation researchers in Antarctica.

Telemedicine applications have increased in recent years, due in part to the advent of mobile computing, which has enabled the deployment of *mHealth*—health-focused applications accessible to the general public. These user-friendly and low-cost applications allow patients to monitor and report health indicators such as blood pressure or blood glucose easily and conveniently. However, for traditional telemedicine applications such as specialist consultation or remote diagnostic procedures, issues remain related to reimbursement for remote services, state licensure of health professionals when the system crosses state borders, patient privacy protection, and government regulations (Thompson 2006). Clinical outcome benefits achieved through various telemedicine applications differ, as do cost savings.

The types of articles published in the *Journal of Telemedicine and Telecare* over the past few years suggest that the number and variety of telemedicine applications continue to increase as technology innovations offer more opportunities. Research on patient satisfaction with telemedicine applications appears to be declining. As computer technology pervades business and social environments, individuals may be more accepting of telemedicine and mHealth applications. Although age is sometimes identified as a barrier to technology acceptance, one nine-month study shows that frail elderly subjects are able to use a web-portal telehealth service to reduce their use of facility-based healthcare (Finkelstein et al. 2011). Subjects needed minimal training to use the web portal, and their self-ratings showed improvement in technology acceptance over the course of the study.

Research involving a US Department of Veterans Affairs cohort showed that patients rated service access and educational components of telehealth programs positively, but they reported frustration with equipment problems and slow responses to requests for assistance (Young et al. 2011). Incorporating routine monitoring of these elements of a telehealth service is pivotal to the long-term success of the service.

The ability to meet data-sharing requirements for telemedicine encounters are emerging as key factors in the sustainability of these e-health systems (Ganguly et al. 2009). Telemedicine providers need access not only to clinical data, such as that extracted from an EHR, but also to research findings and other knowledge-based information. Thus, the data-exchange protocol must address both standard format data and free-text formats.

Computer Applications in Medical Research and Education

Information systems and medical databases are used extensively to support biomedical education and research. Computerized patient records serve as the basis for epidemiological studies of a variety of diseases and their potential linkages to social and environmental factors. In addition, computers are used to support medical, dental, nursing, and allied health education, using such techniques as computer-aided instruction and patient-management simulation.

Computers are an integral component of most medical research projects. Effective project design requires close collaboration among clinicians, biostatisticians, and information systems specialists. Some research projects would not be possible without the high-speed computational capabilities and data-storage capacity of large computer systems. An excellent example is the Human Genome Project, which mapped all the genes of the *Homo sapiens* species. One element of the map detailed all sequences of DNA chemical bases—an astounding three billion pairs. Analytical work of this magnitude is inconceivable without supercomputing capabilities.

Hospitals, medical libraries, and individual clinicians use personal computers to access references to the medical literature and full-text online documents. The most widely used bibliographic databases are available through the National Library of Medicine (www.nlm.nih.gov). Articles from thousands of biomedical journals are indexed, stored in computer files, and available for searching and retrieval using standard medical subject headings and keyword searches. The Internet is used extensively to retrieve clinical information from a wide variety of specialty databases and sponsored websites.

Computers are an important tool for the education of clinicians. Computer-based education for physicians and other health professionals engages the students actively in the learning process and builds foundational skills in preparation for clinical training. Learning activities range from presentation of information to students via the Internet or course management systems to sophisticated simulations of clinical problems. Students are presented initial cues and additional information on request as they proceed through a diagnostic process. Final diagnosis, patient management, and follow-up plans selected by the students are entered, and the system responds with a comparison to the "ideal" solution and critiques the process followed.

Increasingly, computerized mannequins are used to teach clinical skills in a laboratory environment before health professions students are assigned to healthcare organizations for clinical practice. These mannequins also can be used in continuing medical education as a tool for testing new technologies or exploring procedure innovations.

Summary

Most healthcare organizations began using electronic data processing by developing or purchasing financial information systems. Financial applications remain essential, but from a broader perspective, healthcare organizations use computers and information systems to support not only financial activities but also all administrative operations, including human resources management, resource utilization and scheduling, materials management, facilities and project management, and office automation.

As healthcare is delivered more frequently in outpatient and nonhospital settings, development of information systems specific to these delivery sites has accelerated. Typical functions for ambulatory settings include patient scheduling and appointments, electronic medical records and medical management, patient and third-party billing, managed care contract management, and electronic communication with other providers in a network of care. LTC systems support census management, residential care documentation, pharmacy, and other areas of operation in skilled nursing facilities. Home health providers use laptop computers or other remote-access devices to document care at the location where it is provided and to access clinical data from previous encounters.

Applications developed to assist physicians and other providers in the delivery of high-quality care include CDS systems and evidence-based medicine programs. These tools aid in diagnosis and treatment planning and comparing treatment plans with established "best practices" using large databases.

Computers have become an integral component of medical equipment for instrument control, image enhancement, and medical data processing. These foundation applications evolved into sophisticated integration of computer and communications technology in telemedicine applications that support patient care at remote locations.

Information systems are used extensively to support biomedical education and research. Automated databases of patient records support epidemiological studies of disease linkage to social and environmental factors. Computer-assisted instruction and patient-management simulation programs support the education of physicians and other health professionals.

Simply stated, no aspect of healthcare delivery or health services management is untouched by computers and information systems. The computer, in its various forms, has become a ubiquitous tool used by clinicians and managers alike. Technological evolution has brought forth powerful machines whose functional capabilities are optimized through the judicious selection of application software to meet business and care delivery needs.

Web Resources

A number of organizations (through their websites) provide more information on the topics discussed in this chapter:

- *Healthcare Informatics* (www.healthcare-informatics.com) is a magazine that provides information about vendors of information technology products and information systems management services.
- Health Level Seven (HL7) (www.hl7.org) is a leading healthcare standard-developing organization. HL7 is working as a coordinating agent for various active standard-setting groups.
- KLAS Enterprises (www.healthcomputing.com/VendorDirectory) offers information about vendors of software, services, and medical equipment.

Discussion Questions

1. Why are administrative systems more evolved than clinical systems?
2. Why do features of handheld devices make them inappropriate for some medical computing applications?
3. What are the key components of groupware as a resource to the management team?
4. What aspects of clinical applications support quality-management and cost-control programs?
5. Describe various functionalities of a pharmacy information system that can aid in reducing medication errors.
6. Distinguish between the logic used in an expert CDS system and systems that employ probabilistic algorithms.
7. What are some ways that HIT contributes to patient satisfaction?
8. Why has HIT development in some segments of the healthcare industry, such as long-term care, lagged other segments?

9. What challenges do legacy systems pose for enterprise system integration?

10. How are transaction-processing systems employed in financial information systems?

11. What are the key functions of a human resources information system?

12. How can centralized scheduling systems contribute to the financial bottom line?

13. List some of the key drivers and some of the challenges of employing telemedicine applications in a healthcare organization.

14. What are the typical elements of a physician practice management system?

15. Describe the basic documentation requirements for an LTC information system. How do these requirements differ from those for the information system used in an inpatient facility?

STRATEGIC COMPETITIVE ADVANTAGE

HIT PROJECT PORTFOLIO MANAGEMENT

Overview

Healthcare in the United States now consumes more than 17 percent of the country's gross domestic product, yet US residents generally do not live longer nor are they healthier than those in other developed nations that spend less than half that amount on healthcare (Goldman and McGlynn 2005). The reality of these statistics, along with the Institute of Medicine's 1999 report (*To Err Is Human*) on preventable deaths in the United States, has energized the federal and state governments in ways that will continue to put pressure on healthcare organizations. For example, plans for reduced reimbursement rates will put a crimp on the increasing bottom-line pressures to ensure that any investments in capital gain the envisioned returns. Clearly, just by their sheer size—seven-, eight-, or even nine-figure expenditures—electronic health record (EHR) projects (depending on the size of the organization) should automatically create a heightened need for due diligence among healthcare executives; nothing can get an executive fired faster than spending $50 million with nothing to show for that investment.

In their presentation, titled "IT Disasters: The Worst IT Debacles and the Lessons Learned from Them" at the American College of Healthcare Executives Congress on Healthcare Leadership, Hunter and Ciotti (2006) provided ample evidence that risks are associated with large-scale healthcare information technology (HIT) projects. While inadequate planning and foresight are problematic in such projects, the single greatest cause of project failure is poor execution (Bossidy and Charan 2002; Hunter and Ciotti 2006). Furthermore, some studies have suggested that HIT systems may cause, rather than reduce, medical errors (Ash et al. 2007; Han et al. 2005; Koppel et al. 2005). However, a careful reading of the original academic articles shows the obvious system design and implementation problems indicating that medical errors are caused by human error and not the HIT itself.

Exhibit 11.1 depicts the results of a Standish Group study and an American Medical Informatics Association literature review. In the Standish Group (2010) study, only 35 percent of HIT projects reviewed achieved anticipated benefits. Organizations that fall into the category of the 65 percent who failed to achieve benefits often rely on the collective experience of the individuals who have previously implemented HIT at the organization but typically do not employ disciplined project management methodologies, such as those suggested by the Project Management Institute (www.pmi.org; discussed in more detail later in this chapter). Furthermore, in their review of the literature, Kaplan and Harris-Salamone (2009) found that only about 40 percent of HIT projects met their goals.

Healthcare delivery is a complex business with incredibly multifaceted, interdependent workflows, yet the field as a whole has been inexplicably slow to adopt professional project management approaches. Organizations that fall into this category typically implement a "go live" only to find that large

EXHIBIT 11.1
IT Project
Success Rates

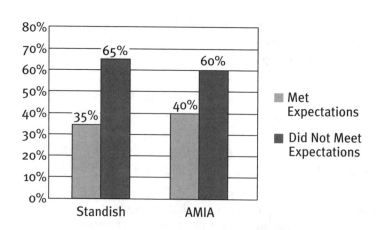

SOURCE: Information from Kaplan and Harris-Salamone (2009) and Standish Group (2011).

stakeholder groups or key workflows have been overlooked. These organizations must then scramble, after implementation, to reengineer processes that easily could have been proactively addressed had the organization followed disciplined project management methodologies.

This chapter provides an overview of HIT project management and encourages healthcare organizations to improve their project success rate by establishing an HIT project portfolio management office.

What Is an HIT Project Portfolio Management Office?

The following terms and their definitions are used in this chapter to clarify concepts related to portfolio management:

- A *project* is a temporary effort to create a unique product, service, or result (PMI 2008).
- *Project management* is the planning, organizing, directing, and controlling of company resources for a relatively short-term objective that has been established to complete specific goals and objectives (Kerzner 2003).
- A *program* is a group of related, often interdependent projects.
- A *portfolio* is a collection of programs and projects.
- *Portfolio management* encompasses managing the collections of programs and projects in a portfolio. This includes weighing the value of each project, or potential project, against desired organizational strategic business and clinical objectives. It also encompasses monitoring active projects to ensure adherence to specified objectives and desired outcomes, balancing the portfolio with other investments of the organization, using resources efficiently, and balancing return on investment with risk (Kaplan 2005).
- A *portfolio management office* (PMO) is a centralized organization dedicated to improving the practice and outcomes of projects via holistic management of all projects.

While definitions can help distinguish concepts, often the terms *project management office, program management office, portfolio management office,* and *project portfolio management office* are used interchangeably in the business press. All imply the professional management and oversight of an organization's entire collection of current projects. PMO, however, specifically refers to the activity of providing investment decision support capabilities to an organization's overall HIT governance structure and processes. The term *project management office* or *program management office* does not necessarily mean that decision support capabilities for these investments are in place. Organizations that use the term *PMO* or *project portfolio management office* are intentionally and accurately referring to a more expansive concept, reflecting the methodology's HIT portfolio investment decision support capabilities (Jeffery and Leliveld 2004). To be consistent, we use the term PMO throughout this chapter. Exhibit 11.2 illustrates how projects, and programs of projects, might interrelate within a typical HIT portfolio.

Individual projects, such as a new inpatient EHR or a new pharmacy system, are grouped into a clinical applications program. Ideally, clinical application projects are led or championed by an influential stakeholder from within the clinical leadership of an organization. Likewise, upgrades of an existing financial budgeting system and implementation of a new human resource system are grouped into a business applications program. Business application projects are ideally led or championed by an influential business stakeholder. Purely infrastructure–type projects, such as a network upgrade or implementation of wireless technology, are grouped into a HIT infrastructure program championed or led by the chief information officer (CIO) or one of the CIO's key directors. All of the projects in all program groupings then make up the entire HIT portfolio that can be professionally managed via formal HIT portfolio management structures and practices—an HIT PMO.

Why Is a PMO Essential?

As indicated earlier in this chapter, some studies have found that 65 percent of HIT projects fail to achieve anticipated benefits (Kaplan and Harris-

EXHIBIT 11.2
HIT Portfolio

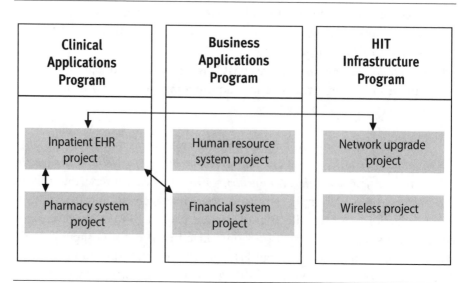

Salamone 2009; Standish Group 2011). One of the primary causes of failed HIT projects is a "silo" project management mentality, which occurs when projects are initiated, planned, and fully executed without an effective consideration of their impact on other, preexisting systems or other parallel projects being planned and executed. As indicated in Exhibit 11.2, contemporary healthcare applications have significant interdependencies that, if not explicitly and deliberately addressed, can have unintended consequences. Exhibit 11.3 provides real-world examples of unintended consequences of HIT projects that were planned and executed in relative isolation.

IT Project	Project Outcome
New Pharmacy System: The pharmacy director sponsored a new best-of-breed pharmacy system project	The pharmacy system project was expertly managed and implemented on time and within budget. Unfortunately, only after the system was implemented did the pharmacist realize that this new proprietary best-of-breed system could not be reliably interfaced with the hospital's preexisting EHR system, which had built-in computerized physician order entry capability. As such, when a provider entered an order for a pharmaceutical into the EHR, that order had to be printed out in the pharmacy and then reentered into the new pharmacy system. From a pure project management standpoint, the project was successful. From an enterprise portfolio standpoint, however, a very inefficient, labor-intensive workflow was created to overcome the lack of integration that this silo-based project management approach created.
Voice Over Internet Protocol (VOIP) Project: A telecommunications director sponsored a switch to digital phone service	The telecommunications director of a large metropolitan hospital system wanted to save millions of dollars annually by switching from a basic traditional phone service model to a VOIP model, whereby the hospital system's existing computer network would be used to provide digital phone service. Unfortunately, the project did not consider the robustness of the existing computer network, which had single points of failure in many of its buildings. The digital phone service was implemented, and soon thereafter, any network outage to one of the buildings affected all phone service for the building. More than an inconvenience, these outages eroded consumer trust and market appeal. Using contingency funds, the hospital system scrambled to re-architect its computer network to provide the level of redundancy and reliability needed to ensure digital phone service. Had a portfolio management approach been taken for this project, computer network inadequacies could have been identified up front and computer network upgrades could have been built into the project plan.

EXHIBIT 11.3
Examples of HIT Projects That Did Not Follow an HIT Portfolio Management Approach

While the examples described in Exhibit 11.3 may seem to be obvious, common-sense mistakes, they are not uncommon because in reality healthcare delivery organizations have thousands of cross-departmental interrelated workflows that must be considered when embarking on a new HIT project. Exhibit 11.4 depicts sample high-level application interfaces that are in place at a typical academic medical center that is representative of any medium to large integrated delivery system. This graphic conveys an incredibly complex web that relies heavily on interfacing applications wherever possible. The sheer volume of interdependencies shown in this exhibit clearly makes a case that individual projects or programs of applications should not be managed in silos but rather in a professional PMO focused on successfully achieving envisioned benefits of particular projects.

In many ways, allowing informal, silo-based project management to occur in a healthcare organization is somewhat like attempting to minimize collisions at an airport without the benefit of a flight control tower. Not incidentally, Exhibit 11.4 resembles a typical major airline hub city with flights coming and going from all points on the compass; yet it depicts a real organization's current applications and how each is interfaced and interrelated. This level of interrelatedness strongly suggests the need for a professional control tower to manage HIT projects. In fact, Gartner Research suggests that "three

EXHIBIT 11.4

Example of Typical Hospital Application Interfaces

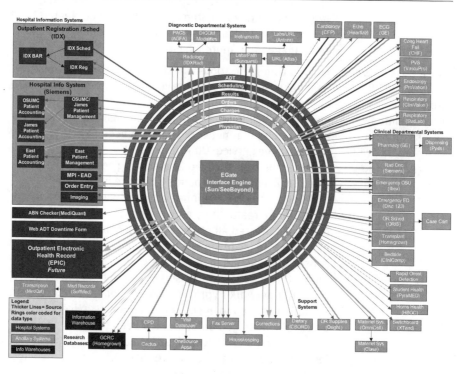

out of four successful $500,000-plus projects will be planned and tracked with project office support, while three out of four failed projects will not" (Light et al. 2005). An organization's ability to successfully and efficiently implement large HIT projects increases as its project management maturity moves from no professionally managed projects to simple project management to program management and ultimately to portfolio management.

Typically, as an organization's HIT project management matures, its overall cost of HIT projects decreases significantly and the success rate of these projects increases substantially. A nonintuitive overall time savings occurs as well, although one would suspect that it would take more time to accomplish the additional work of identifying and tracking interdependencies with other projects across the portfolio of projects. However, Kendall and Rollins (2003) suggest that this additional planning time, which is marginal, actually reduces the number of surprises and "gotchas" that occur later when unforeseen interdependencies invariably crop up in projects that are run in a more informal, silo approach, thus decreasing overall project time. One of the main causes of time delays in projects is *scope creep*—when the original agreed-on requirements for a system are continually expanded by the project sponsors. With project management methodologies in place, added or new requirements are collected and saved for a future version of the system so that the original system scope can be implemented within the established time frames.

The next section addresses project management methodologies. Thereafter, managing the collection of projects is discussed, and the suggestion is reiterated that a PMO is a logical organizational response to the increasing HIT complexity in healthcare organizations.

Project Management

Project management entails the following five processes (PMI 2008):

1. *Project initiation:* launch of a process that can result in the authorization of a new project
2. *Project planning:* definition of the objectives, scope, and plan of action to achieve the desired outcomes
3. *Project execution:* actions to complete the work defined in the project planning process
4. *Project monitoring and controlling:* measurements designed to assess how well a project is being executed per the budget and deliverables as well as to alert project managers to potential corrective actions that might be necessary from time to time

5. *Project closing:* actions to formally terminate all activities associated with the project either by delivering a finished product or by ceasing effort on a canceled project

Professionalizing project management at a healthcare delivery organization means that each HIT project should follow these five key processes. While project management frameworks are important, hiring professionally trained and ideally credentialed project managers is equally important. A number of project management credentialing organizations exist, including the Project Management Institute (PMI), which offers both the Project Management Professional (PMP) certification and the Program Management Professional certification. The PMP certification ensures that an individual has mastered a requisite body of knowledge on project management (see Exhibit 11.5 for a list of applicable knowledge areas) and has at least 60 months of project management experience. Furthermore, survey data suggest that increasing the number of individuals within the organization who have professional project management skills and experience and following an explicit HIT project management process framework raise the likelihood that the project will be a success (Lee 2006; Taylor 2004); see Exhibit 11.6.

Project Management Tools

A number of project management applications are available that provide the automated support to manage projects more professionally. While not intended to be an exhaustive list, the following are applications that can provide automation to support the five project management processes outlined earlier; many of these applications also carry the higher-level program/portfolio management capabilities discussed later in this chapter:

- Clarity (Computer Associates)
- Changepoint (Compuware)
- Project (Microsoft)
- Project Portfolio Management (Planview)
- Primavera P6 (Oracle)

Standardizing HIT operations on a set of project and portfolio management tools provides a common way to establish the processes and business rules that an organization must follow for managing projects. For instance, a healthcare organization's applications group uses one tool (say, Microsoft Project software), the infrastructure group uses a different tool (say, Oracle's Primavera P6), and the informatics and analytics group uses no tool at all. Because there is no visibility into the total number of projects going on

Project Management Knowledge Area	Individuals Must Know How To
Project integration management	Develop project charter Develop project management plan Direct and manage project execution Monitor and control project work Perform integrated change control Close project or phase
Project scope management	Collect requirements Define scope Create work breakdown structure Verify scope Control scope
Project time management	Define activities Sequence activities Estimate activity resources Estimate activity durations Develop schedule Control schedule
Project cost management	Estimate costs Determine budget Control costs
Project quality management	Plan quality Perform quality assurance Perform quality control
Project HR management	Develop human resource plan Acquire project team Develop project team Manage project team
Project communications management	Identify stakeholders Plan communications Distribute information Manage stakeholder expectations Report performance
Project risk management	Plan risk management Identify risks Perform qualitative analysis Perform quantitative analysis Plan risk responses Monitor and control risks
Project procurement management	Plan procurements Conduct procurements Administer procurements Close procurements

EXHIBIT 11.5
Project Management Knowledge Areas

SOURCE: Information from Project Management Institute (2008).

EXHIBIT 11.6
Benefits of HIT
PMO

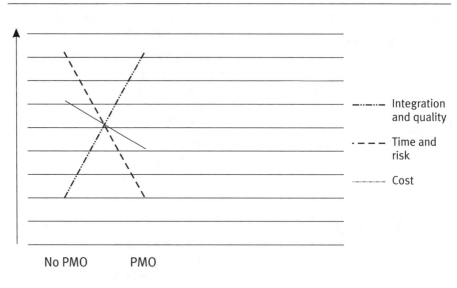

EXHIBIT 11.6
Benefits of HIT
PMO

Integration and quality

Time and risk

Cost

No PMO   PMO

among these groups, it becomes incredibly difficult to establish standardization of project management processes that is a prerequisite for managing interdependencies between projects; thus, it is difficult to achieve program or portfolio management capabilities.

Entire textbooks have been written on project management (e.g., Coplan and Masuda 2011) and the tools that support it. For illustrative purposes, we discuss project plans and Gantt charts as examples of key artifacts that are easily developed from within most project management/portfolio management tools.

Project Plans and Gantt Charts

All project management applications should have the ability to create a project plan and display it in a way that easily shows task interdependencies. Exhibit 11.7 shows a simple example of a Gantt chart for some tasks in an infrastructure project of a hospital system. This list of tasks is known as a *work breakdown structure* in project management parlance. Note how the interdependencies are clearly visible by the linking arrows that show which tasks must be fully completed before their successor tasks can begin. Other tasks without these interdependencies can be accomplished in parallel (i.e., they have no interdependencies but must nevertheless be accomplished to complete the project). Project management applications have the ability to collapse these tasks—these are all of the tasks that have predecessor (tasks that must be completed before the next tasks can be started) or successor (tasks that cannot begin until certain tasks have been completed) interdependencies—into the critical path of a project (see Exhibit 11.8). The reason critical

EXHIBIT 11.7
Project Plan in Gantt Chart Format

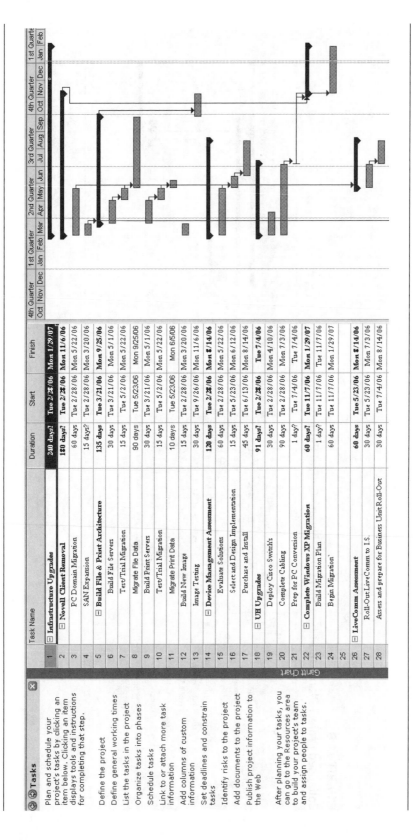

	Task Name	Duration	Start	Finish
1	☐ **Infrastructure Upgrades**	**240 days?**	**Tue 2/28/06**	**Mon 1/29/07**
2	☐ **Novell Client Removal**	**180 days?**	**Tue 2/28/06**	**Mon 11/6/06**
3	PC Domain Migration	60 days	Tue 2/28/06	Mon 5/22/06
4	SAN Expansion	15 days?	Tue 2/28/06	Mon 3/20/06
5	☐ **Build File & Print Architecture**	**135 days**	**Tue 3/21/06**	**Mon 9/25/06**
6	Build File Servers	30 days	Tue 3/21/06	Mon 5/1/06
7	Test/Trial Migration	15 days	Tue 5/2/06	Mon 5/22/06
8	Migrate File Data	90 days	Tue 5/23/06	Mon 9/25/06
9	Build Print Servers	30 days	Tue 3/21/06	Mon 5/1/06
10	Test/Trial Migration	15 days	Tue 5/2/06	Mon 5/22/06
11	Migrate Print Data	10 days	Tue 5/23/06	Mon 6/5/06
12	Build New Image	15 days	Tue 2/28/06	Mon 3/20/06
13	Image Testing	30 days	Tue 9/26/06	Mon 11/6/06
14	☐ **Device Management Assessment**	**120 days**	**Tue 2/28/06**	**Mon 8/14/06**
15	Evaluate Solutions	60 days	Tue 2/28/06	Mon 5/22/06
16	Select and Design Implementation	15 days	Tue 5/23/06	Mon 6/12/06
17	Purchase and Install	45 days	Tue 6/13/06	Mon 8/14/06
18	☐ **UH Upgrades**	**91 days?**	**Tue 2/28/06**	**Tue 7/4/06**
19	Deploy Cisco Switch's	30 days	Tue 2/28/06	Mon 4/10/06
20	Complete Cabling	90 days	Tue 2/28/06	Mon 7/3/06
21	Prep for PC Conversion	1 day?	Tue 7/4/06	Tue 7/4/06
22	☐ **Complete Windows XP Migration**	**60 days?**	**Tue 11/7/06**	**Mon 1/29/07**
23	Build Migration Plan	1 day?	Tue 11/7/06	Tue 11/7/06
24	Begin Migration`	60 days	Tue 11/7/06	Mon 1/29/07
25				
26	☐ **LiveComm Assessment**	**60 days**	**Tue 5/23/06**	**Mon 8/14/06**
27	Roll-Out LiveComm to I.S.	30 days	Tue 5/23/06	Mon 7/3/06
28	Assess and prepare for Business Unit-Roll-Out	30 days	Tue 7/4/06	Mon 8/14/06

Tasks

Plan and schedule your project's tasks by clicking an item below. Clicking an item displays tools and instructions for completing that step.

Define the project

Define general working times

List the tasks in the project

Organize tasks into phases

Schedule tasks

Link to or attach more task information

Add columns of custom information

Set deadlines and constrain tasks

Identify risks to the project

Add documents to the project

Publish project information to the Web

After planning your tasks, you can go to the Resources area to build your project's team and assign people to tasks.

EXHIBIT 11.8
Collapsed Project Plan Gantt Chart Showing Only the Critical Path

	Task Name	Duration	Start	Finish
1	⊟ **Infrastructure Upgrades**	**240 days?**	**Tue 2/28/06**	**Mon 1/29/07**
2	⊟ **Novell Client Removal**	**180 days?**	**Tue 2/28/06**	**Mon 11/6/06**
4	SAN Expansion	15 days?	Tue 2/28/06	Mon 3/20/06
5	⊟ **Build File & Print Architecture**	**135 days**	**Tue 3/21/06**	**Mon 9/25/06**
6	Build File Servers	30 days	Tue 3/21/06	Mon 5/1/06
7	Test/Trial Migration	15 days	Tue 5/2/06	Mon 5/22/06
8	Migrate File Data	90 days	Tue 5/23/06	Mon 9/25/06
13	Image Testing	30 days	Tue 9/26/06	Mon 11/6/06
22	⊟ **Complete Windows XP Migration**	**60 days?**	**Tue 11/7/06**	**Mon 1/29/07**
24	Begin Migration	60 days	Tue 11/7/06	Mon 1/29/07

path analysis is important is that it provides a forecast of the shortest possible time in which the overall project can be completed.

Program Management

As noted earlier, organizations that put in place program management capabilities have moved beyond managing individual projects to managing the interrelationships between projects and/or preexisting applications and systems. While managing this level of complexity takes slightly longer to plan up front, the extra time expended is recovered during the execution phase of the project in the form of reduced surprises and cost overruns associated with unforeseen interdependencies. In essence, the critical dependency analysis and management depicted in exhibits 11.7 and 11.8 are simply extended beyond a single project to interdependencies that exist within a particular program of projects or even across the HIT portfolio (Exhibit 11.2).

Portfolio Management

Along with the professional project management expertise described in the previous sections, organizations that employ a portfolio management approach also have tightly coupled HIT governance (essentially, making decisions about which information technology to invest in and which not to invest in) with its PMO (Smaltz, Carpenter, and Saltz 2007). In other words, think of project and/or program management as ensuring that things are done right within a particular project, whereas portfolio management concerns itself with doing the right kinds of projects that align with the organization's overall strategic goals and objectives. This distinction is why a PMO must work hand-in-hand with an organization's HIT governance structure (covered in Chapter 5). Illustrating this point is Exhibit 11.9, which shows a HIT portfolio of all the projects that are "in flight" at a for-profit healthcare organization. Prior to its annual HIT capital budget process, the particular organization, using the knowledge gained from professionally managing its portfolio of current HIT projects, put together a profile of all of the current HIT projects already in flight and rated them on the basis of value and risk. The organization further labeled each quadrant. The lower left quadrant, which represents low-value and high-risk HIT projects, is labeled "Think Twice (or More)." The upper right quadrant represents HIT projects that are deemed to both be of high value and have low risk associated with implementation; this quadrant is labeled "Ideal." The size of the bubbles in Exhibit 11.9 denotes the size in relative dollars of each individual project. Projects are categorized into nondiscretionary projects (e.g., some projects are mandated by law, such as the Sarbanes-Oxley Act) and discretionary projects. Much like an investor reviewing a portfolio of stocks before deciding which to divest and which to add to, an organization developing a graphic

EXHIBIT 11.9
Illustrative HIT
Portfolio

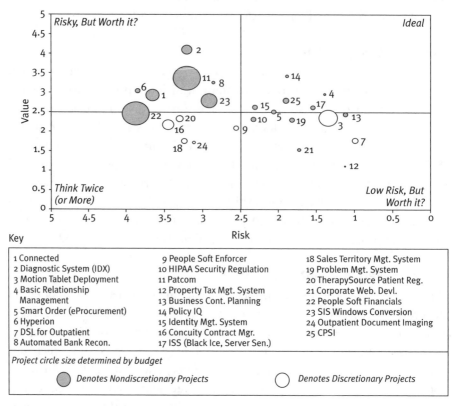

Key

1 Connected	9 People Soft Enforcer	18 Sales Territory Mgt. System
2 Diagnostic System (IDX)	10 HIPAA Security Regulation	19 Problem Mgt. System
3 Motion Tablet Deployment	11 Patcom	20 TherapySource Patient Reg.
4 Basic Relationship	12 Property Tax Mgt. System	21 Corporate Web. Devl.
Management	13 Business Cont. Planning	22 People Soft Financials
5 Smart Order (eProcurement)	14 Policy IQ	23 SIS Windows Conversion
6 Hyperion	15 Identity Mgt. System	24 Outpatient Document Imaging
7 DSL for Outpatient	16 Concuity Contract Mgr.	25 CPSI
8 Automated Bank Recon.	17 ISS (Black Ice, Server Sen.)	

Project circle size determined by budget

⬤ *Denotes Nondiscretionary Projects*   ◯ *Denotes Discretionary Projects*

SOURCE: Carpenter (2005). Used with permission.

such as Exhibit 11.9 gains a powerful and succinct decision-support means to evaluate proposed HIT projects.

In addition to decision support, an HIT portfolio management capability also provides regular portfolio status reports to the HIT governance of an organization. For instance, an HIT portfolio dashboard is typically created—sometimes via one of the project/portfolio management applications and sometimes via an organization's overall quality or other enterprise dashboard tools—to give leadership a view of project progress. Exhibit 11.10 is a sample of one such view, showing all in-flight projects of the organization (listed in Exhibit 11.9) grouped by strategic categories that are important to the organization along with the dollar amounts budgeted for each category. The graph on the left of this exhibit, titled "Portfolio by Category," depicts the monthly expenditures of each project category. The graph on the right of this exhibit, titled "Resource by Category," depicts the amount of full-time equivalent resources being expended on each project category.

While an HIT portfolio dashboard can be set up to provide status along any number of dimensions, its greatest impact comes in providing strategic views into the myriad projects the organization is working on to benefit HIT governance decision making. In the examples provided in exhibits 11.9 and 11.10, this for-profit healthcare organization is trying to balance strategically the need for greater regulatory compliance with the Sarbanes-Oxley Act and other legislation with the need for revenue growth. Therefore, the dashboard is designed to quickly provide a view within the past three quarters and the next six quarters of the amount of money being (or slated to be) invested in compliance-related projects, operational effectiveness projects, and projects the organization hopes will generate increased revenue. While illustrative and not intended to be a definitive example, this example makes the point that organizations must be able to produce flexible data representations (like Exhibit 11.9) on the entire portfolio of HIT projects to aid their HIT governance bodies. Such data are essential to making informed investment decisions and monitoring progress.

EXHIBIT 11.10

Sample HIT Portfolio Dashboard

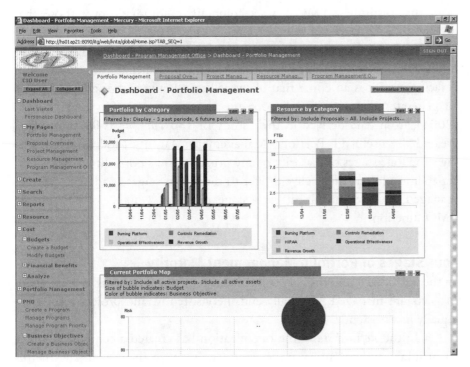

SOURCE: Carpenter (2005). Used with permission.

The PMO

Generally, these high-functioning portfolio management capabilities are being formalized in many leading healthcare organizations via the establishment of an HIT PMO. Typically, the functions of a PMO include but are not limited to the following:

- Issuing regular *communications* to project stakeholders and the rest of the organization regarding progress or status, programs of projects, and the entire portfolio
- Providing authoritative *management and oversight* of all projects within the portfolio
- Serving as *staff support to the HIT governance* of the organization, including performing portfolio analyses as requested by HIT governance and recommending HIT investments
- Creating *metrics and dashboards* to facilitate transparency

These tasks can be accomplished without putting in place a formal PMO, but a number of consultants and researchers suggest that organizations that institute a PMO have a competitive advantage over those that do not (Cooke-Davies, Crawford, and Lechler 2009; Jeffery and Leliveld 2004; Kaplan 2005; Light et al. 2005). Do note that establishing a PMO is not a quick fix to whatever project management challenge the organization is facing, and it is an effort that likely will take between two and four years to generate significant benefits for the organization. Jeffery and Leliveld (2004), from data derived in their study of 130 *Fortune* 1000 companies, created the useful IT Portfolio Management Maturity Model, which outlines the four stages of maturity of any organization's portfolio management capabilities. Jeffery and Leliveld refer to these four stages as ad hoc, defined, managed, and synchronized; each stage indicates a higher, more capable PMO function.

Four Stages of Portfolio Management Maturity

In the *ad hoc stage,* no formal project management capability is in place at all. Projects are managed informally and inconsistently, and project results are equally inconsistent.

In the *defined stage*, the organization has created a centralized entity to maintain and inventory projects and to manage them centrally. In this stage, applications and infrastructure are well defined and documented.

In the *managed stage*, the organization has created processes for vetting and rationalizing or ranking projects on the basis of key strategic criteria.

Furthermore, investment decisions employ financial metrics to help prioritize projects (e.g., return on investment, return on assets, net present value) and conduct at least annual reviews with business unit leadership on how well the HIT portfolio is aligned with overall organizational strategies.

In the *synchronized stage*, organizations conduct much more frequent evaluations of the HIT portfolio with business unit leaders and include a consistent assessment of returns versus risks in their project portfolios. Typically, organizations at the synchronized level of HIT portfolio management maturity have created PMO scorecards or dashboards that serve to transparently communicate project status and value. They also consistently conduct post-project benefits realization assessments to see if benefits envisioned prior to the project's adoption are achieved.

Since Jeffery and Leliveld (2004) articulated this maturity model, there has been considerable debate within the project management community about the best framework to use for assessing an organization's project/program/portfolio management maturity (Lianying, Jing, and Xinxing 2012; Pasian 2011; PMI 2008). Each framework suggests more complex and granular approaches for assessing an organization's project management capabilities. While the debate continues, Jeffery and Leliveld's model continues to provide HIT leaders and professionals with a simple, quick way of assessing the maturity of their organization's HIT portfolio management capabilities.

Summary

This chapter makes the case that many HIT projects generally do not achieve the benefits envisioned and that implementing professional portfolio management capabilities is an important first step toward mitigating this project risk. Furthermore, identifying and managing the cross-project interdependencies that a portfolio management approach embodies is an important second step toward mitigating project risk. Finally, implementing an HIT PMO that is tightly coupled with an organization's HIT governance structures and processes and that provides the full complement of capabilities outlined in Jeffery and Leliveld's (2004) IT Portfolio Management Maturity Model represents the greatest return on HIT investments for a healthcare organization.

Web Resources

A number of organizations (through their websites) provide more information on the topics discussed in this chapter:

- *CIO* magazine, Project Management section (www.cio.com/topic /3198/Project_Management). *CIO Magazine,* a leading publication of senior IT executive practices, provides a web resource on project management.
- Computer Associates, Clarity Project and Portfolio Management software (www.ca.com/us/products/detail/ca-clarity-ppm.aspx). This is an example of a vendor that provides project and portfolio management software.
- Compuware, Changepoint Business Portfolio Management software (www.compuware.com/business-portfolio-management). Another example of a vendor that provides project and portfolio management software.
- Healthcare Information and Management Systems Society, Project Management Special Interest Group (www.himss.org/get-involved /sigs/project-management?navItemNumber=12549).
- Microsoft, Project software (www.microsoft.com/project/en-us /project-management.aspx). Another example of a vendor that provides project and portfolio management software.
- Planview, Project Portfolio Management software (www.planview.com /products/enterprise/project-portfolio-management). This is another example of a vendor that provides project and portfolio management software.
- Project Management Institute (PMI; www.pmi.org). Check out what PMI offers:
    1. PMI Healthcare Community of Practice (http://healthcare .vc.pmi.org/Public/Home.aspx), a web space reference for practitioners in the field of project management.
    2. PMI Information Systems Community of Practice (http://is.vc .pmi.org/Public/Home.aspx), a web space reference site for practitioners in the field of information systems.
- Oracle, Primavera P6 Enterprise Project Portfolio Management software (www.oracle.com/us/products/applications/primavera/over view/index.html). This is yet another example of a vendor that provides project and portfolio management software.

Discussion Questions

1. Discuss some of the primary reasons an HIT implementation project might fail in a healthcare organization.

2. What are the main differences between HIT project management, HIT program management, and HIT portfolio management?

3. What are the five processes of project management?

4. What requirements should be considered when selecting project management tools for an organization?

5. Why are project metrics and portfolio dashboards important to HIT governance?

6. List and describe the major roles and functions of the PMO.

7. Which two project management knowledge areas described in Exhibit 11.5 do you consider to be the most important? Why?

8. What actions/changes are necessary within an organization to reach the synchronized stage of maturity of Jeffery and Leliveld's IT Portfolio Management Maturity Model?

9. Even with the development of a PMO, will there be instances in which an HIT venture fails? Explain your rationale.

THE KNOWLEDGE-ENABLED ORGANIZATION

Learning Objectives

1. Describe the impact of knowledge on quality of care.
2. Articulate the differences between knowledge and information.
3. Define sensemaking, and describe how it can be applied to healthcare organizations.
4. Define knowledge management.
5. Articulate what it means to "bake in" knowledge into organizational workflows, and provide some examples of how that is being done in the healthcare field.
6. List some reasons that healthcare organizations invest in enterprise data warehousing, data mining, and data analytics capabilities.

Overview

The Institute of Medicine (IOM) 1999 report, *To Err Is Human*, suggests that each year up to 98,000 patients in the United States die as a direct result of errors made in the course of their care. More recent studies (e.g., Health-grades 2009) indicate that the actual number of deaths attributable to medical errors may be significantly higher than the rate initially proposed by the IOM. A key contributing cause of these errors, according to the IOM report, is a lack of relevant information. A follow-up IOM report released in 2001 (*Crossing the Quality Chasm*) specifically recommends significant investments in healthcare information technology (HIT) to achieve its six goals of making healthcare safe, effective, patient centered, timely, efficient, and equitable. In 2009, the American Recovery and Reinvestment Act went a step further by providing significant financial incentives to healthcare organizations that meaningfully use electronic health record (EHR) systems to deliver patient care.

While information technology has great potential, a solution to the quality problem transcends simple information. The complexity of healthcare delivery has increased as diagnostic and therapeutic technologies have advanced. Another factor that contributes to the complexity of delivering patient care is the exponential expansion of medical knowledge, making it virtually impossible for a physician to stay abreast of the latest medical information (AMA 2006). Compounding this problem is that many physicians perceive that the impact of managed care practices has essentially limited the amount of time they could spend with a patient and the amount of cognitive time they could spend thinking about diagnoses and treatment options for any given patient (Morrison and Smith 2000).

These dynamics create increasing decision complexity, which affects what a caregiver notices and what a caregiver ignores. Weick (1995) notes that "information load is a complex mixture of the quantity, ambiguity, and variety of information that people are forced to process. As [information] load increases, people take increasingly strong steps to manage it. They begin with omission, and then move to greater tolerance of error, queuing, filtering, abstracting, using multiple channels, escape, and end with chunking." Weick's seminal work suggests that to adequately overcome complexity and information load, organizations must put in place deliberate systems of *sensemaking*—the ability to more accurately make sense of any given situation. Leading healthcare organizations are adopting sensemaking strategies to reduce medical errors and increase operational efficiency. Knowledge management principles and practices adopted in a sensemaking environment help optimize decision making with the limited time and ambiguous information available to contemporary providers (Middleton et al. 2004).

Knowledge Management

While a relatively new concept to healthcare delivery organizations, knowledge management is being successfully used by many other industries, particularly industries that gain from reusing knowledge (e.g., consulting firms) or quickly leveraging new discoveries into new products and services (e.g., manufacturing research and development). From Peter Senge's (1990) *The Fifth Discipline* to Nonaka and Takeuchi's (1995) *The Knowledge Creating Company* to Davenport and Prusak's (1998) *Working Knowledge*, ample resources are available to inform the healthcare field about the basics of knowledge management and how to apply its principles within a complex organizational setting. The key underlying tenet of the seminal knowledge management literature is that when individuals within organizations have the knowledge they need to be able to make decisions and accomplish their individual jobs, organizational efficiency and effectiveness are significantly improved. Often, however, healthcare workers do not have key information, and errors and suboptimal outcomes may follow.

Knowledge management is the organizational practice of explicitly and deliberately building, renewing, and applying relevant intellectual assets to maximize an enterprise's effectiveness (Wiig 2000). Knowledge management practices seek to leverage as much of the information and knowledge that exists within and beyond an organization as possible. Smaltz and Cunningham (2005, 126) suggest that "this knowledge can either be in explicit form (such as in databases, spreadsheets, presentation slides, documents, or other media) or in tacit form (such as the 'know-how' in an individual's head). The task of knowledge managers is to explicitly and deliberately build the organizational processes and toolsets that bring this knowledge asset to bear on the thousands of daily tactical and strategic decisions that are made each day in a healthcare organization."

Building the Knowledge-Enabled Healthcare Organization

One mistake many healthcare organizations make is that they expect to achieve better decision making, more efficient operations, and better healthcare outcomes by simply providing more and more data to caregivers and administrators. As noted by Weick (1995), such approaches merely increase the information load on caregivers, thereby making it more difficult to arrive at quality decisions. In response, leading healthcare organizations are taking systematic and deliberate steps to reduce the information load on caregivers by focusing attention on the data and information that truly matter in a given situation. They accomplish this primarily by using the following two practices:

1. *Baking in*, or embedding, knowledge into clinical and administrative workflows. This may be done via alerts, reminders, evidence-based order sets, and "click through" capability to relevant medical literature and evidence.
2. Achieving excellence in data warehousing, data mining, and analytics. This excellence is often evidenced through front-line patient safety dashboards, real-time process and outcomes reporting, and real-time feedback loops. An example is between patient care systems such as an electronic medical record (EMR) and the organization's data warehouse.

Knowledge-Enabled Workflows

A typical twenty-first century healthcare organization has thousands of workflows. Some examples of workflows include the process of admitting a patient to the hospital, scheduling a patient appointment in an outpatient clinic, and assessing a patient's condition in the emergency department. On the surface, these seem fairly innocuous examples, but consider the implications of missing information, too much information, or ambiguous information on any of these workflows. Being alerted that a patient is allergic to amoxicillin, is currently already taking a beta-blocker for an unrelated condition, or is epileptic can make a profound difference in the treatment plan initiated by the caregiver team (not to mention the patient outcome). Exhibit 12.1 provides some examples of how healthcare organizations are baking in knowledge into their workflows to increase patient safety and ensure more quality outcomes for the services they provide.

While not infallible, the practice of placing relevant knowledge directly within the workflow creates an organizational system that will maximize quality decision making, reduce medical errors, and significantly increase the quality of care provided to patients (Bates et al. 1998; Berner and La Lande 2007).

EXHIBIT 12.1
Baking-In
Healthcare
Knowledge
with Workflow
Examples

Types of Baked-In Knowledge	Workflow Example
Alerts	Within an electronic medical record (EMR) system, an alert is triggered when a provider orders a new drug for a patient that interacts negatively with another drug that either the physician has ordered previously or the patient is already taking
Reminders	On a nursing unit, a nurse is reminded that a patient is due for another dose of a particular medication at a prescribed time
Evidence	Within an EMR system, providing click-through capability to access relevant medical literature (often via an electronic subscription service) pertinent to the current patient situation
Order sets	Within an EMR system, physicians often place orders for various drugs or treatments (Creating order sets is the practice of pre-populating orders into groups that evidence has shown to be effective together; rather than having to place individual orders, a physician may select an entire order set.)
Automatic billing codes	During an outpatient visit, E&M (evaluation and management) codes are automatically generated to facilitate billing via information that the caregiver team annotates in the EMR

Excellence in Data Warehousing, Data Mining, and Analytics

Contemporary healthcare organizations produce mass quantities of data often housed within siloed, transaction-based systems. For instance, vast quantities of test results sit in a typical hospital laboratory system; vast quantities of drug orders for various patients at various points in time sit in a pharmacy system; and a growing body of text reports and notes describing signs, symptoms, and diagnoses for various patients sit in an EMR. To aid organizational efforts to holistically assess patient outcomes, improve patient safety, and enhance organizational efficiencies, these data must be aggregated into a data warehouse to facilitate analyses, thereby aiding continuous process improvement efforts. Smaltz and Cunningham (2005, 118) note that

> enterprise data warehouses essentially provide a homogeneous location for the data that heterogeneously resides in your various information systems.... The way an enterprise data warehouse typically functions is that data collected from the main transaction-based systems (appointing and scheduling, laboratory, pharmacy, and the like) is copied over to the data warehouse for use in organizational analyses and performance measurement activities. Once in the data warehouse, it serves as the one-stop shopping for management engineering studies, operations research studies, clinical process studies, and other decision support processes. Most recently, enterprise data warehouses have enabled the new field of data mining (large variable data set correlation and associative studies).

Exhibit 12.2 depicts a typical hospital data warehouse. Data from various source systems are acquired and transferred to the data warehouse. The data integration is accomplished via a process commonly known as *extraction, transformation, and load* (ETL). Because the data formats within the source systems on the left of Exhibit 12.2 are often quite heterogeneous, the ETL process transforms the data into homogeneous data fields for ease of management and further analysis. When data-quality errors are encountered during the extraction and transformation stages, action is taken to improve the data quality within the source system, as opposed to within the data warehouse itself. The actual data warehouse may be organized into logical groups of data marts. A *data mart* is a subset of the data that resides within a data warehouse, often organized into logical groupings. In this example, the data warehouse is made up of business, clinical, research, and external (benchmarking) data marts.

The organization benefits from the data warehouse by being able to accomplish a variety of data queries and multidimensional analyses and can

EXHIBIT 12.2

Notional Depiction of a Data Warehouse

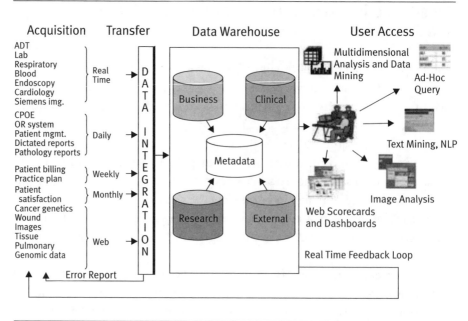

support management dashboards and scorecards designed to focus organizational attention on a metrics-driven approaches to improvement. Pioneering healthcare organizations are also creating real-time feedback loops whereby novel groupings of data from the data warehouse are fed back into source systems (often via web portals) to facilitate real-time quality improvements.

Smaltz and Cunningham (2005, 115) note that

> most organizations would agree that realization of investments in HIT fall[s] short when attempting to truly assess population health, to manage disease processes within that population, to analyze variation in practice patterns among physicians, to determine the efficacy of long-term health promotion programs, to gauge the benefit of outsourcing to other healthcare providers, or, in some cases, to gain a true picture of their own organizations' performance in spite of the mounds of data available to do so. Interestingly, the HIT functionality (for the most part) currently exists to create these capabilities. However, responsibility for ensuring that the HIT assets are used effectively and efficiently has primarily fallen on users who, in general, know little about the systems or their full capabilities (beyond what they need to know to accomplish transactions within their responsibility), making it impossible to achieve full realization of HIT benefits. While some might call for more training or for vendors to make information systems easier to use (which certainly is beneficial), *organizations cannot avoid investing in people, processes and capabilities that are expressly focused on leveraging enterprise-wide data, information and knowledge . . . if they want to truly achieve and sustain superior clinical and business results.*

The Health Information Technology for Economic and Clinical Health Act (HITECH) Act of 2009 and the incentives it provides for healthcare organizations to not only invest in but also meaningfully use an EHR has dramatically increased investment in HIT. When organizations make these investment decisions, they also typically invest in the requisite people and process redesign to gain full benefit from the applications that they implement. Ironically, our anecdotal observations suggest that few healthcare delivery organizations are adequately investing in the people and processes needed to leverage the data these systems create. As profit margins continue to be challenged by increasingly difficult reimbursement mechanisms, data warehousing, data mining, and analytics will increasingly become vital in efforts to analyze business and clinical processes and outcomes and to maximize efficiencies and effectiveness (Smaltz and Cunningham 2005).

Summary

Medical knowledge is increasing at a rate impossible for physicians and caregivers to comprehend and retain. Furthermore, physicians and caregivers are often faced with limited time to make clinical decisions with imperfect information about their patients. The practice of knowledge management attempts to systematically and deliberately take steps to reduce the information load on physicians and caregivers by focusing attention on the data and information that truly matter in a given situation. Knowledge management also attempts to create organizational competencies that leverage the hordes of data produced from myriad healthcare applications. Healthcare delivery organizations' knowledge management foci are typically in two key areas:

1. Baking in knowledge into clinical and administrative workflows
2. Achieving excellence in data warehousing, data mining, and data analytics

While quality in the delivery of healthcare has been highlighted as a systemic problem within the US healthcare system, organizations can—at least in part—overcome such systemic problems by investing in resources focused on building a knowledge-enabled organization. In fact, Garets and Lazerow (2012) suggest that healthcare organizations can expect to enjoy increasing levels of competitive advantage to the extent that they empower their employees at all levels with integrated information to drive organizational performance improvement. Healthcare organizations are well served to invest more resources focused on creating a knowledge-enabling core competency.

Web Resources

A number of organizations (through their websites) provide more information on the topics discussed in this chapter:

- Brint Institute, Knowledge Management Think Tank Discussions Archives (www.brint.com/km). This website is a virtual knowledge management community of practice that provides a plethora of information on the field of knowledge management.
- eKnowledge Center (www.eknowledgecenter.com). The eKnowledge Center provides online training to knowledge management practitioners and certifications in knowledge management.
- Google Scholar, index of knowledge management articles (http:// scholar.google.com/scholar?hl=en&q=Knowledge%20Management). This is a list of scholarly articles indexed by Google Scholar.
- KM World (www.kmworld.com). This is a publisher of knowledge management, content management, and document management material.
- Knowledge Management Professional Society (KMPro; www.kmpro .org). KMPro is a professional association for knowledge management practitioners. It offers both reference information and certifications in knowledge management.
- The Data Warehouse Institute (http://tdwi.org). This organization provides education, training, and certifications in the field of data warehousing and business intelligence.

Discussion Questions

1. What is the impact of knowledge on quality of care?
2. What, if any, are the major differences between knowledge and information?
3. What is sensemaking, and how can it be applied to healthcare organizations?
4. Define knowledge management.
5. What does it mean to bake in knowledge into organizational workflows?
6. What are some of the ways that knowledge can be baked into information technology–enabled workflows?
7. Why should an organization invest in enterprise data warehousing, data mining, and data analytics capabilities?

HIT VALUE ANALYSIS

Learning Objectives

1. Specify why making healthcare information technology (HIT) investment decisions on the basis of realized value rather than on "anecdote, inference, and opinion" leads to better outcomes.
2. Describe five changes that make today's HIT investment decisions more challenging than in the past.
3. Provide examples of HIT costs and outcomes changes that will "always" be adopted and examples that will "never" be adopted.
4. Analyze how the major techniques used for evaluation of an HIT investment differ.
5. List the eight key steps in cost evaluation.
6. Analyze why certain types of HIT applications are less likely to be performed.
7. Describe value realization and total cost of ownership methodologies.

Overview

Up to this point in the book, the discussions surrounding healthcare information technology (HIT) have explicitly recognized that the organization, financing, and delivery of healthcare services are different from those of other goods and services. While we consider this to be fundamentally true, some aspects of healthcare, especially HIT, should adhere to core business processes. HIT can be considered an input into the "production" process just as are inputs of nursing time, allied health staff, medical supplies, and physician services. In that context, the decisions regarding how much and what type of HIT inputs to use should fall under a valuation paradigm. Johnston, Pan, and Middleton (2002) make this point strongly in their argument for finding value from HIT.

Firmly establishing value in many healthcare investments has proven to be a challenge, however. Clinical technologies have increasingly been subject to critical valuation, or benefits received relative to costs incurred, and this notion has taken hold for HIT as well (Board 2004; Bower 2005; Buntin et al. 2011; Miller et al. 2005; Wiley and Daniel 2006). Issues related to data collection, methodology, and application make the realization of value from and widespread use of evidence-based management a challenge. The health economics literature is replete with methodologies of cost, cost–benefit, and cost-effectiveness analyses and quality-adjusted life years (e.g., Chaudhry et al. 2006; Gold et al. 1996; Rahimi and Vimarlund 2007; Shekelle, Morton, and Keeler 2006; Simon and Simon 2006; Warner and Luce 1982). Most of these studies involve developing the methodology for assessing complex medical applications, and only a few are applied. In addition, large organizations have become sources for clinical intervention evaluations (see University HealthSystem Consortium at www.uhc.edu or Blue Cross and Blue Shield Technology Evaluation Center at www.bcbs.com/betterknowledge/tec). Surprisingly, only a few studies look specifically at HIT interventions (e.g., Chaudhry et al. 2006; Featherly et al. 2007; Rahimi and Vimarlund 2007; Shekelle, Morton, and Keeler 2006; Simon and Simon 2006). Some earlier studies still serve the literature well (e.g., Glandon and Shapiro 1988). The Center for Information Technology Leadership (www.citl.org) now serves as one of the sources of information regarding HIT value.

Because of the complexity of the problem and the lack of comprehensive data, healthcare executives have largely been forced to make decisions about HIT investments on the basis of cursory evidence at best and instinct or hope at worst. In the words of Johnston, Pan, and Middleton (2002), HIT decisions are often based on "anecdote, inference, and opinion." Inevitably, this approach produces decisions that may not yield the hoped-for benefits. As a result, HIT may fall short in addressing the problems plaguing healthcare.

This is not totally unexpected, however. A host of problems arise from performing these analyses including the following:

- Need for complex (econometric) techniques rather than straightforward finance and accounting techniques to find meaningful results (Meyer and Degoulet 2008)
- Indirect measurement of benefits because of the interdependent nature of the production process and because benefits are found in areas not expected (Bower 2005; Encinosa and Bae 2011; Featherly et al. 2007)
- Physician and other clinicians' resistance to change once cost data are delivered (Asch, Hershey, and Ubel 2003)
- Indication from the market that some portions of HIT investments are not appropriate (If people do not realize the value, why should we force them to use it? [Loomis et al. 2002])

As organizations struggle to meet patient and community health needs and improve quality with tight budgets, performing a strict value assessment of all investments has become even more important. To give some idea of the magnitude of the issue at an individual hospital level, according to an American Hospital Association (AHA 2007) survey, in 2006, the median hospital spent $5,556 per bed for health information technology capital. This translates to more than $1 million in capital expenditures for a 200-bed hospital. Among the hospitals responding to the survey, 54 percent reported that capital costs were a significant barrier to information technology adoption, and 32 percent reported that operating costs were a significant barrier to adoption. Financial barriers exceeded interoperability, acceptability by clinical staff, availability of qualified staff, and inadequate technology in importance as perceived barriers to adoption. By 2011, capital costs per bed had increased to at least $6,300 per bed using survey data and author's calculations (*Trustee* 2011). However, the estimates from this *Trustee* article suggest that capital spending on HIT declined in recent years, so note that HIT spending is hard to forecast for some of the reasons discussed in Chapter 4. The diffusion of HIT workers across an organization makes budget estimates less precise. In 2012, 14 percent of HIT leaders participating in the annual HIMSS survey cited financial factors as a barrier to implementing HIT in their organization, a concern second only to adequate staffing—cited by 22 percent of respondents as the top barrier. Both vendor ability to deliver and difficulty in end user acceptance were named as significant barriers as well, selected by 12 percent and 9 percent of respondents, respectively (HIMSS 2012a, Figure 12).

Even as the government and competitive pressures induce healthcare delivery organizations to implement interoperable electronic health records (EHRs) that enable the exchange of information within and across institutions, these organizations must still focus on value creation. Early evidence indicates that the financial benefits of interoperable EHRs to the healthcare system may be substantial. Walker and colleagues (2005) estimate that health information exchange (HIE) and interoperability, when fully implemented, may generate upwards of $77 billion in savings to the US healthcare system. Providers will come to expect electronic HIE. They increasingly work in healthcare delivery teams consisting of physicians, nurses, pharmacists, therapists, and others who require a real-time exchange of information. The Health Information Technology for Health and Clinical Health (HITECH) Act provides significant incentives to providers that fully implement an HIE. Value has not been identified yet, and some analysts (e.g., Vest and Gamm 2010) recommend that organizations examine the partially effective past efforts to facilitate HIE for evidence that the potential benefits may be less than estimated. Interestingly, according to the 2012 HIMSS survey data (Figure 18), while 49 percent of hospital leaders said they participated in an HIE, 26 percent had no plans to participate, 22 percent had an HIE in their area but did not participate, and 2 percent were unfamiliar with HIE.

Supported by the health reform legislation, consumers will demand new delivery modes for their care and expect coordination of care across provider segments. Consequently, the ability to assess value will be crucial for the HIT leader of the future, and information technology will play a vital role in that value delivery.

This chapter first outlines why the evaluation problem is more complex today because of the systems nature of healthcare delivery. Then, it presents what is known about how HIT investments are analyzed and provides the steps for conducting these analyses. Next, it details value realization as a method to implement evaluation. Last, it presents selected findings from cost-evaluation studies.

Systems Challenges

Despite its costs, at one level, HIT is essential in the provision of high-quality care in today's environment. However, technology acquisition is not an all-or-nothing proposition. Questions of scale, scope, application, integration, and timing must be addressed, all of which make the decision complex. Do you wait another year? Do you purchase and install some applications and not others? How do you ensure that the appropriate mix of information technologies is selected? Furthermore, once that set of decisions is made, how do you implement so that costs stay at the expected level and the benefits promised are actually realized? In the face of these questions, some have come to challenge the wisdom of assumed value and even the benefits of HIT investments (e.g., Carr 2003; Koppel 2005; Koppel et al. 2005; Loomis et al. 2002).

If these considerations did not make this problem difficult enough, the interdependence of providers in a healthcare "system" complicates the decision further. As detailed in Chapter 2, problems of cost, quality, and access plague those responsible for healthcare delivery. In a general discussion regarding the transformation of the US healthcare system, Adams and colleagues (2007) identify the following five features that make today's challenges different from challenges in the past:

1. Globalization
2. Consumerism
3. Aging and overweight populations

4. Diseases that are more expensive to treat

5. New medical technologies and treatments

To respond successfully to these challenges, Adams and colleagues argue that value decisions must extend beyond an individual organization's considerations to the perspective of society as a whole. For example, medical tourism may become common as the financial incentives for care delivered outside of the United States could eventually drive select care overseas (see Exhibit 13.1).

Adams and colleagues' recommendations for successful transformation of the healthcare system include many features, but most important, they argue that there will be different perspectives on value. The US healthcare system will transform from one that emphasizes individual value and cost containment to one with an emphasis on balancing "stakeholder value across dimensions (cost, quality, access, and choice)" (Adams et al. 2007, 42). The latter emphasis will usher in a transformation from the current state of data management to electronic, evidence-based, standard, shared, and interoperable information (Adams et al. 2007). Similarly, Enthoven and Tollen (2005) make the point that to address cost and quality concerns, rather than introduce competition to the healthcare market, healthcare organizations need to consider moving away from market changes that foster independent competing business units. In their opinion, to capture potential cost savings and quality improvements, the US government should encourage organizations within local and regional markets to form "integrated delivery systems, with incentives for teams of professionals to provide coordinated, efficient, evidence-based care, supported by state-of-the-art information technology" (Enthoven and Tollen 2005, 420).

Procedure	US	Mexico	Costa Rica	Thailand
Appendectomy	$17,600	$ 15,136	$ 15,312	N/A
Angioplasty	$23,900	$13,384	N/A	$12,848
Heart bypass	$52,500	N/A	$27,300	$10,384
Hip replacement	$25,000	$ 11,250	$12,750	$ 8,448
Knee replacement	$24,500	$ 11,515	$ 13,198	$ 9,152
Dentures	$ 2,700	$ 1,782	$ 2,214	N/A
...ectomy	$25,200	$20,664	$21,672	$14,080
	$25,300	$ 15,180	$ 16,192	$ 7,392

EXHIBIT 13.1
Approximate Costs of Key Procedures in Four Countries from a Single Source

...llmedicaltourism.com.

Evaluation Problem

At the most fundamental level, business decisions faced by the chief information officer (CIO), and indirectly by the CEO and board of trustees, come down to a challenge of deciding among competing alternatives. The questions they must ask are as follows: Does the investment in HIT increase, have no effect on, or decrease organizational outcomes? Does it increase, have no effect on, or decrease the costs to the organization?

Exhibit 13.2 presents a simple paradigm that can effectively support HIT decisions. The matrix consists of nine cells or potential outcome/cost combinations, and, in some cells, the decision to adopt the technology or not to adopt it is straightforward. For example, if adopting the technology results in a reduction in outcomes and an increase in costs (cell 3), most CIOs will not adopt (never). Similarly, if outcomes improve with the new technology and costs are reduced (scenario 7), the decision to adopt is straightforward (always). Combinations of costs and outcomes that place the organization in scenarios 2, 3, or 6 are *never* adopted. Similarly, combinations of costs and outcomes that place the organization in scenarios 4, 7, or 8 are *always* adopted.

The interesting cases involve combinations of costs and outcomes that place the organization on the diagonal in scenarios 1, 5, or 9. For these cases, a methodology must be put in place to more rigorously measure the magnitude of the changes in outcomes and the magnitude of the changes in costs. Formal benefit–cost or cost-effectiveness analyses need to be applied to assess the relative changes for these three cases: both outcomes and costs increase, neither benefits nor costs change, and both benefits and costs decrease.

Benefit–Cost and Cost-Effectiveness Analyses

A number of studies have documented the use of conventional benefit–cost, cost-effectiveness, or cost–utility analysis in healthcare (e.g., Gold et al. 1996). The discussions that follow are not significantly concerned with differentiating these techniques, as a full history of the concepts is beyond the scope of this book. In simple terms, *benefit–cost analyses* are applied when all aspects of the costs related to a technology and benefits of that technology

EXHIBIT 13.2
Technology Cost and Outcome Effect Decision Matrix

Cost Effect	Outcome Effect		
	Improve	No Change	Worsen
Increase	1 ?????	2 Never	3 Never
No change	4 Always	5 ?????	6 Never
Decrease	7 Always	8 Always	9 ?????

are measured in monetary terms. The outcome from these analyses might be presented as $3 in benefits for every $1 in cost ($3/$1). The decision calculus then enables leadership to select among alternatives that have the highest ratio.

For many healthcare applications, some of the outcomes or benefits may be difficult or objectionable to put into financial terms. Loss of life, for example, can be quantified in financial terms (Viscusi 2004), but not everyone is comfortable with making those assessments. *Cost-effectiveness analyses* were developed for technologies and resulted in outcomes that could not be quantified (Weinstein and Stason 1977). For example, one might estimate the costs associated with extending life for an additional year. The outcome from these analyses might be presented as $10,000 cost per life year saved ($10,000/life year). In this case, considering alternative technologies, leadership would adopt the technology with the *lowest* cost per life year saved.

Cost–utility analysis extends this measurement challenge even further by recognizing that the quality of life year extended might not always be the same. That realization led to a host of attempts to adjust the life years saved by some notion of the utility, value, or quality of that life (see, for example, the findings on the Centers for Disease Control and Prevention's Health-Related Quality of Life website at www.cdc.gov/hrqol/index.htm). For example, if the outcome is an additional year of life, but the patient spends that year in pain or confined to a nursing home bed, the value of that life year might not be as great as nine months of pain-free or fully functional extended life.

The key to using any of these formal methods of cost evaluation is to follow a series of eight steps (see Glandon and Shapiro 1988; Gold et al. 1996; Warner and Luce 1982).

Steps in Using Cost-Evaluation Methods

While this step may be obvious to many, clearly identifying study objectives may be the most important step in the analysis. Without knowing precisely what the organization desires or what the proposed HIT application or technology is designed to do, the outcomes of the evaluation are meaningless. Essentially, the decision comes down to whether the organization is looking narrowly at the financial benefits and costs associated with the decision or considering broader organizational or social benefits and costs. From the perspective of information technology, social costs include those incurred by physicians or others who are not employees of the organization but whose opinions matter to decision makers. An otherwise strong HIT system may fail if the burden on the users is not fully measured.

Step 1: Identify Study Objectives

Step 2: Specify the Alternatives

The relevant alternatives to the proposed technology must be clearly articulated; otherwise, a valid decision cannot be attained. Make the decision relative to the best alternative to ensure that the optimal choice is made. Not using credible alternatives in judging the proposed technology invites the risk of participants losing faith in the outcomes. A common error is to compare a proposed HIT solution with the status quo; the status quo is often not relevant when adopting an EHR, for example. Comparisons should be required among alternative vendors rather than with the current state of health record management.

Step 3: Develop a Framework for Analysis

The analysis framework is often called the *theoretical framework* or theoretical model, and one might have a tendency to ignore this step. Developing the framework is important, however, because it puts the technology into the broader systems context and defines how the inputs to the technology are related and how the outcomes are used by the system. It also forces an understanding of how the technology affects the total healthcare delivery system so that the direct and indirect (unintended consequences) costs and benefits to the system can be clearly identified and measured (Han et al. 2005). Returning to the EHR example, the theoretical framework forces a full understanding of how the information flows from the bedside or the physician's office to the electronic record; how that information is stored, catalogued, and retrieved from the record; and what the information's end uses are designed to be. Without that full understanding, crucial components of costs and benefits might be ignored or shortchanged.

Step 4: Measure Costs

Cost assessment is essential to the benefit–cost analysis. The identification and measurement of costs is relatively straightforward for big-ticket items such as direct labor, equipment, and supplies, but fully identifying indirect or opportunity costs associated with the intervention takes more time. The concept of *total cost of ownership* is an operational device designed to aid in defining and collecting relevant startup (one time) and recurring costs (Hickman and Kusche 2006; Smaltz and Berner 2007). The EHR might shift some of the burden of data collection, analysis, and reporting. Unless that added burden results in easily measurable increases in time or supply use, it can often be overlooked. Management, in particular, can easily be affected by added data availability. The electronic record facilitates more analysis in an attempt to make better evidence-based decisions. While this may result in benefits associated with better decision making, it may also result in added time spent understanding the data that are generated. Managers may find they spend more time preparing and poring over reports at the expense of other tasks.

As with cost identification, good evaluation requires clear identification of all benefits associated with the technology. Ignoring key benefits can clearly lead to underestimating the net effect of technology. Johnston, Pan, and Middleton (2002) argue that many researchers take a narrow view of benefits, or, in their term, *HIT value*. They argue that one should consider organizational, financial, and clinical benefits. Identifying these benefits is facilitated if the framework for analysis is done correctly. A related issue with regard to benefits is that they must be realized and not necessarily speculative, assumed, or hypothetical.

Step 5: Measure Benefits

Most HIT projects have a pattern of costs and benefits that varies over the product's lifecycle. Typically, costs are incurred early in a project cycle as resources are expended to purchase equipment, hire staff, and train staff. Conversely, the benefits or value to the organization accrue over time. Understanding that cycle with respect to the organization's technology is important for making valid comparisons. Although the CIO or HIT decision maker may not be as concerned with the timing issue as others in the healthcare organization, the timing of incurred benefits and costs cannot be ignored. In fact, considering alternatives with the same net costs and benefits, one should select that project with the distribution of costs skewed toward the future rather than that project with the distribution of benefits skewed toward the present.

Step 6: Factor-in Lifecycle and Discounting

By the nature of HIT investments, uncertainty exists regarding the estimates of both their costs and their value or benefits. Despite leadership's best efforts, they may find that these estimates are inaccurate. For example, with the EHR, physicians may not readily adopt the new technologies and systems as planned. In these cases, the costs of developing and implementing the system are the same, but the measured benefits are much lower. One never assumes exceedingly high levels of avoidance by the medical staff. If physicians do not adopt, the evaluation of the EHR most likely appears unsatisfactory. To deal with uncertainty, most look at the estimates being used and develop a best-case scenario and a worst-case scenario. For example, in the EHR example, assume benefits with 80 percent of the medical staff fully participating. To test the best case, estimate benefits with 90 percent medical staff participation (base estimate + 10 percent). To test the worst case, estimate benefits with 70 percent medical staff participation (base estimate −10 percent). This process is often called *sensitivity analysis*. If performing a sensitivity analysis yields estimates that do not change the overall evaluation of the technology, then confidence has been added to the decision. If at extreme values the overall evaluation of the technology changes, return to the framework and assumptions to be certain they are accurate.

Step 7: Deal with Uncertainty

**Step 8:
Consider Equity**

This step has its origins in the federal government's use of benefit–cost analysis for evaluating alternative government interventions. However, it has application to individual healthcare organizations as well. Equity considerations require examination of not just what the costs and benefits are for the organization but also who receives those benefits and costs. Again from the perspective of the EHR, if the benefits accrue to the institution, its employees, and its patients, but the costs are largely borne by those involved in using the technology (physicians), the EHR strategy is likely to fail (Landro 2003). For social investment decisions, consider compensating those who bear the costs from the gains made in the use of the technology. Healthcare organizations have no way to compensate cost bearers, and legal restrictions may limit their compensation.

Challenges to Evaluation

Despite the prevalence of HIT mechanisms in place in healthcare organizations, much evidence exists that HIT value is not easy to attain or ensure. Early assessments of the "state of the art" (Glandon and Shapiro 1988) suggested that more work was needed in this area. High-profile failures occurred, such as at Cedars-Sinai Medical Center in Los Angeles, which ended its effort to convert to a computerized physician order entry (CPOE) system in January 2003 (Chin 2003). The cause of this extreme failure is uncertain. Failure most probably occurs at the implementation stage, although failure of that magnitude may have had many causes.

In the late 1980s, some key findings on reasons for poor evaluations of technology suggested why HIT value did not always ensue from these significant investments. First, much of the technology was selected for the wrong reasons, such as keeping up with the competition. While there might be good reasons to adopt the technology that the competition is using, that alone is not sufficient reason to implement a HIT system or application. Second, knowledge, time, and money prohibited adequate evaluation. The CIO and his or her managers just might have been too busy to spend the time conducting evaluations to determine value from the investment. Third, in many cases, the technology in place was determined to be a poor decision, which might help in future decisions but has no impact on the original decision going forward. This "water under the bridge" argument might keep leaders who are living in the past from investigating prior failures seriously (Glandon and Shapiro 1988).

Related to these items are the following two fundamental impediments to maximizing HIT value:

1. *Documentation.* The comprehensive, reliable data on the clinical or business outcomes related to the technology and the true, full costs

associated with selecting, purchasing, implementing, hiring staff, training staff, training users, and so forth are difficult to obtain, synthesize, and report. It takes time and money to determine if the value from HIT investments actually exists. More on this issue, called the *total cost of ownership*, is presented in the next section.

2. *Interdependence.* Even if data have been defined and collected, the pervasive nature of the influence of many HIT investments across functional areas in the organization makes determination of value difficult at best. Many systems have both direct and indirect cost and outcome effects across a wide portion of the organization; thus, assigning value to a particular investment is a major undertaking.

Glandon and Buck (1994) identified these fundamental challenges to effectively maximize value from HIT investments. They developed a model of information systems that separates application and function (see Exhibit 13.3) and suggests where more rigorous evaluation might exist.

Assessing and ensuring value at the operational systems level has the greatest chance of success. Investments to improve admissions, discharge, and transfer (ADT) or general ledger applications have a greater chance of clearly linking the technology change to a measurable outcome. The well-defined and limited scope of such application reduces the severity of the measurement challenges. Outcomes at the operational level are generally characterized as intermediate compared with outcomes of the healthcare organization as a whole. For example, ADT outcomes might include time to admit a patient to a bed from the emergency department as an intermediate outcome. This

Information Requirement	Function	
	Clinical	**Business**
External systems	Physician recruitment and retention Contracting	Legal actions Cost containment
Administrative systems	Case mix Incomplete chart reporting Care planning Patient scheduling	Absence and turnover control Revenue statistics Wage and salary planning Capital spending
Operational systems	Admission, discharge, and transfer Census reporting	Inventory control General ledger Accounts payable

EXHIBIT 13.3
Information Systems by Function and Information Requirement

SOURCE: Glandon and Buck (1994). Adapted with permission from Sage Publications, Thousand Oaks, California.

outcome may depend on the ADT system, but ultimate outcome of patient mortality, morbidity, or satisfaction is less likely to be influenced by the ADT system.

Investments applied to administrative systems are less clear in terms of value assessment. These systems influence the efficiency and effectiveness of institutional operations and often contain some of the quantifiable elements inherent in operational systems. However, they often apply to cross-functional areas within the organization, making their impact more difficult to quantify. In administrative systems, then, it is less clear than in operational systems that outcomes, benefits, and costs are attributable to the new technology. Outcomes for administrative systems are generally intermediate, as are the outcomes for operational applications, but should apply more broadly than operational systems. For example, systems designed to improve incomplete chart reporting can have somewhat measurable outcomes, such as delinquent report rates. This outcome has broader impact because medical staff, nursing, ancillary systems, and quality assurance and accreditation preparation all bear costs or benefit from changes in this outcome.

Finally, investments applied to strategic planning have the greatest difficulty with respect to value determination. All of the inputs used in these systems are cross-functional, which implies that data must be gathered from diverse units across the institution and often from outside of the institution. Outcomes are generally final from the perspective of the healthcare organization as a whole; thus, they are very difficult to measure, and attribution is always a challenge. For example, systems to support physician recruitment might be expected to lead to greater market share and improved physician retention. However, many external factors influence these outcomes, leading to greater uncertainty with respect to the value of this type of HIT investment. For example, you might have improved physician recruitment by operating a well-functioning system. However, your market share and physician retention may suffer because a specialty hospital moved into your market and siphoned off key physicians and associated patients. The outcomes are poor from the organization's perspective.

Probably the best example of this type of challenge is with the introduction of the EHR strategy. Smaltz and Berner (2007) outline the interrelated nature of benefits and challenges the EHR system faces. Because EHR is not a thing but a comprehensive strategy, it is difficult to value. It is an "organizational, cultural transformation project that just happens to have a technology component" (Smaltz and Berner 2007, 16). Examination of just the benefits section of an EHR strategy described by these authors reveals how investment in this process spans the organization and creates difficulties in financial documentation. The descriptions in Exhibit 13.4 by major benefit

Category	Subcategory	Description Example of Impact
Improve efficiency		Improve efficiency of the clinical patient care–related processes
	Access to information	Getting information when and where it is needed
	Organization of the data	Patient data entered one time
	Claims processing	By allowing the clinical data to drive billing processes
Improve monitoring		Enables individual provider profiles of performance as well as aggregate profiles
Improve clinical processes		Real-time clinical decision support
	Quality improvement	Clinical and financial outcomes can be more easily monitored and linked
	Disease management	Aggregate data across patients

EXHIBIT 13.4
Descriptions of EHR Benefits by Category: Demonstration of System Nature of EHR

SOURCE: Smaltz and Berner (2007). Reprinted with permission from Health Administration Press, Chicago.

category and subcategory demonstrate that benefits are not confined to a single operational unit.

Value Realization

The IT Governance Institute (2006, 5) developed a multipart initiative to support HIT value realization in response to a perceived need for "organizations to optimize the realisation of value" from investments (see Chapter 5 for more background on HIT governance). The comprehensive framework assists users in measuring, monitoring, and maximizing realized value from HIT investments. Rather than a simple "cookbook" approach, this framework employs a holistic approach to value realization. While not fundamentally different from the benefit–cost analysis and cost-effectiveness analysis methodologies described earlier, this framework is more attuned to practicing HIT leadership's decision making.

The IT Governance Institute approach starts by asking the following four questions, posed originally by Thorp (2003):

1. *Strategic question: Are we doing the right thing?* Is the investment aligned with a broader business vision, is it consistent with established principles, and does it contribute to the strategic objectives?

2. *Architecture question: Are we doing it the right way?* Is the investment aligned with existing information technology architecture and consistent with ongoing architecture principles?

3. *Value question: Are we getting the benefits?* Do you have a clear understanding of the expected benefits, and do you have a process for realizing the benefits?

4. *Delivery question: Are we getting it done the right way?* Do you have effective and disciplined management, delivery, and change management processes with technical and business resources to deliver the promise of the technology investment?

In the context of these four questions, the Governance Institute uses a three-part strategy to maximize return on HIT investment (the first two elements are developed in chapters 5 and 11, and the third is discussed below):

1. *Value governance.* Optimizes the value of an organization's information technology–enabled investments by establishing the governance, monitoring, and control framework; providing strategic direction for the investments; and defining the investment portfolio characteristics (see Chapter 5)

2. *Portfolio management.* Ensures that an organization's overall portfolio of information technology–enabled investments is aligned with and contributing optimal value to its strategic objectives by establishing and managing resource profiles, defining investment thresholds, evaluating and prioritizing new investments, managing the overall portfolio, and monitoring and reporting on portfolio performance (see Chapter 11)

3. *Investment management.* Ensures that HIT investments deliver outcomes at reasonable costs while also managing associated risk

To accomplish the investment management aspect of obtaining a return on HIT investment, the IT Governance Institute proposes that the organization engage in an eight-step process. In this framework, implementing the investment management process requires detailed information gathering; assessment of benefits, costs, and risks; selecting the investment vehicle; and monitoring outcomes. This process is geared to the corporate environment, as opposed to the government or social perspective. These eight steps by the IT Governance Institute (2006) are outlined in Exhibit 13.5 and detailed in the following sections.

EXHIBIT 13.5
Steps in Information Technology Business Case Development

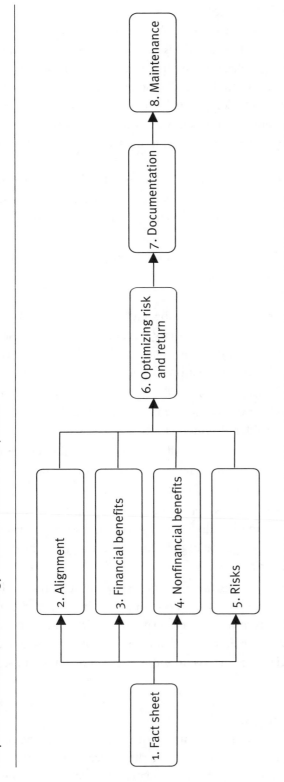

SOURCE: *Enterprise Value: Governance of IT Investments, the Business Case*, IT Governance Institute, © 2006. All rights reserved. Used by permission.

Step 1: Building the Fact Sheet

The first step in the process is to gather all of the information relevant for making the appropriate HIT business decision. The IT Governance Institute provides a model form for collecting the necessary data, but our experience suggests that each organization should implement a collection form that works in its environment. The key point is that no category of information can be ignored. At a minimum, the following categories need to be assembled (IT Governance Institute's equivalent terms are given in parentheses):

- *Congruence (Alignment)*. The investment must be consistent with documented business strategy (see Chapter 5), current HIT management practices, and government regulatory constraints (current and anticipated).
- *Business outcomes*. The investment must deliver an organizational need to achieve intermediate and final outcomes. These outcomes need to be documented and measurable.
- *Financial benefits*. Input for financial benefits should document cost savings, revenue enhancements, capacity/volume growth, and risk mitigation from the investment decision. These include the tangible revenue enhancements or cost reductions in capital, operations, or risk.
- *Indirect benefits (Nonfinancial benefits)*. As in the benefit–cost assessment, some benefits are not easily quantified in financial terms but must be seriously considered nonetheless.
- *Costs (Resources and expenditures)*. All categories of equipment, human resources, supplies, consultants, and other resources necessary for the HIT investment must be documented.
- *Sensitivity (Risk)*. Alternatives that quantify the risk in the investment must be identified. Understanding the best-case and worst-case scenarios for the investment helps the organization select an investment that meets its tolerance for risk.
4. *Model (Assumptions and constraints)*. Understanding how the HIT investment accomplishes the desired outcomes, with associated benefits and costs, helps to determine the reasonableness of the subsequent analyses. The logic of the empirical claims for outcomes, benefits, and costs depends crucially on the assumptions employed. These must be articulated clearly.

Step 2: Alignment Analysis

Investment alternatives abound, necessitating decision making. The selected option needs to optimize net benefits from the scarce resources available. Alignment helps to ensure that the HIT-related investments support the organization's strategic business objectives. This might include direct contribution to the objectives of the current organization or to the broader system or contribution to a future vision for the organization. The investment must also be consistent with existing enterprise architecture. Assuming that this architecture has been selected as a guideline to achieve the current vision, each investment must be chosen carefully so as not to move away from that guideline.

Step 3: Financial Benefits Analysis

To gain acceptance in the healthcare corporate environment, HIT investments must pass conventional financial analysis constraints. Discounting of financial benefits and costs is an essential technique. The final decision requires the project to have a positive discounted net value (positive net present value or NPV) and perhaps have better NPV than alternative investments so that the organization selects the best investment.

Step 4: Nonfinancial Benefits Analysis

The nonfinancial aspects of business processes must also be considered, especially in not-for-profit healthcare organizations. Building positive relations with constituencies external to the HIT function may create value for the organization. Alternatively, negative relations can destroy value. Consideration of the external or indirect effects of the investment may not fully offset poor financial considerations but may influence a decision that is otherwise close.

Step 5: Risk Analysis

Not every organization tolerates risk in the same way, and not all investment opportunities carry the same risks. Assessing and documenting these risks in outcomes, financial benefits, and resource use or costs are integral steps in the value-assessment process. Both delivery risk and benefits risk are inherent in any HIT investment. One must ask if the investment delivers on the anticipated business processes, human resources, technology, and organizational changes being proposed. Likewise, the outcomes and financial benefits promised may not, in fact, occur. In simple terms, the HIT investment may not perform as promised. The IT Governance Institute (2006) provides many examples of both delivery and benefits risks.

Step 6: Optimizing Risk and Return

As stated in Chapter 11, the program planning office (portfolio management office) must assess and review the HIT investment proposal in the context of other applications and broad business needs. The key is that all proposals have the same sets of information collected and reported and that assessment is done in a comparable manner. The best decision emerges if valid comparisons are made by those with the incentive to maximize value to the organization.

Step 7: Documenting Business Case

Nothing can be more important than transparency in decision making. Documentation of data and information, assessment techniques, and findings all add to the open framework for decisions. This "open architecture" helps to create a culture of critical assessment that is so important to good decision making. The tendency to not reveal information as a mechanism to protect those making the decision may lead to poorer outcomes and to greater consequences should those outcomes fail to meet standards.

Step 8: Feedback Mechanism

The single view of HIT investment value as presented by the value-realization effort is a necessary first step for healthcare organizations, but HIT investment needs, organizational priorities, staffing constraints, and other environmental changes occur continuously. The information collected, assumptions made, benefits observed, and costs incurred should be reviewed periodically throughout the lifecycle of the investment. While many decisions cannot be undone, mid-course adjustments in investment scale and scope are often possible. If the organization veers off course as a result of an investment, having a feedback mechanism enables the organization to adjust to minimize loss. CPOE provides a good example of the potential value of feedback. Faced with resistance to the widespread adoption of this technology, an organization could apply a temporary solution of implementing it in only some parts of the organization; that is, identify clinical areas or key supportive medical staff leaders and implement only in select areas. This prevents some of the resistance and presents the areas more likely to be successful. Full implementation might occur later, but the costly failure of the entire project could be avoided.

To close this discussion, a number of investigators and thought leaders have found that the methods for realizing HIT value are often difficult to implement. As Johnston, Pan, and Middleton (2002) suggest, HIT investment decisions continue to rely on "anecdote, inference, and opinion" rather than evidence. They argue that HIT leadership must support a comprehensive assessment of value using existing data. Toward that end, Bates and colleagues (2003) propose the "ten commandments" to follow for effective clinical decision support. While specifically interested in making evidence-based medicine a reality, these commandments also enhance HIT value realization. Four of the ten commandments are particularly important for HIT value and are as follows (Bates et al. 2003):

1. *Be aware that speed is everything.* Providers will not accept a system that does not respond quickly to their inquiries. System design for rapid access appears to be essential for information technology effectiveness.

2. *Fit into the user's workflow.* The HIT investment must support the providers' and other users' current practice processes to be readily accepted. They will not use a system that does not fit seamlessly.

3. *Keep in mind that simple interventions work best.* The HIT investment with grand plans to alter the practice of medicine may not be as effective as a simple solution.

4. *Monitor impact, get feedback, and respond.* The feedback mechanism appears to be essential for success. Even the best systems may not integrate in the manner anticipated; thus, being flexible and adaptable may be keys to success.

HIT Value Findings

Impact of Specific HIT Investments on Patients

Many studies have been conducted on specific HIT investment value recognition, and in this section we feature three studies that illustrate this process. A common characteristic of these studies is that they tend to report only narrow analyses of the effects of HIT investments. The desire for academic rigor results in such narrow scope. HIT managers need broader evaluations to make decisions for the organization; therefore, two additional studies report organizational value of HIT investments.

The first study, by Hillestad and colleagues (2005), presented a national simulation of the potential cost savings from HIT investments—specifically, adoption of an electronic medical record (EMR). Exhibit 13.6, from the Hillestad and colleagues study, suggested that in the near term, savings may total as much as $21.3 billion per year (year 5), more of which was derived from inpatient care than from outpatient care. Once adoption reached the anticipated 90 percent, savings could amount to more than $77 billion per year (again, more of this savings was derived from inpatient care). The savings in inpatient care came from reductions in length of stay followed by reductions in nursing time. On the outpatient side, most of the savings came from reduced/appropriate drug use.

In addition to these cost savings, benefits or value from HIT investments were derived from improved patient safety and health outcomes. Hillestad and colleagues (2005) estimated that the safety benefits of CPOE were seen at the national level for both inpatient and outpatient care. Inpatient care savings resulting from an estimated 200,000 adverse drug events (ADEs) eliminated amounted to $1 billion per year once fully implemented.

EXHIBIT 13.6
Short-Term
and Long-
Term Annual
Cost Savings
from HIT, by
Selected Major
Categories

	Short Term Year 5 (in billions)	Percent of Total	Long Term Year 15 (in billions)	Percent of Total
Outpatient				
Transcription	$ 0.4	1.9	$ 1.7	2.2
Chart pulls	$ 0.4	1.9	$ 1.5	1.9
Laboratory tests	$ 0.5	2.3	$ 2.0	2.6
Drug usage	$ 3.0	14.1	$ 11.0	14.2
Radiology	$ 0.8	3.8	$ 3.3	4.3
Total output savings	$ 5.2	24.4	$20.4	26.3
Inpatient				
Nursing time	$ 3.4	16.0	$13.7	17.7
Laboratory tests	$ 0.8	3.8	$ 2.6	3.4
Drug usage	$ 1.0	4.7	$ 3.5	4.5
Length of stay	$10.1	47.4	$34.7	44.8
Medical records	$ 0.7	3.3	$ 2.4	3.1
Total input savings	$16.1	75.6	$57.1	73.7
Total HIT savings	$21.3	100.0	$77.4	100.0

NOTE: Numbers and percentages do not sum to totals because of rounding.
SOURCE: Hillestad et al. (2005). Used with permission from Project HOPE, Milwood, Virginia.

Outpatient care savings resulting from an estimated two million ADEs avoided amounted to $3.5 billion per year. In both settings, the bulk of the study participants were older than age 65, thus the findings might not be generalizable to other participants. Featherly and colleagues (2007) also found that EMR benefits were largely indirect and came from workflow improvements and reductions in medical mishaps.

Near-term preventive care can benefit from HIT intervention as well. This study generated estimates for two vaccination programs (influenza and pneumococcal vaccinations) and three screening programs (breast cancer, cervical cancer, and colorectal cancer screenings). The findings were highly positive from a health outcome perspective and depended heavily on assumptions regarding current compliance rates in the defined population, compliance rates for the specific vaccination and screening programs, and costs. Taking the midpoints of the estimated effects, pneumococcal vaccination resulted in a median reduction of 21,000 deaths per year (15,000 to 27,000), 2.25 million median bed days eliminated (1.5 million to 3.0 million), and

150,000 median workdays restored (100,000 to 200,000). These effects came at a program cost of about $90 million per year. At the same time, however, the program generated median financial benefits estimated at $750 million per year ($500 million to $1 billion).

The second study, by Pizziferri and colleagues (2005), examined the issue of an EHR and physician clinic time with patients. The study broke time down into a number of key components so that the total time and contributing factors to any time change could be examined. Overall, Pizziferri and colleagues found no difference in time spent in direct care, indirect care (reading, writing, or other activities), administrative activities, or miscellaneous activities. From a value perspective, this is only one small consideration but an important element with regard to physician acceptance of the EMR. Pizziferri and colleagues recommended that future investigations examine the impact of the EMR on nonclinic time spent.

The third study, by Poissant and colleagues (2005), involved a comprehensive review of research examining physician and nurse documentation time as a result of implementation of an EHR. Generally, Poissant and colleagues reported that neither bedside nor central nursing station use of EHR reduced nursing documentation time by more than 20 percent. Physician documentation time increased by 17 percent for bedside technology and by more than 200 percent for central nursing station terminals. This analysis of time impact raised some significant questions regarding system impact. This study did not examine the cost of the EHR or the direct cost impact.

Consistent with the assertion that HIT leadership must reach out to the entire organization in its efforts to invest in HIT, studies are now being published that assess the value of HIT investments in terms of their impact on the organization as a whole.

Impact of HIT Investments on Organizations

Iansiti and colleagues (2005) demonstrate that HIT matters at least in mid-size firms. Their research does not measure the impact of any specific technology intervention or even overall dollars spent. It uses an index of what "IT actually does for a business" to measure impact. Iansiti and colleagues created an IT scorecard to assess HIT capability in the functional areas of sales/marketing, finance, operations, empowered professionals, and information technology infrastructure. They found that greater capability generates business process scalability, which enables firms to do the following:

- Improve process knowledge and standardization
- Streamline operations, allowing the firm to grow without expanding the labor force

- Become flexible enough to take advantage of or respond to new opportunities
- Enhance management's access to critical business indicators used in decision making

Similarly, Menachemi and colleagues (2006) demonstrate a robust relationship between HIT adoption and hospital financial performance, at least for hospitals in Florida. Their findings suggest that overall and operational improvement followed from information technology adoption. This outcome was observed for their categories of clinical, administrative, and strategic information technology.

Summary

HIT should adhere to core business processes. In that context, the decisions regarding how much and what types of HIT resources an organization uses should fall under a valuation paradigm. Finding value in any healthcare investment has proven to be a challenge, however, because data collection, methodology, and application make the use of evidence-based management difficult. Because of the complexity of the problem and the lack of comprehensive data, healthcare executives have largely been forced to make decisions about HIT investments on the basis of cursory evidence at best and occasionally on the basis of instinct or hope at worst. As a result, HIT may fall short in helping to address the problems plaguing healthcare.

The median hospital spent at least $6,300 per bed on HIT in 2011. From a HIT leadership perspective, however, HIT is essential for the provision of high-quality care in today's environment, so they must face the decision to invest in HIT. Many factors make such decisions difficult, including the scaling of information technology and the systems nature of information technology. For example, technology acquisition is not an all-or-nothing proposition; questions of scale, scope, application, integration, and timing are involved. The interdependence of providers in a healthcare "system" complicates the decision further. Healthcare delivery organizations implement interoperable EHRs to enable the exchange of information across venues while still focusing on value creation.

Early evidence from HIT investment studies indicates that EHRs, HIEs, clinical decision support systems, and a host of other technologies have the potential to improve care and contain or lower costs. However, value has not been identified and the potential benefits may be less than estimated. Furthermore, not all HIT leaders are yet fully behind HIT implementation. Providers will come to expect electronic information exchange as they increasingly work in teams that require a real-time exchange of information. The incentives offered by the HITECH Act are intended to encourage widespread adoption of HIE and other HIT technologies, but impediments still exist. The 2012 HIMSS survey data suggested that many HIT leaders face barriers and remain reluctant to facilitating or implementing an HIE.

Business decisions faced by the CIO—and indirectly by the CEO and board—come down to a challenge of deciding among competing alternatives, leading to the evaluation challenge. The questions that must be asked are whether the HIT investment increases or decreases organizational outcomes, and whether it increases or decreases costs to the organization. Economists have frameworks for assisting in making these decisions, called benefit–cost analyses, cost-effectiveness analyses, and cost–utility analyses. Further, business models suggest a similar evaluation process for value realization that consists of conceptualizing, capturing, analyzing, and reporting detailed financial and nonfinancial information. In addition, the IT Governance Institute (2006) has developed a detailed value-realization process that can direct HIT leadership to achieve their goals.

A number of challenges hinder the efforts to maximize the value of HIT investments, including lack of proper, detailed documentation of key information and conceptual problems of assigning benefits and costs to a particular investment. These investments garner benefits from and impose costs throughout the organization, thus posing problems of assignment to uniquely evaluate the net effect of any single investment. These effects are now extending even outside of the confines of the traditional organizational entity. Obtaining that data and generating reliable estimates of net value are problematic at best.

Web Resources

A number of organizations (through their websites) provide more information on the topics discussed in this chapter:

- Blue Cross and Blue Shield's Technology Evaluation Center (www.bcbs.com/betterknowledge/tec/) and University HealthSystem Consortium (www.uhc.edu). These websites provide information on cost analyses for healthcare technologies.
- Center for Information Technology Leadership (www.citl.org). This website provides specific HIT intervention evaluations.
- Centers for Disease Control and Prevention's Health-Related Quality of Life (www.cdc.gov/hrqol/index.htm). This website provides quality-of-life measurements.

Discussion Questions

1. Explain why obtaining value from HIT investments is so important in today's healthcare environment.

2. How valid and reliable do you think HIT investment decisions are currently? Why?

3. What is the system nature of healthcare, and why does it affect value estimation?

4. What do you think will drive adoption of interoperable EHRs—cost savings or consumer preferences? Why?

5. What is the evaluation problem faced by HIT investment decision makers? Why does the matrix in Exhibit 13.2 help in understanding that problem?

6. Why do we not observe examples of all of the cells in Exhibit 13.2?

7. Compare and contrast benefit–cost, cost-effectiveness, and cost–utility analyses. Which do you prefer, and why?

8. List and assess the eight steps in conducting benefit–cost analysis, cost-effectiveness analysis, or cost–utility analysis.

9. What is value realization? In what ways is it similar to and different from economic evaluation techniques?

10. Explain the four questions proposed by the IT Governance Institute, and explain why they are important.

11. Describe how the nature of the HIT investment application affects the quality and nature of the value determination.

REFERENCES

Adams, J., E. Mounib, A. Pai, N. Stuart, R. Thomas, and P. Tomaszewicz. 2007. "Healthcare 2015: Win–Win or Lose–Lose? A Portrait and a Path to Successful Transformation." IBM Global Business Services, IBM Institute for Business Value. Accessed January 4, 2008. www-931.ibm.com/tela/servlet/Asset/169464/Healthcare2015-Win-win_or_lose-lose.pdf.

Agarwal, R., and V. Sambamurthy. 2002. "Principles and Models for Organizing the IT Function." *MIS Quarterly Executive* 1 (1): 1–16.

Agency for Healthcare Research and Quality (AHRQ). 2005. AHRQ Archives, Electronic Newsletter. Published October 14, 2005, Issue #181. http://archive.ahrq.gov/news/enews/enews181.htm.

———. 2004. "Secretary Announces New Health Information Technology Strategic Framework." Published July. www.ahrq.gov/about/hitframe.htm.

Al-Haddad, M., J. Friedlin, J. Kesterson, J. Waters, J. Aguilar-Saavedra, and C. Schmidt. 2010. "Natural Language Processing for the Development of a Clinical Registry: A Validation Study in Intraductal Papillary Mucinous Neoplasms." *The Official Journal of the International Hepato Pancreato Biliary Association* 12 (10): 688–95.

Amatayakul, M. 2007. "Managing Information Privacy & Security in Healthcare: Setting Standards in Healthcare Information." HIMSS Privacy and Security Toolkit. Published January 1. www.himss.org/content/files/CPRIToolkit/version6/v7/D09_Setting_Standards_in_Healthcare_Information.pdf.

American College of Healthcare Executives (ACHE). 2008. "Access to Healthcare." Policy statement. Approved by the Board of Governors of the American College of Healthcare Executives, November 10, 2008. www.ache.org/policy/access.cfm.

American Hospital Association (AHA). 2010. "Detailed Summary of 2010 Health Care Reform Legislation." Legislative Advisory, April 19. Chicago: AHA.

———. 2007. *Continued Progress: Hospital Use of Information Technology.* Chicago: American Hospital Association.

American Medical Association (AMA). 2006. *Preliminary Report on the American Medical Association Initiative to Transform Medical Education.* Accessed June 28, 2007. www.ama-assn.org/ama1/pub/upload/mm/377/2006results.pdf.

American National Standards Institute (ANSI). 2005. "New Healthcare Information Technology Standards Panel Formed Under Contract from DHHS." News and Publications. Published October 6. www.ansi.org/news_publications /news_story.aspx?menuid=7&articleid=1054.

Anderson, G., B. Frogner, R. Johns, and U. Reinhardt. 2006. "Health Care Spending and Use of Information Technology in OECD Countries." *Health Affairs* 25 (3): 819–31.

Anderson, B., and D. Peris. 2007. "Capacity Management of Computer Resources Through Performance Analysis." ISACA. Accessed May 4. www.isaca.org /Content/ContentGroups/InfoBytes/19981/Capacity_Management_of _Computing_Resources_Through_Performance_Analysis.htm.

Anton, J. 2001. *Call Center Performance Benchmark Report.* No. 1347. West Lafayette, IN: Purdue Research Foundation.

Appari, A., E. Carian, E. Johnson, and D. Anthony. 2012. "Medication Administration Quality and Health Information Technology: A National Study of US Hospitals." *Journal of the American Medical Informatics Association* 19: 360–67.

Applied Health Informatics Learning and Assessment. n.d. "IT Leader: Macro Roles and Competencies." Accessed March 22, 2013. www.nihi.ca/hi/ahimacro roles.php?id=1&MenuItemID=5.

Aron, D., and L. Pogach. 2009. "Transparency Standards for Diabetes Performance Measures." *Journal of the American Medical Association* 301: 210–12.

Arrow, K. 1963. "Uncertainty and the Welfare Economics of Medical Care." *American Economic Review* 52: 941–73.

Asch, D., J. Hershey, and P. Ubel. 2003. "How Physicians React to Cost-Effectiveness Information." *LDI Issue Brief* 8 (9).

Ash, J. S., D. F. Sittig, E. G. Poon, K. Guappone, E. Campbell, and R. H. Dykstra. 2007. "The Extent and Importance of Unintended Consequences Related to Computerized Provider Order Entry." *Journal of the American Medical Informatics Association* 14 (4): 415–23.

Austin, C. J., K. D. Hornberger, and J. E. Shmerling. 2000. "Managing Information Resources: A Study of Ten Healthcare Organizations." *Journal of Healthcare Management* 45 (4): 229–39.

Austin, C. J., J. M. Trimm, and P. M. Sobczak. 1995. "Information Systems and Strategic Management." *Health Care Management Review* 20 (3): 26–33.

Ayanian, J. Z., J. S. Weissman, E. C. Schneider, J. A. Ginsburg, and A. M. Zaslavsky. 2000. "Unmet Health Needs of Uninsured Adults in the United States." *Journal of the American Medical Association* 284 (16): 2061–69.

Babitch, L. A. 2009. "Solving the Interoperability Puzzle: A Guide to Data Interchange Between Hospitals and Physician Practices." *Journal of Medical Practice Management* 24 (6): 372–75.

Baicker, K., and A. Chandra. 2004. "Medicare Spending, the Physician Workforce, and Beneficiaries' Quality of Care." *Health Affairs.* Accessed June 20, 2012. http://content.healthaffairs.org/content/early/2004/04/07/hlthaff.w4 .184.short.

Baron, R. 2007. "Quality Improvement with an Electronic Health Record: Achievable, but Not Automatic." *Annals of Internal Medicine* 147: 549–52.

Baschab, J., and J. Piot. 2003. *The Executive's Guide to Information Technology.* Hoboken, NJ: John Wiley and Sons.

Bates, D. W., G. J. Kuperman, S. Wang, T. Gandhi, A. Kittler, L. Volk, C. Spurr, R. Khorasani, M. Tanasijevic, and B. Middleton. 2003. "Ten Commandments for Effective Clinical Decision Support: Making the Practice of Evidence-Based Medicine a Reality." *Journal of the American Medical Informatics Association* 10 (6): 523–30.

Bates, D., L. Leape, D. Cullen, N. Laird, L. Petersen, J. Teich, E. Burdick, M. Hickey, S. Kleefield, B. Shea, M. Vander Vliet, and D. Seger. 1998. "Effect of Computerized Physician Order Entry and a Team Intervention on Prevention of Serious Medication Errors." *Journal of the American Medical Association* 280 (15): 1311–16.

Baucus, M. 2005. "Looking at the U.S. Healthcare System in the Rear-View Mirror." *Health Affairs* Web Exclusives. Published November 16. http://content .healthaffairs.org/cgi/content/abstract /hlthaff.w5.544v1.

Beeler, G. W. 2001. "The Crucial Role of Standards." *Healthcare Informatics* 18 (2): 98–104.

Bell, K. 2012. "From the Chair: Evaluating HIT Beyond EHR Certification." *Electronic Health Record Information and News.* Published November 19. Accessed April 7, 2013. http://ehrdecisions.com/.

Berner, E., and T. La Lande. 2007. "Overview of Clinical Decision Support Systems." In *Clinical Decision Support Systems*, 2nd ed., edited by E. Berner. New York: Springer.

Berner, E. S., T. K. Houston, M. N. Ray, J. J. Allison, G. R. Heudebert, W. W. Chatham, J. I. Kennedy, G. L. Glandon, P. A. Norton, M. A. Crawford, and R. D. Maisiak. 2006. "Improving Ambulatory Prescribing Safety with a Handheld Decision Support System: A Randomized Controlled Trial." *Journal of the American Medical Informatics Association* 13 (2): 171–79.

Bigalke, J., B. Copeland, and P. Keckley. 2011. "I'm OK, You're OK . . . But Will We Be All Right?" Deloitte Review 9. Accessed December 14. http:// dupress.com/articles/im-ok-youre-ok-but-will-we-be-all-right-innovations -in-addressing-health-care-reform/?ind=0.

Black, A., J. Car, C. Pagliari, C. Anandan, K. Cresswell, T. Bokun, B. McKinstry, R. Procter, A. Majeed, and A. Sheikh. 2011. "The Impact of eHealth on the Quality and Safety of Health Care: A Systematic Overview." *PLoS Medicine* 8 (1): e1000387.

Blanchet, K. 2005. "Innovative Programs in Telemedicine." *Telemedicine and e-Health* 11 (2): 116–23.

Blitstein, R. 2012. "IT Governance: Bureaucratic Logjam or Business Enabler? Business Technology Strategies." *Executive Update* 15 (10): 1–3.

Blumenthal, D. 2006. *Health Information Technology: What Is the Federal Government's Role?* The Commonwealth Fund Commission on a High Performance Health System #907. New York: Commonwealth Fund.

Blumenthal, D., and M. Tavenner. 2010. "The 'Meaningful Use' Regulation for Electronic Health Records." *New England Journal of Medicine* 363 (6): 501–04.

Board, A. 2004. *Prioritizing IT Investments: Toward a Disciplined Approach amid Heightened Competition for Capital.* New York: Advisory Board Company.

Book, E. L. 2005. "Health Insurance Trends Are Contributing to Growing Healthcare Inequality." *Health Affairs* Web Exclusives. Published December 6. http://content.healthaffairs.org/cgi/content/abstract/hlthaff.w5.577v1.

Bossidy, L., and R. Charan. 2002. *Execution: The Discipline of Getting Things Done.* New York: Crown Business.

Bower, A. 2005. *The Diffusion and Value of Healthcare Information Technology.* Santa Monica, CA: Rand Corporation.

Boyd, D., and N. Ellison. 2007. "Social Network Sites: Definition, History, and Scholarship." *Journal of Computer-Mediated Communication* 13: 210–30.

Boyd, J. 2005. "The Grass Is Greener? Outsourcing and the Merits of Marriage." In *The CEO–CIO Partnership: Harnessing the Value of Information Technology in Healthcare,* edited by D. Smaltz, J. Glaser, R. Skinner, and T. Cunningham III. Chicago: Healthcare Information and Management Systems Society.

Bradley, C., D. Neumark, L. Shickle, and N. Farrell. 2008. "Differences in Breast Cancer Diagnosis and Treatment: Experiences of Insured and Uninsured Women in a Safety Net Setting." *Inquiry* 45 (3): 323–39.

Breen, C., and L. M. Rodrigues. 2001. "Implementing a Data Warehouse at Inglis Innovative Services." *Journal of Healthcare Information Management* 15 (2): 87–97.

Briggs, B. 2002. "Is the Future in the Palm of Your Hand?" *Health Data Management* 10 (1): 44–62.

Broadbent, M., and E. Kitzis. 2005. *The New CIO Leader: Setting the Agenda and Delivering Results.* Boston: Harvard Business School Press.

Brown, A., and G. Grant. 2005. "Framing the Frameworks: A Review of IT Governance Research." *Communication of the Association for Information Systems* 15: 696–712.

Brynjolfsson, E., and L. Hitt. 2000. "Beyond Computation: Information Technology, Organizational Transformation and Business Performance." *Journal of Economic Perspectives* 14 (4): 23–48.

Buntin, M., M. Burke, M. Hoaglin, and D. Blumenthal. 2011. "The Benefits of Information Technology: A Review of the Recent Literature Shows Predominantly Positive Results." *Health Affairs* 30 (3): 464–71.

Bush, G. 2006. "Executive Order: Promoting Quality and Efficient Health Care in Federal Government Administered or Sponsored Health Care Programs."

Published August 22. http://georgewbush-whitehouse.archives.gov/news
/releases/2006/08/20060822-2.html.

Carpenter, R. 2005. "IT Governance." Guest lecture, presented to the University of
Alabama at Birmingham, January 8.

Carr, N. 2003. "IT Doesn't Matter." *Harvard Business Review* 81 (5): 41–49.

Center for Organization, Leadership, and Management Research. 2006. "A Paradigm Shift for Managers and Researchers: Evidence-Based Management."
Accessed December 28, 2007. www.colmr.research.va.gov/mgmt_research
_in_va/framework/evidence.cfm.

Centers for Medicare & Medicaid Services (CMS). n.d.(a). "Medicare and Medicaid
EHR Incentive Program Basics." Updated January 30, 2013. www.cms.gov
/Regulations-and-Guidance/Legislation/EHRIncentivePrograms/Basics
.html.

———. n.d.(b). "HIPAA—General Information." Accessed December 1, 2011. www
.cms.gov.

———. n.d.(c). "Medicare Inpatient Hospital Dashboard." www.cms.gov/Research
-Statistics-Data-and-Systems/Statistics-Trends-and-Reports/Dashboard
/CMS-Dashboard-Medicare-Inpatient-Hospital-Dashboard.html?agree=yes.

———. 2013. "Data and Data Programs." Modified April 4. www.cms.gov/Regula
tions-and-Guidance/Legislation/EHRIncentivePrograms/DataAndReports
.html.

———. 2012a. "Accountable Care Organizations (ACOs): General Information."
Center for Medicare & Medicaid Innovation. Accessed April 2012. www
.innovations.cms.gov/initiatives/ACO/index.html.

———. 2012b. "National Health Expenditure Tables: Historical." Accessed Janu-
ary 9, 2013. www.cms.gov/Research-Statistics-Data-and-Systems/Statistics
-Trends-and-Reports/NationalHealthExpendData/NationalHealthAccounts
Historical.html.

———. 2010a. *Medicare and Medicaid EHR Incentive Program: Meaningful
Use Stage 1 Requirements Overview.* Accessed May 15. www.cms.gov/Reg
ulations-and-Guidance/Legislation/EHRIncentivePrograms/Downloads
/MU_Stage1_ReqOverview.pdf.

———. 2010b. "Flow Chart: Determine Eligibility for Medicare and Medicaid
Electronic Health Record (EHR) Incentive Programs." Published Sep-
tember. www.cms.gov/MLNProducts/Downloads/Eligibility_Flow_Chart
-ICN905343.pdf.

———. 2005a. "HIPAA: Overview." Accessed January 2, 2008. www.cms.hhs.gov
/HIPAAGenInfo/01_Overview.asp.

———. 2005b. "Health Insurance Portability and Accountability Act of 1996:
Summary of Administrative Simplification Provisions." Accessed January 2,
2008. www.cms.hhs.gov/HIPAAGenInfo/Downloads/SummaryofAdminis
trativeSimplificationProvisions.pdf.

———. 2005c. "National Provider Identifier Activities Begin in 2005." Accessed January 2, 2008. www.cms.hhs.gov/NationalProvIdentStand/Downloads /NPIdearprovider.pdf.

———. 2005d. "Transactions and Code Sets Regulations." Accessed January 2, 2008. www.cms.hhs.gov/TransactionCodeSetsStands/.

———. 2005e. "Privacy Act of 1974: Overview." Accessed January 2, 2008. www .cms.hhs.gov/PrivacyActof1974/.

Chan, K., J. Fowles, and J. Weiner. 2010. "Electronic Health Records and Reliability and Validity of Quality Measures: A Review of the Literature." *Medical Care Research and Review* 67 (5): 503–27.

Chaudhry, B., J. Wang, S. Wu, M. Maglione, W. Mojica, E. Roth, S. C. Morton, and P. G. Shekelle. 2006. "Systematic Review: Impact of Health Information Technology on Quality, Efficiency and Costs of Medical Care." *Annals of Internal Medicine* 144 (10): 742–52.

Chesney, J. 2005. "IT Contracts, Negotiation, and Outsourcing: Let's Make a Deal." Seminar in Healthcare Administration Executive Program, University of Alabama at Birmingham, January 14.

Chin, T. 2003. "Doctors Pull Plug on Paperless System." *AMNews*. Published February 17. www.ama-assn.org/amednews/2003/02/17/bil20217.htm.

Ciccolini, C., and M. McDermott. 2005. "Leveraging the ITIL Service Support Framework." ITSM Watch. Accessed August 23, 2012. www.itsmwatch .com/itil/article.php/3348501/Leveraging-the-ITIL-Service-Support -Framework.htm.

Ciotti, V., and T. Birch. 2005. "How Does Your IT Department Stack Up?" *Healthcare Financial Management* 59 (1): 44–49.

Clancy, C., and J. Eisenberg. 1998. "Outcomes Research: Measuring the End Results of Healthcare." *Science* 282 (5387): 245–46.

Clarke, L. 2004. "What's the Plan?" *Harvard Business Review* 82 (6): 21–22.

College of Healthcare Information Management Education (CHIME). 2013. "CHIME CIO Compensation Survey Reveals Base Salary and Reimbursement Influencers for Healthcare's Top IT Executives." Accessed March 28. www.cio-chime.org/chime/press/surveys/pdf/CHIME_2012_CIO_Salary _Survey_Report.pdf.

Collen, M. F. 1995. *A History of Medical Informatics in the United States: 1950–1990.* Indianapolis, IN: BooksCraft, Inc.

Collins, S., and K. Davis. 2006. "Transparency in Health Care: The Time Has Come." The Commonwealth Fund. Published March 15. www.common wealthfund.org/Publications/Testimonies/2006/Mar/Transparency-in-Health-Care--The-Time-Has-Come.aspx.

Commonwealth Fund. 2006. *Why Not the Best? Results from a National Scorecard on US Health System Performance.* Commonwealth Fund Commission on a High Performance Health System. New York: Commonwealth Fund.

Conn, J. 2007. "IT Guru Says Some E-vendor Contracts Violate Privacy." *Modern Healthcare.* Accessed January 10, 2008. www.modernhealthcare.com/apps /pbcs.dll/article?AID=/20070719/FREE/70719007/0/FRONTPAGE.

Cooke-Davies, T., L. Crawford, and T. Lechler. 2009. "Project Management Systems: Moving Project Management from an Operational to a Strategic Discipline." *Project Management Journal* 40 (1): 110–23.

Coplan, S., and D. Masuda. 2011. *Project Management for Healthcare Information Technology.* New York: McGraw-Hill Company.

Cuellar, A., and P. Gertler. 2003. "Trends in Hospital Consolidation: The Formation of Local Systems." *Health Affairs* 22 (6): 77–87.

Cummings, L. A., and R. Magnusson. 2001. "Genetic Privacy and Academic Medicine: The Oregon Experience." *Academic Medicine* 76 (11): 1089–93.

Cutler, D. M., A. B. Rosen, and S. Vijan. 2006. "The Value of Medical Spending in the United States, 1960–2000." *New England Journal of Medicine* 355 (9): 920–27.

Davenport, T., and L. Prusak. 1998. *Working Knowledge.* Boston: Harvard Business School Press.

Davis, D., and K. Having. 2006. "Compliance with HIPAA Security Standards in U.S. Hospitals." *Journal of Healthcare Information Management* 20 (2): 108–15.

Davis, K., C. Schoen, S. Schoenbaum, A. M. Audet, M. Doty, and K. Tenney. 2004. *Mirror, Mirror on the Wall: Looking at the Quality of American Healthcare Through the Patient's Lens.* Report no. 683 (January). New York: Commonwealth Fund.

Davis, M. 2009. *The State of U.S. Hospitals Relative to Achieving Meaningful Use Measurements.* Chicago: HIMSS Analytics.

Davis, M. A., and R. J. Pavur. 2011. "The Relationship Between Office System Tools and Evidence-Based Care in Primary Care Physician Practice." *Health Services Management Research* 24 (3): 107–13.

De Angelo, M. 2000. "Internet Solution Provides Important Component in Reducing Medical Errors." *Health Management Technology* 21 (2): 20–21.

DeFord, D., and D. Porter. 2005. "To Centralize or Decentralize? That Is the Question." In *The CEO–CIO Partnership: Harnessing the Value of Information Technology in Healthcare,* edited by D. Smaltz, J. Glaser, R. Skinner, and T. Cunningham III. Chicago: Healthcare Information and Management Systems Society.

Deloitte Center for Health Solutions. 2007. "Health Care Price Transparency: A Strategic Perspective for State Government Leaders." Accessed October 2012. www.deloitte.com/assets/Dcom-UnitedStates/Local%20Assets/Doc uments/us_chs_pricetransparency_031307.pdf.

DeNavas-Walt, C., B. Proctor, and J. Smith. 2012. *Income, Poverty, and Health Insurance Coverage in the United States: 2011.* Washington, DC: US Census Bureau. Also available at www.census.gov/prod/2012pubs/p60-243.pdf.

———. 2011. *Income, Poverty, and Health Insurance Coverage in the United States: 2010.* Washington, DC: US Census Bureau.

Denis, D. 2001. "Twenty-Five Years of Corporate Governance Research . . . and Counting." *Review of Financial Economics* 10 (3): 191–212.

Diamond, D. 2012. "How Wal-Mart May Have Just Changed the Game on Health Care." *California Healthline.* Published October 17. www.californiahealth line.org/road-to-reform/2012/how-wal-mart-may-have-just-changed-the -game-on-health-care.aspx.

Diamond, G., and S. Kaul. 2008. "The Disconnect Between Practice Guidelines and Clinical Practice—Stressed Out." *Journal of the American Medical Association* 300 (15): 1817–19.

Dick, R. S., E. B. Steen, and D. E. Detmer (eds.). 1997. *The Computer-Based Patient Record: An Essential Technology for Health Care,* revised edition. Washington, DC: National Academies Press.

Doheny, K. 2009. "Deadly Medical Errors Still Plague the U.S." WebMD. Published May 19. www.webmd.com/healthy-aging/news/20090519/deadly-medical -errors-still-plague-us.

Dolan, T. G. 2006. "Contracting for ASP Services: When Signing On for the Benefits, Remember to Manage the Risks." *Journal of AHIMA* 77 (5): 48–50.

Donabedian, A. (ed.). 2002. *An Introduction to Quality Assurance in Health Care.* Cambridge, MA: Oxford University Press.

———. 1988. "The Quality of Care: How Can It Be Assessed?" *Journal of the American Medical Association* 260: 1743–48.

———. 1980. *The Definition of Quality and Approaches to Its Assessment.* Ann Arbor, MI: Health Administration Press.

———. 1966. "Evaluating the Quality of Medical Care." *The Milbank Memorial Fund Quarterly* 44 (3): 166–206.

Doolan, D., and D. Bates. 2002. "Computerized Physician Order Entry Systems in Hospitals: Mandates and Incentives." *Health Affairs* 21 (4): 180–88.

Dorenfest Institute for HIT Research and Education. 2006. *The Financial Systems Hospital IT Market, 1998–2005.* Chicago: HIMSS Foundation.

Downing, G. J., S. N. Boyle, S. M. Brinner, and J. A. Osheroff. 2009. "Information Management to Enable Personalized Medicine: Stakeholder Roles in Building Clinical Decision Support." *BMC Medical Informatics and Decision Making* 9 (44): doi: 10.1186/1472-6947-9-44.

Dunn, R. 2006. "A Quick Scan of Bar Coding." *Journal of AHIMA* 77 (1): 50–54.

Edwards, A., I. Hollin, J. Barry, and S. Kachnowski. 2010. "Barriers to Cross-Institutional Health Information Exchange: A Literature Review." *Journal of Healthcare Information Management* 23 (3): 22–34.

Egleson, N., J. H. Kang, D. Collymore, W. Esmond, L. Gonzalez, P. Pong, and L. Sherman. 2010. "A Health Center Controlled Network's Experience in Ambulatory Care EHR Implementation." *Journal of Health Information Management* 24 (2): 28–33.

Elliott, V. 2012. "Large Companies Try Domestic Medical Tourism." Amednews .com. Published January 9. www.ama-assn.org/amednews/2012/01/09/bis b0109.htm.

Ellwood, P. M. 2003. "Crossing the Health Policy Chasm: Pathways to Healthy Outcomes." Accessed December 28, 2007. www.ppionline.org/ppi_ci.cfm ?knlgAreaID=111&subsecID=138&contentID=251324.

EMRapproved.com. 2012. "Selecting an EMR or HIT Consulting Service." Accessed November 11. www.emrapproved.com/emr-consulting-services.php.

Encinosa, W., and J. Bae. 2011. "Health Information Technology and Its Effects on Hospital Costs, Outcomes, and Patient Safety." *Inquiry* 48 (4): 288–303.

Engel, M. 2007. "Mix-Up Breaches Confidentiality of Dozens in State AIDS Program." *Los Angeles Times,* March 3.

Enthoven, A. C., and S. J. Singer. 1996. "Managed Competition and California's Health Care Economy." *Health Affairs* 15 (1): 39–57.

Enthoven, A., and L. Tollen. 2005. "Competition in Health Care: It Takes Systems to Pursue Quality and Efficiency." *Health Affairs* Web Exclusive (W5-420-433). Accessed January 4, 2008. http://content.healthaffairs.org/cgi/con tent/abstract/hlthaff.w5.420.

Epipheo Studios. n.d. "What Is Google Chrome?" Accessed June 6, 2012. www .youtube.com/watch?v=0QRO3gKj3qw.

Evans, R., S. Pestotnik, D. Classen, T. Clemmer, L. Weaver, J. Orme, J. Lloyd, and J. Burke. 1998. "A Computer-Assisted Management Program for Antibiotics and Other Antiinfective Agents." *New England Journal of Medicine* 338 (4): 232–38.

Families USA. 2012. Dying *for Coverage: The Deadly Consequences of Being Uninsured.* New York: Families USA.

Farah, J. 2004. "Taking the Complexity Out of Release Management." *CM Crossroads.* Accessed April 25, 2007. www.cmcrossroads.com/content/view/6741 /135/.

Farkas, D., A. Greenbaum, V. Singhal, and J. Cosgrove. 2012. "Effect of Insurance Status on the Stage of Breast and Colorectal Cancers in a Safety-Net Hospital." *The American Journal of Managed Care* 18 (2): SP65–SP70.

Featherly, K., D. Garets, M. Davis, P. Wise, and P. Becker. 2007. "Sharpening the Case for Returns on Investment from Clinical Information Systems." *Healthcare Quarterly* 10 (1): 101–10.

Federal Communications Commission (FCC). 2012. "Findings and Recommendations: Improving Care Delivery Through Enhanced Communications Among Providers, Patients and Payers." mHealth Task Force. Draft published September 4. www2.itif.org/2012-mhealth-taskforce-recommendations.pdf.

Feinson, C. 2004. "Current Issues in Access to Healthcare." Medscape Public Health, Medscape Education. Accessed June 2012. www.medscape.org /viewarticle/466706.

Feldstein, P. J. 2001. *The Politics of Health Legislation: An Economic Perspective.* Chicago: Health Administration Press.

Ferranti, M. 2007. "Head of IT Finance." *CIO Magazine* 20: 16.

Field, T. 1998. "Shop Talk: Goodyear's Debra Walker on Leveraging Business-Side Experience in IS." *CIO Magazine* (11) 16: 80.

Finkelstein, S. M., S. M. Speedie, X. Zhou, S. Potthoff, and E. R. Ratner. 2011. "Perception, Satisfaction, and Utilization of the VALUE Home Telehealth Service." *Journal of Telemedicine and Telecare* 17: doi: 10.1258/jtt.2011.101208.

Fisher, E., J. Bynum, and J. Skinner. 2009. "Slowing the Growth of Health Care Costs—Lessons from Regional Variation." *New England Journal of Medicine* 360: 849–52.

Fisher, E., D. Wennberg, T. Stukel, D. Gottlieb, F. Lucas, and E. Pinder. 2003. "The Implications of Regional Variations in Medicare Spending. Part 1: The Content, Quality, and Accessibility of Care." *Annals of Internal Medicine* 138: 273–87.

Flores, J. A., and A. Dodier. 2005. "HIPAA: Past, Present, and Future Implications for Nurses." *Online Journal of Issues in Nursing* 10 (2): 5.

Ford, E., N. Menachemi, and M. Phillips. 2009. "Resistance Is Futile: But It Is Slowing the Pace of EHR Adoption Nonetheless." *Journal of the American Medical Informatics Association* 16 (3): 274–81.

———. 2006. "Predicting the Adoption of Electronic Health Records by Physicians: When Will Healthcare Be Paperless?" *Journal of the American Medical Informatics Association* 13 (1): 106–12.

Ford, E., N. Menachemi, T. Huerta, and F. Yu. 2010. "Hospital IT Adoption Strategies Associated with Implementation Success: Implications for Achieving Meaningful Use." *Journal of Healthcare Management* 55 (3): 175–88.

Gabler, J. M. 2001. "Linking Business Values to IT Investments." *Health Management Technology* 22 (2): 76–77.

Gamble, K. 2012. "healthsystemCIO.com Survey Says CIOs Just Want to Be Players, No Matter Who's Boss." healthsystemCIO.com. Accessed September 18. http://healthsystemcio.com/2012/09/26/healthsystemcio-com-survey.

Ganguly, S., P. Kataria, R. Juric, A. Ertas, and M. M. Tanik. 2009. "Sharing Information and Data Across E-Health Systems." *Telemedicine and e-Health* 15 (5): doi: 10.1089/tmj.2008.0149.

Garets, D., and M. Davis. 2006. "Electronic Medical Records vs. Electronic Health Records: Yes There Is a Difference." A HIMSS Analytics™ White Paper. Accessed May 17, 2012. www.himssanalytics.org/docs/WP_EMR_EHR.pdf.

Garets, D., and R. Lazerow. 2012. "An IT Blueprint for Accountable Care: Assessing the IT Implications for Emerging Payment Models." Healthcare Information and Management Systems Society Annual Conference, Las Vegas, Nevada, February 20.

Garg, A., N. Adhikari, H. McDonald, P. Rosas-Arellano, P. Devereaux, J. Beyene, J. Sam, and R. Haynes. 2005. "Effects of Computerized Clinical Decision Support Systems on Practitioner Performance and Patient Outcomes." *Journal of the American Medical Association* 293 (10): 1223–38.

Gartner, Inc. 2001. "Describing the Capability Maturity Model." Accessed February 9, 2007. www.e-strategy.ubc.ca/_shared/assets/MeasureIT-Gartners CMMmodel1278.pdf.

Gauthier, A., and M. Serber. 2005. *A Need to Transform the U.S. Healthcare System: Improving Access, Quality, and Efficiency.* New York: Commonwealth Fund.

Gawande, A. 2010. "Now What?" Talk of the Town column. *New Yorker.* Accessed April 21, 2011. www.newyorker.com/talk/comment/2010/04/05/1004 05taco_talk_gawande.

———. 2009. "The Cost Conundrum." *New Yorker,* June 1. Also available at www .newyorker.com/reporting/2009/06/01/090601fa_fact_gawande.

Gilchrist, J., M. Frize, E. Bariciak, and D. Townsend. 2008. "Integration of New Technology in a Legacy System for Collecting Medical Data—Challenges and Lessons Learned." *Engineering in Medicine and Biology Society, Conference Proceedings Annual International Conference of the IEEE* (1557-170X). doi: 10.1109/IEMBS.2008.4650167.

Gillespie, G. 2001. "Wireless Catching Up, Catching On in Health Care." *Health Data Management* 9 (8): 26–34.

Gilmer, T., and R. Kronick. 2005. "It's the Premiums, Stupid: Projections of the Uninsured Through 2013." *Health Affairs* Web Exclusives. Accessed January 4, 2008. http://content.healthaffairs.org/cgi/reprint/hlthaff.w5.43v1?max toshow=&HITS=10&hits=10&RESULTFORMAT=&author1=Gilmer&and orexactfulltext=and&searchid=1&FIRSTINDEX=0&resourcetype=HWCIT.

Ginsburg, P. B. 2005. "Competition in Healthcare: Its Evolution Over the Past Decade." *Health Affairs (Millwood)* 24 (6): 1512–22.

Glandon, G. L., and T. Buck. 1994. "Cost–Benefit Analysis of Medical Information Systems: A Critique." In *Evaluating Health Care Information Systems: Methods and Applications,* edited by J. Anderson, C. Aydin, and S. Jay. Thousand Oaks, CA: Sage Publications.

Glandon, G. L., and R. J. Shapiro. 1988. "Benefit–Cost Analysis of Hospital Information Systems: The State of the (Non) Art." *Journal of Health & Human Resources Administration* 11 (1): 30–92.

Glaser, J. 2002. *The Strategic Application of Information Technology in Health Care Organizations,* 2nd ed. San Francisco: Jossey-Bass.

Glaser, J., and D. Garets. 2005. "Where's the Beef? Part 1: Getting Value from Your IT Investments." In *The CEO–CIO Partnership: Harnessing the Value of Information Technology in Healthcare,* edited by D. Smaltz, J. Glaser, R. Skinner, and T. Cunningham III. Chicago: Healthcare Information and Management Systems Society.

Goedert, J. 2004. "How to Select the Right Consulting Firm." *HealthData Management*. Published August 1. www.healthdatamanagement.com/issues/2004 0801/10036-1.html?zkPrintable=1&nopagination=1.

Gold, M., J. Siegel, L. Russell, and M. Weinstein. 1996. *Cost-Effectiveness in Health and Medicine*. New York: Oxford University Press.

Goldman, D., and E. McGlynn. 2005. *U.S. Health Care: Facts About Cost, Access and Quality*. Santa Monica, CA: Rand Corporation.

Goldsmith, J. A. 1980. "The Healthcare Market: Can Hospitals Survive?" *Harvard Business Review* 58 (5): 100–12.

Goldsmith, J., D. Blumenthal, and W. Rishel. 2003. "Federal Health Information Policy: A Case of Arrested Development." *Health Affairs (Millwood)* 22 (4): 44–55.

Gostin, L. O., J. G. Hodge, and R. O. Valdiserri. 2001. "Informational Privacy and the Public's Health: The Model State Public Health Privacy Act." *American Journal of Public Health* 91 (9): 1388–92.

Gottlieb, D. F. 2010. "Regulatory Compliance: The Regulatory Framework for Qualifying EHR Donations." *Healthcare Informatics* 27 (7): 36–39.

Grajek, S., and W. Cunningham. 2007. *ITIL: An Effective Methodology of Managing IT Services*. EDUCAUSE Annual Conference, October 27. Seattle, Washington.

Guevara, J., L. Hall, and E. Stegman. 2011. "IT Key Metrics Data 2012. Key Infrastructure Measures: End-User Computing Analysis. Current Year." Research Note G00226871. Stamford, CT: Gartner Research.

Hagland, M. 2001. "CIO of the Year." *Healthcare Informatics* 18 (4): 18–19.

Hali, M. 2007. "A/R Outsourcing—Coming of Age in the New Millennium." Accessed September 9. www.lowdso.com/Articles1.html.

Halpern, M., J. Bian, E. Ward, N. Schrag, and A. Chen. 2007. "Insurance Status and Stage of Cancer at Diagnosis Among Women with Breast Cancer." *Cancer* 110 (2): 403–11.

Han, Y. Y., J. A. Carcillo, S. T. Venkataraman, R. S. Clark, R. S. Watson, T. C. Nguyen, H. Bayir, and R. A. Orr. 2005. "Unexpected Increased Mortality After Implementation of a Commercially Sold Computerized Physician Order Entry System." *Pediatrics* 116 (6): 1506–12.

Handler, T. 2006. "Magic Quadrant for North American Enterprise CPR, 2006." Research ID # G00137829. Stamford, CT: Gartner Industry.

———. 2005. "Enterprise CPT Systems Are Nearing the Generation 3 Milestone." Research ID # G00125960. Stamford, CT: Gartner Industry.

———. 2004. "Building Blocks for the Future: Implementing a CPR." Gartner Healthcare Mini Symposium, College of Healthcare Information Management Executives, La Jolla, California, October 26.

Harris, J., and K. Keywood. 2001. "Ignorance, Information, and Autonomy." *Theory of Medical Bioethics* 22 (5): 415–36.

Haseley, S., and J. Brucker. 2012. "Assessing IT Governance: Considerations for Internal Audit." *Journal of the Association for Healthcare Internal Auditors* 31 (2): 54–58.

Hayden, M. 2001. *Sams Teach Yourself Networking in 24 Hours.* Indianapolis, IN: Sams Publishing.

Healthcare Information and Management Systems Society (HIMSS). 2012a. *23rd Annual HIMSS Leadership Survey, Final Report: Healthcare Senior IT Executive.* Chicago: HIMSS. Also available at www.himss.org/content/files/2012 FINAL%20Leadership%20Survey%20with%20Cover.pdf.

———. 2012b. "Electronic Health Record." Accessed February 14. www.himss.org /ASP/topics_ehr.asp.

———. 2012c. "Computerized Provider Order Entry (CPOE) Wiki." Accessed May 31. https://himsscpoewiki.pbworks.com/w/page/10258531/FrontPage.

———. 2006a. *Seventeenth Annual HIMSS Leadership Survey. Final Report: Healthcare CIO.* Sponsored by ACS Healthcare Solutions. Chicago: HIMSS.

———. 2006b. *2006 HIMSS Compensation Survey Results.* Accessed December 6, 2007. www.himss.org/surveys/compensation/ASP/memberIndex.asp.

———. 2005a. *Sixteenth Annual HIMSS Leadership Survey.* Sponsored by Superior Consultant. Chicago: HIMSS.

———. 2005b. "New Healthcare Information Technology Standards Panel Formed under Contract by DHHS." Published October 6. www.himss.org/ASP /ContentRedirector.asp?ContentID=65351.

———. 2002. *Thirteenth Annual HIMSS Leadership Survey.* Chicago: HIMSS.

———. 1996. *Seventh Annual HIMSS Leadership Survey.* Chicago: HIMSS.

Healthgrades. 2009. "The Sixth Annual Healthgrades Patient Safety in American Hospitals Study." Accessed February 6, 2012. www.healthgrades.com/business/img/PatientSafetyInAmericanHospitalsStudy2009.pdf.

Health Informatics. 2012. "Controlled Medical Vocabularies–CMV." Accessed May 31. http://healthinformatics.wikispaces.com/Controlled+Medical+Vocabularies+-+CMV.

HealthIT.gov. n.d. "What Is Meaningful Use?" Accessed May 22, 2012. www .healthit.gov/policy-researchers-implementers/meaningful-use.

Health Privacy Project. 2007. "Health Privacy Stories." Accessed July 1. www.health privacy.org/usr_doc/Privacystories.pdf.

Hensley, S. 1997. "Outsourcing Moves Into New Territory." *Modern Healthcare* 27 (2): 39–43.

Herman, D., G. Scalzi, and R. Kropf. 2011. *Managing Healthcare IS Supply and Demand: IT Governance Remains a Top Organizational Challenge.* IT Governance Best Practices. Wheat Ridge, CO: Aspen Systems, Inc.

Heubusch, K. 2006. "Interoperability: What It Means, Why It Matters." *Journal of AHIMA* 77 (1): 26–30.

Hicken, V. N., S. N. Thornton, and R. A. Rocha. 2004. "Integration Challenges of Clinical Information Systems Developed Without a Shared Data Dictionary." *Studies in Health Technology and Informatics* 107 (Part 2): 1053–57.

Hickman, G., and K. Kusche. 2006. "Building the EHR Total Cost of Ownership (TCO) Model." Healthcare Information and Management Systems Society Webinar, Chicago, April 27.

Hicks, J. 2009. "Highlighting Devices." *Modern Healthcare* 39 (26): C8.

Hiles, A. 1992. "Surviving a Computer Disaster." *Computing and Control Engineering Journal* 3 (3): 133–35.

Hill, L. 2006. "How Automated Access Verification Can Help Health Organizations Demonstrate HIPAA Compliance: A Case Study." *Journal of Healthcare Information Management* 20 (2): 116–22.

Hillestad, R., J. Bigelow, A. Bower, F. Girosi, R. Meili, R. Scoville, and R. Taylor. 2005. "Can Electronic Medical Record Systems Transform Health Care? Potential Health Benefits, Savings, and Costs." *Health Affairs* 24 (5): 1103–17.

Hiltzik, M. 2012. "Her Case Shows Why Healthcare Privacy Laws Exist." *Los Angeles Times.* Accessed March 15, 2013. http://articles.latimes.com/2012/jan/04/business/la-fi-hiltzik-20120104.

HIMSS Analytics. 2012a. *Essentials of the U.S. Hospital IT Market,* 7th ed. Chicago: Healthcare Information and Management Systems Society. Also available at www.himssanalytics.org/docs/20-signposts-12r.pdf.

———. 2012b. "U.S. EMR Adoption Model^SM Trends." Accessed May 31. www.himssanalytics.org/docs/HA_EMRAM_Overview_Eng%20011812.pdf.

———. 2005. *Annual Report of the US Hospital IT Market.* Chicago: Healthcare Information and Management Systems Society.

HIPAA Survival Guide. 2013. "HIPAA Privacy Rule Checklist Under HITECH." Accessed March 14. http://store.hipaasurvivalguide.com/checklists.html.

Hoerbst, A., W. Hackl, R. Blomer, and E. Ammenwerth. 2011. "The Status of IT Service Management in Health Care—ITIL in Selected European Countries." *BMC Medical Informatics and Decision Making* 11 (76): 1–12. Accessed March 1, 2013. www.biomedcentral.com/content/pdf/1472-6947-11-76.pdf.

Hook, J., E. Pan, J. Adler-Milstein, D. Bu, and J. Walker. 2006. "The Value of Healthcare Information Exchange and Interoperability in New York State." *AMIA Annual Symposium Proceedings* 953. Accessed December 31, 2007. www.pubmedcentral.nih.gov/articlerender.fcgi?tool=pubmed&pubmedid=17238572.

Houser, S., H. Houser, and R. Shewchuk. 2007. "Assessing the Effects of the HIPAA Privacy Rule on Release of Patient Information by Healthcare Facilities." *Perspectives in Health Information Management* 4 (1): 1–11.

Hsiao, C., E. Hing, T. Socey, and B. Cai. 2011. "Electronic Health Record Systems and Intent to Apply for Meaningful Use Incentives Among Office-based

Physician Practices: United States, 2001–2011." No. 79, November. Atlanta: National Center for Health Statistics and Centers for Disease Control and Prevention.

Hunter, D. P., and V. Ciotti. 2006. "IT Disasters: The Worst Debacles and Lessons Learned from Them." *Healthcare Executive* 21 (5): 8–12.

Iansiti, M., G. Favaloro, J. Utzechneider, and G. Richards. 2005. "Why IT Matters in Midsized Firms." Harvard Business School Working Paper Series No. 06-013. Accessed March 2013. www.hbs.edu/faculty/Publication%20Files/06-013 .pdf.

India Knowledge@Wharton. 2011. "Healthy Business: Will Medical Tourism Be India's Next Big Industry?" Accessed June 20, 2012. http://knowledge .wharton.upenn.edu/india/article.cfm?articleid=4615.

Institute of Medicine (IOM). 2010. *The Healthcare Imperative: Lowering Costs and Improving Outcomes: Workshop Series Summary.* Washington, DC: National Academies Press.

———. 2009. *Initial National Priorities for Comparative Effectiveness Research.* Washington, DC: National Academies Press.

———. 2003. *Hidden Costs, Value Lost: Uninsurance in America.* Washington, DC: National Academies Press.

———. 2001. *Crossing the Quality Chasm: A New Health System for the 21st Century.* Washington, DC: National Academies Press.

———. 1999. *To Err Is Human: Building a Safer Health System.* Washington, DC: National Academies Press.

International Health Terminology Standards Development Organisation (IHTSDO). 2012. "SNOMED CT." Accessed April 3, 2013. www.ihtsdo.org/snomed-ct/.

Internet World Stats. 2011. "Internet Usage Statistics for the Americas." Accessed December 9. www.internetworldstats.com.

IT Governance Institute. 2006. *Enterprise Value: Governance of IT Investments, the Business Case.* Rolling Meadows, IL: IT Governance Institute.

———. 2005. *CoBit 4.0.* Rolling Meadows, IL: IT Governance Institute.

IT Service Management Forum (itSMF). 2004. *An Introductory Overview of ITIL.* Version 1.0a. London: Office of Government Commerce.

———. 2001. *IT Service Management.* Version 2.1.b. London: Office of Government Commerce.

———. 2000. *Best Practice for Service Support.* London: Office of Government Commerce.

Jamal, A., K. McKenzie, and M. Clark. 2009. "The Impact of Health Information Technology on the Quality of Medical and Health Care: A Systematic Review." *Journal of Health Information Management* 38 (3): 26–37.

Jeffery, M., and I. Leliveld. 2004. "Best Practices in IT Portfolio Management." *Sloan Management Review* 45 (3): 41–49.

Jha, A., D. Doolan, D. Grandt, T. Scott, and D. Bates. 2008. "The Use of Health Information Technology in Seven Nations." *International Journal of Medical Informatics* 77: 848–54.

Johnson, W. 2005. "The Planning Cycle." *Journal of Healthcare Information Management* 19 (3): 56–64.

Johnston, D., E. Pan, and B. Middleton. 2002. *Finding the Value in Healthcare Information Technologies.* Boston: Center for Information Technology Leadership.

Johnston, D., E. Pan, B. Middleton, J. Walker, and D. Bates. 2003. "The Value of Computerized Provider Order Entry in Ambulatory Settings." Accessed September 1, 2006. http://citl.org/research/ACPOE_Executive_Preview.pdf.

Journal of AHIMA. 2011. "Practice Brief: Managing Nontext Media in Healthcare Practices." *Journal of AHIMA* 82 (11): 54–58.

Kaiser. 2012. *Building ACO Foundations: Lessons from Kaiser Permanente's Integrated Delivery Model: Case Study.* Danvers, MA: HealthLeaders Media Rounds.

Kaplan, J. 2005. *Strategic IT Portfolio Management: Governing Enterprise Transformation.* Waltham, MA: Pittiglio Rabin Todd and McGrath, Inc.

Kaplan, B., and D. Harris-Salamone. 2009. "Health IT Success and Failure: Recommendations from Literature and an AMIA Workshop." *Journal of the American Medical Informatics Association* 16 (3): 291–99.

Kapoor, R., J. Fuchs, C. Lutz, and A. Jain. 2006. "A Model for Extending Physician-Specific Process Measures to the Advanced Practice Nurses." *AMIA Annual Symposium Proceedings,* 975.

Kaushal, R., K. N. Barker, and D. W. Bates. 2001. "How Can Information Technology Improve Patient Safety and Reduce Medication Errors in Children's Healthcare?" *Archives of Pediatric Adolescent Medicine* 155 (9): 1002–7.

Kaushal, R., A. K. Jha, C. Franz, J. Glaser, K. D. Shetty, T. Jaggi, B. Middleton, G. J. Kuperman, R. Khorasani, M. Tanasijevic, D. W. Bates, and Brigham and Women's Hospital CPOE Working Group. 2006. "Return on Investment for a Computerized Order Entry System." *Journal of the American Medical Informatics Association* 13 (3): 261–66.

Kellerman, A., and S. Jones. 2013. "What It Will Take to Achieve the As-Yet-Unfulfilled Promises of Health Information Technology." *Health Affairs* 32 (1): 63–68.

Kendall, G., and S. Rollins. 2003. *Advanced Project Portfolio Management and the PMO: Multiplying ROI at Warp Speed.* Boca Raton, FL: J. Ross Publishing and International Institute of Learning.

Kerzner, H. 2003. *Project Management: A Systems Approach to Planning, Scheduling, and Controlling,* 8th ed. Hoboken, NJ: Wiley and Sons.

Kim, G. 2006. "Unplanned Work Is Silently Killing IT Departments." *Computerworld.* Accessed January 29, 2007. www.computerworld.com/action/article.do?command=viewArticleBasic&articleId=110242.

Kleinke, J. D. 2005. "Dot-Gov: Market Failure and the Creation of a National Health Information Technology System." *Health Affairs (Millwood)* 24 (5): 1246–62.

Koppel, R. 2005. "Computerized Physician Order Entry Systems: The Right Prescription?" *LDI Issue Brief* 10 (5): 1–4.

Koppel, R., J. P. Metlay, A. Cohen, B. Abaluck, A. R. Localio, S. E. Kimmel, and B. L. Strom. 2005. "Role of Computerized Physician Order Entry Systems in Facilitating Medication Errors." *Journal of the American Medical Association* 293 (10): 1197–203.

Kovner, A. R., D. J. Fine, and R. D'Aquila. 2009. *Evidence-Based Management in Healthcare*. Chicago: Health Administration Press.

Kraatz, A. S., C. M. Lyons, and J. Thompkinson. 2010. "Strategy and Governance for Successful Implementation of an Enterprise-wide Ambulatory EMR." *Journal of Healthcare Information Management* 24 (2): 34–40.

Kramer, S. 2006. "The Secrets of Successful CIOs. Top CIOs Talk About What It Takes to Lead So Others Want to Follow." *Healthcare Informatics* 23 (10): 24–30.

Kuperman, G., A. Boyer, C. Cole, B. Forman, P. Stetson, and M. Cooper. 2006. "Using IT to Improve Quality at New York-Presbyterian Hospital: A Requirement-Driven Strategic Planning Process." *AMIA Annual Symposium Proceedings*, 449–53.

Kutscher, B. 2012. "Expertise on Call." ModernHealthcare.com. Accessed March 29, 2013. www.modernhealthcare.com/article/20120901/MAGAZINE /309019954.

Landro, L. 2003. "Doctors Need Incentives to Embrace Technology." Accessed March 1, 2006. http://online.wsj.com/article/sb105777796472723600 .html.

Landry, M. D., and W. J. Sibbald. 2001. "From Data to Evidence: Evaluative Methods in Evidence-Based Medicine." *Respiratory Care* 46 (11): 1226–35.

Lang, R. D. 2006. "Patient Safety and IT: A Need for Incentives." *Journal of Healthcare Information Management* 20 (4): 2–4.

Lau, R. K., and M. Catchpole. 2001. "Improving Data Collection and Information Retrieval for Monitoring Sexual Health." *International Journal of STD and AIDS* 12 (1): 8–13.

Leapfrog Group. 2002. "The Leapfrog Group Expands Patient Safety Improvement Initiative Into 12 New Regions." Press release, April 22.

Lee, W. 2006. *The Effect of PMO on IT Project Management: A Summary of Survey Data Results*. Research Report. Honolulu: Hawaii Pacific University.

Legnick-Hall, C. A., and M. L. Legnick-Hall. 2006. "HR, ERP, and Knowledge for Competitive Advantage." *Human Resource Management* 45 (2): 179–94.

Lianying, Z., H. Jing, and Z. Xinxing. 2012. "The Project Management Maturity Model and Application Based on PRINCE2." 2012 International Workshop on Information and Electronics Engineering. *Procedia Engineering* 29: 3691–97.

Library of Congress. 2002. "Corporate and Auditing Accountability, Responsibility, and Transparency Act of 2002." HR 3763. Accessed March 3, 2008. http://thomas.loc.gov/cgi-bin/query/D?c107:3:./temp/~c10 7gMRwC9.

Light, M., M. Hotle, D. Stang, and J. Heine. 2005. *Project Management Office: The IT Control Tower.* No. G00132836. Stamford, CT: Gartner.

Lohman, P. 1996. "Measure Consultant's Objectivity and Character Before Contracting." *Health Management Technology* (July): 31.

Loomis, G. A., J. S. Ries, R. M. Saywell, Jr., and N. R. Thakker. 2002. "If Electronic Medical Records Are So Great, Why Aren't Family Physicians Using Them?" *Journal of Family Practice* 51 (7): 636–41.

Lutchen, M. 2004. *Managing IT as a Business: A Survival Guide for CEOs.* Hoboken, NJ: PricewaterhouseCoopers and John Wiley and Sons.

Lutchen, M., and A. Collins. 2005. "IT Governance in Healthcare Setting: Reinventing the Healthcare Industry." *Journal of Healthcare Compliance* 7 (6): 27–30.

Marietti, C. 2002. "HIPAA: Blueprint for Privacy and Security." *Healthcare Informatics* 19 (1): 55–60.

Markle Foundation. 2012. *Markle Connecting for Health Common Framework: Resources for Implementing Private and Secure Health Information Exchange.* Accessed May 10, 2013. www.markle.org/health/marklecommon-framework.

———. 2004. *Achieving Electronic Connectivity in Healthcare: A Preliminary Roadmap from the Nation's Public and Private-Sector Healthcare Leaders.* Accessed December 31, 2007. www.connectingforhealth.org/resources/cfh_aech_roadmap_072004.pdf.

Maslow, A. 1970. *Motivation and Personality,* 2nd ed. New York: Harper and Row.

McGitten, J., K. Potter, J. Guevara, L. Hall, and E. Stegman. 2013. "IT Metrics: IT Spending and Staffing Report, 2013." Research Note G00248502. Cambridge, MA: Gartner Research.

McNickle, M. 2012. "Top 10 Data Security Breaches in 2012." *Healthcare Finance News.* Accessed August 13. www.healthcarefinancenews.com/news/top-10-data-security-breaches-2012.

Medical Tourism Corporation. 2012. "Medical Tourism: What Is It?" Accessed June 20. www.medicaltourismco.com.

Menachemi, N., D. Burke, M. Diana, and R. Brooks. 2005. "Characteristics of Hospitals That Outsource Information System Functions." *Journal of Healthcare Information Management* 191 (1): 63–69.

Menachemi, N., J. Burkhardt, R. Shewchuk, D. Burke, and R. Brooks. 2006. "Hospital Information Technology and Positive Financial Performance: A Different Approach to Finding an ROI." *Journal of Healthcare Management* 51 (1): 40–58.

Menning, W., and R. Carpenter. 2005. "Who's Minding the Store? Effective IT Governance." In *The CEO–CIO Partnership: Harnessing the Value of Information Technology in Healthcare*, edited by D. Smaltz, J. Glaser, R. Skinner, and T. Cunningham III. Chicago: Healthcare Information and Management Systems Society.

Mercy Hospital. 2009. "Mercy Recognized as Being the Top 0.5 percent of Automated Hospitals in the U.S.: Implemented 21 Cerner Millennium Solutions in 14 Months." *Globe News Wire*. Accessed March 29, 2013. www.globenews wire.com/news-release/2009/04/03/394426/161742/en/Mercy-Hos pital-Medical-Center-Reaches-HIMSS-Stage-6-Using-Cerner-Millennium -Solutions.html.

Metzger, J., M. Ame, and J. Rhoads. 2010. "Hospital Quality Reporting: The Hidden Requirements in Meaningful Use." Computer Sciences Corporation. Accessed June 20, 2012. http://assets1.csc.com/health_services/down loads/CSC_Hospital_Quality_Reporting_Hidden_Requirements.pdf.

Meyer, R., and P. Degoulet. 2008. "Assessing the Capital Efficiency of Healthcare Information Technologies: An Econometric Perspective." *IMIA Yearbook of Medical Informatics*, 114–27.

Meyer, J., and J. Ingold. 2012. "Source: Psychiatrist Rejected Offer to Put James Holmes on Psych Hold." *The Denver Post*. Accessed March 15, 2013. www .denverpost.com/breakingnews/ci_22129860/cu-expected-release-nearly-3 -800-emails-referencing.

Middleton, B., G. Christopherson, R. Rocha, and D. Smaltz. 2004. "Knowledge Management in Clinical Systems: Principles and Pragmatics." Paper presented at the International Medical Informatics Association Medinfo 2004 Conference, San Francisco, September 11.

Miller, H. 2009. *How to Create Accountable Care Organizations*. Pittsburgh: Center for Healthcare Quality and Payment Reform.

Miller, R. H., C. West, T. M. Brown, I. Sim, and C. Ganchoff. 2005. "The Value of Electronic Health Records in Solo or Small Group Practices." *Health Affairs* 24 (5): 1127–37.

Mitchell, R. L. 2009. "Confidence in the Cloud." *Computerworld* 43 (23): 28, 30–31.

Monohan, T. 2001. "And an ASP Is . . .?" *Healthcare Informatics* 18 (2): 54–56.

Moreira, M. 2004. "ABCs of Release Management." *CM Crossroads*. Accessed April 25, 2007. www.cmcrossroads.com/content/view/6735/158/.

Morrissey, J. 1996. "CIO Pay Averages $110,000 a Year." *Modern Healthcare* 26 (10): 122–124.

Morrisey, M., J. Alexander, L. Burns, and V. Johnson. 1996. "Managed Care and Physician–Hospital Integration." *Health Affairs* 15 (4): 62–73.

Morrison, I., and R. Smith. 2000. "Hamster Health Care: Time to Stop Running Faster and Redesign Health Care." *British Medical Journal* 321: 1541–42.

Moskowitz, D., and T. Bodenheimer. 2011. "Moving from Evidence-Based Medicine to Evidence-Based Health." *Journal of General Internal Medicine* 26 (6): 658–60.

mThink. 2003. "Selecting a Clinical IT Vendor." Accessed April 2, 2013. http:// mthink.com/dev/mthink/content/selecting-clinical-it-vendor.

Murphy, P. 2011. "The Vendor Selection Process." Working paper. Houston: Encore Health Resources.

National Alliance for Health Information Technology. 2007. "What Is Interoperability?" Work Products, National Alliance for Health Information Technology. Accessed December 11. www.nahit.org/cms/index.php?option=com_content &task=view&id=220&Itemid=115.

National Institute of Standards and Technology (NIST). 2010. "Cloud Computing Forum & Workshop." Updated February 15, 2012. http://csrc.nist.gov /groups/SNS/cloud-computing.

National Library of Medicine (NLM). 2012. "Unified Medical Language System (UMLS)." Accessed June 5. www.nlm.nih.gov/research/umls/.

———. 2004. "National Library of Medicine Functional Statement." Accessed June 5, 2012. www.nlm.nih.gov/about/functstatement.html.

National Training and Dissemination Center. 2012. "Component 5: History of Health Information Technology in the U.S." Health IT Workforce Curriculum Components. Office of the National Coordinator for Health Information Technology. www.onc-ntdc.org.

Nelson, S. 2006. "Privacy and Medical Information on the Internet." *Respiratory Care* 51 (2): 183–87.

Ng, H. S., M. L. Sim, C. M. Tan, and C. C. Wong. 2006. "Wireless Technologies for Telemedicine." *BT Technology Journal* 24 (2): 130–37.

Nonaka, I., and H. Takeuchi. 1995. *The Knowledge Creating Company*. Oxford, UK: Oxford University Press.

Oas, B. 2001. "Integration: Organizations Streamline the Business of Healthcare by Joining Disparate Systems." *Healthcare Informatics* 18 (2): 58–60.

O'Connor, K. 2005. "Minimize Large-Scale IT Project Risk Through Effective Contracting Strategies." *Journal of Healthcare Information Management* 19 (2): 16–18.

Office of Government Commerce (OGC). 2005. *Best Practices for Service Support*, 10th impression. London: Office of Government Commerce.

Office of National Coordinator for Health Information Technology (ONCHIT). 2012a. "Electronic Health Records and Meaningful Use." US Department of Health & Human Services. Accessed March 12. http://healthit.hhs.gov /portal/server.pt/communityhealthit_hhs_gov__meaningful_use_announce ment/2996.

———. 2012b. "Certified Health IT Product List." US Department of Health & Human Services. Accessed April 2. http://oncchpl.force.com/ehrcert.

———. 2011. *Federal Health Information Technology Strategic Plan, 2011–2015.* Washington, DC: US Government Printing Office.

Oliner, S. D., and D. E. Sichel. 2000. "The Resurgence of Growth in the Late 1990s: Is Information Technology the Story?" *Journal of Economic Perspectives* 14 (4): 3–22.

Olson, L. A., S. G. Peters, and J. B. Stewart. 1998. "Security and Confidentiality in an Electronic Medical Record." *Healthcare Information Management* 12 (1): 27–37.

O'Neill, J., and D. O'Neill. 2009. *Who Are the Uninsured? An Analysis of America's Uninsured Population, Their Characteristics, and Their Health.* Washington, DC: Employee Policy Institute.

Oravec, J. A. 2001. "On the Proper Use of the Internet: Self-Help Medical Information and On-Line Healthcare." *Journal of Health and Social Policy* 14 (1): 37–60.

Organisation for Economic Co-operation and Development (OECD). 2007. *OECD Health Data, 2007.* Paris: OECD.

Osheroff, J. A., E. A. Pifer, D. F. Sittig, R. A. Jenders, and J. M. Teich. 2005. "Improving Outcomes with Clinical Decision Support: An Implementer's Guide." HIMSS Workbook. www.himss.org/asp/topics_cds_workbook.asp ?faid=108&tid=14.

Panangala, S. V., and D. J. Jansen. 2013. "Departments of Defense and Veterans Affairs: Status of the Integrated Electronic Health Records (iEHR)." Congressional Research Service. Published February 26. www.hsdl.org/?view &did=731928.

Pasian, B. 2011. "Factors for Designing a Second Generation of Project Management Maturity Models." 2011 PMI Global Congress, Dallas, October 22–25.

Peel, D. 2007. "Will Violating Privacy Preserve Mass Murder?" *Modern Healthcare.* Accessed January 4, 2008. http://modernhealthcare.com/apps/pbcs.dll /article?AID=/20070427/FREE/70426007.

Perelman, D. 2007. "Bridging the CEO–CIO Gap." eWeek. Published February 9. www.eweek.com/c/a/IT-Infrastructure/Bridging-the-CEOCIO-Gap.

Petersen, L. A., L. D. Woodard, T. Urech, C. Daw, and S. Sookanan. 2006. "Does Pay-for-Performance Improve the Quality of Health Care?" *Annals of Internal Medicine* 145 (4): 265–72.

Pfeffer, J., and R. I. Sutton. 2006. "Evidence-Based Management." *Harvard Business Review* 84 (1): 62–74, 133.

Phrase Finder. 2011. "Beware of Greeks Bearing Gifts." Accessed December 22. www.phrases.org.uk/meanings/beware-of-greeks-bearing-gifts.html.

Pizziferri, L., A. Kittler, L. Volka, M. Honourb, S. Guptaa, S. Wang, T. Wang, M. Q. Lippincott, Q. Lia, and D. W. Bates. 2005. "Primary Care Physician Time Utilization Before and After Implementation of an Electronic Health Record: A Time-Motion Study." *Journal of Biomedical Informatics* 38: 176–88.

Poissant, L., J. Pereira, R. Tamblyn, and Y. Kawasumi. 2005. "The Impact of Electronic Health Records on Time Efficiency of Physicians and Nurses: A Systematic Review." *Journal of the American Medical Informatics Association* 12 (5): 505–16.

Poon, E. G., A. K. Jha, M. Christino, M. M. Honour, R. Fernandopulle, B. Middleton, J. Newhouse, L. Leape, D. W. Bates, D. Blumenthal, and R. Kaushal. 2006. "Assessing the Level of Healthcare Information Technology Adoption in the United States: A Snapshot." *BMC Medical Informatics and Decision Making* 6: 1.

Poterba, J. 1996. "Government Intervention in the Markets for Education and Health Care: How and Why?" In *Individual and Social Responsibility: Child Care, Education, Medical Care, and Long-Term Care in America*, edited by V. Fuchs. Chicago: University of Chicago Press.

Presidential Initiatives. 2006. "Consolidated Health Informatics." Accessed January 1, 2007. www.whitehouse.gov/omb/egov/c-3-6-chi.html.

PricewaterhouseCoopers Health Research Institute. 2012. *Social Media "Likes" Healthcare: From Marketing to Social Business.* Copyright 2012–2013. www.pwc.com/us/en/health-industries/publications/health-care-social-media.jhtml.

Project Management Institute (PMI). 2008. *A Guide to the Project Management Body of Knowledge (PMBOK Guide)*, 4th ed. Newtown Square, PA: Project Management Institute.

Rahimi, B., and V. Vimarlund. 2007. "Methods to Evaluate Health Information Systems in Healthcare Settings: A Literature Review." *Journal of Medical Systems* (5): 397–432.

Raths, D. 2006. "Making ERP Work: Healthcare Providers Are Taking a Closer Look at Enterprise Resource Planning." *Healthcare Informatics* 23 (6): 16.

Reckmann, M., J. Westbrook, Y. Koh, C. Lo, and R. Day. 2009. "Does Computerized Provider Order Entry Reduce Prescribing Errors for Hospital Inpatients? A Systematic Review." *Journal of the American Medical Informatics Association* 16 (5): 613–23.

Recovery.gov. n.d. "The Recovery Act." Recovery.gov. Accessed May 24, 2012. www.recovery.gov/About/Pages/The_Act.aspx.

Reece, R. L. 2000. "A New Industrial Order for Physicians: A Talk with Jeff C. Goldsmith, Ph.D." *Physician Executive* 26 (1): 16–19.

Regenstrief Institute. 2012. "Logical Observation Identifiers Names and Codes (LOINC)." Accessed Mary 31. http://loinc.org.

Robeznieks, A. 2006a. "Another Computer with VA Data Goes Missing." *HIT Strategist*, August 8.

———. 2006b. "Leavitt Surveys Road to Interoperability." *Modern Healthcare.* Published October 30. www.modernhealthcare.com/apps/pbcs.dll/article?AID=/20061030/FREE/61030014/1029/newsletter 02.

Robinson, P. 2011. "Hybrid SharePoint Environments with Office 365." Microsoft white paper. Accessed January 20, 2012. www.microsoft.com/download/en /details.aspx?displaylang=en&id=27580.

Rockart, J. F. 1979. "Chief Executives Define Their Own Data Needs." *Harvard Business Review* 57 (2): 81–84.

Rooney, J., and L. Vanden Heuvel. 2004. "Root Cause Analysis for Beginners." *Quality Progress* 37 (7): 45–53.

Rosen, S. 1969. "Electronic Computers: A Historical Survey." *Computing Surveys* 1 (1): 7–36.

Rosenfeld, S., S. Koss, and S. Siler. 2007. "Privacy, Security and the Regional Health Information Organization." California Healthcare Foundation. Accessed August 1. www.chcf.org/documents/chronicdisease/RHIOPrivacy Security .pdf.

Rosenthal, M., and J. Camillus. 2007. *How Four Purchasers Designed and Implemented Quality-Based Purchasing Activities: Lessons from the Field*. Agency for Healthcare Research and Quality Pub. No. 07-RG008. Washington, DC: AHRQ.

Rosenthal, M., and A. Dudley. 2007. "Pay for Performance: Will the Latest Payment Trend Improve Care?" *Journal of the American Medical Association* 297 (7): 740–44.

Rosenthal, M., B. Landon, S. L. Normand, R. Frank, and A. Epstein. 2006. "Pay for Performance in Commercial HMOs." *New England Journal of Medicine* 355: 1895–1902.

Rowland, D. 2007. "Healthcare in New Orleans: Before and After Katrina." Testimony before the Subcommittee on Oversight and Investigations, Committee on Energy and Commerce, and United States House of Representatives. Accessed May 14. www.kff.org/uninsured/upload/7624.pdf.

Saad, L. 2009. "Most Urgent U.S. Health Problem Still Access to Healthcare." Gallup Politics. Published November 23; Accessed May 12, 2012. www.gallup .com/poll/124460/urgent-health-problem-access-healthcare.aspx.

Salkever, A. 2004. "A Paperless Health-Care System?" *Business Week*, July 7. Accessed 31, 2007. www.businessweek.com/technology/content/jul2004/ tc2004077_8164_tc_171.htm.

Sambamurthy, V., and R. Zmud. 1999. "Arrangements for Information Technology Governance: A Theory of Multiple Contingencies." *MIS Quarterly* 23 (2): 261–90.

Santerre, R. E., and S. P. Neun. 2004. *Health Economics: Theories, Insights, and Industry Studies*. Mason, OH: Thompson South-Western.

Schess, Z. 2002. "Tapped-Out IT Shops Concentrate on Capacity Management." *Computerworld*. Accessed April 25, 2007. www.snwonline.com/implement /tapped_out_02-18-2002.asp?article_id=99.

Schick, S. 2001. "IT Departments Fall Short on Services." *Computing Canada* 27 (1): 4.

Schiff, J. 2010. "Grid Computing and the Future of Cloud Computing." Accessed December 9, 2011. www.enterprisestorageforum.com.

Schmeida, M. 2005. "Health Insurance Portability and Accountability Act of 1996: Just an Incremental Step in Reshaping Government." *Online Journal of Issues in Nursing* 11 (1): 7.

Schoen, C., and S. How. 2011. "National Scorecard on U.S. Health System Performance, 2011, Chartpack." Accessed June 20, 2012. www.commonwealth fund.org/~/media/Files/Publications/In%20the%20Literature/2006/Sep/U%20S%20%20Health%20System%20Performance%20%20A%20National%20Scorecard/955_Schoen_nat_scorecard_US_hlt_sys_performance_co%20pdf.pdf.

Schwartz, E. 2005. "The End of the CIO? Reality Check." Accessed December 14, 2007. www.infoworld.com/article/05/10/18/43OPreality_1.html.

Scottsdale Institute and HIMSS Analytics. 2005. *Healthcare Leaders Report: The Changing Landscape of Healthcare IT Management and Governance.* Chicago: HIMSS Analytics.

Senge, P. 1990. *The Fifth Discipline: The Art & Practice of the Learning Organization.* New York: Doubleday.

Shekelle, P. G., S. C. Morton, and E. B. Keeler. 2006. *Costs and Benefits of Health Information Technology.* Evidence Report/Technology Assessment #132. Prepared for Agency for Healthcare Research and Quality #06-E006. Rockville, MD: AHRQ.

Shortliffe, E. 2005. "Strategic Action in Health Information Technology: Why the Obvious Has Taken So Long." *Health Affairs* 24 (5): 1222–33.

Sidorov, J. 2006. "It Ain't Necessarily So: The Electronic Health Record and the Unlikely Prospect of Reducing Healthcare Costs." *Health Affairs* 25 (4): 1079–85.

Siemens Medical Solutions. 2005. "Proven Outcomes: Jefferson Regional Medical Center Case Study." Accessed November 5, 2006. www.out sourcing-requests.com/common/sponsors/70899/Proven_Outcomes.pdf.

Siep, T. 2007. "Bluetooth Bolsters UWB Performance." *Microwaves and RF* 46 (2): 86–89.

Simborg, D. 2010. "Consumer Empowerment Versus Consumer Populism in Healthcare IT." *Journal of the American Medical Informatics Association* 17: 370–72.

Simborg, D., D. Detmer, and E. Berner. 2013. "The Wave Has Finally Broken: Now What?" *Journal of the American Medical Informatics Association* [in press]: doi: 10.1136/amiajnl-2012-001508.

Simon, S. J., and J. Simon. 2006. "An Examination of the Financial Feasibility of Electronic Medical Records (EMRs): A Case Study of Tangible and Intangible Benefits." *International Journal of Electronic Healthcare* 2 (2): 185–200.

Singleton, J., E. McLean, and E. Altman. 1988. "Measuring Information Systems Performance: Experience with the Management by Results System at Security Pacific Bank." *MIS Quarterly* 12 (2): 325–37.

Sislo, W. 2002. "What Works: Reaping the Benefits of Wireless." *Health Management Technology* 23 (2): 50.

Slovensky, D. J., J. M. Trimm, R. L. Garrie, and P. E. Paustian. 2006. *Information Management, Volume 6 of the Medical Practice Management Body of Knowledge Review.* Englewood, CO: Medical Group Management Association.

Smaltz, D., and E. Berner. 2007. *The Executive's Guide to Electronic Health Records.* Chicago: Health Administration Press.

Smaltz, D., R. Carpenter, and J. Saltz. 2007. "Effective IT Governance in Healthcare Organisations: A Tale of Two Organisations." *International Journal of Healthcare Technology and Management* 8 (1–2): 20–41.

Smaltz, D., and T. Cunningham III. 2005. "Data Rich, Information Poor: Building a Knowledge-Enabled Organization." In *The CEO–CIO Partnership: Harnessing the Value of Information Technology in Healthcare,* edited by D. Smaltz, J. Glaser, R. Skinner, and T. Cunningham III. Chicago: Healthcare Information and Management Systems Society.

Smaltz, D., V. Sambamurthy, and R. Agarwal. 2006. "The Antecedents of CIO Role Effectiveness in Organizations: An Empirical Study in the Healthcare Sector." *IEEE Transactions on Engineering Management* 53 (2): 207–22.

Smaltz, D., J. Glaser, R. Skinner, and T. Cunningham III (eds.). 2005a. *The CEO–CIO Partnership: Harnessing the Value of Information Technology in Healthcare.* Chicago: Healthcare Information and Management Systems Society.

Smaltz, D., R. Branzell, D. Hoidal, M. Murphy, S. Spooner, R. Stacey, and M. Waldrum. 2005b. "The CEO–CIO Relationship: A Roundtable Discussion." In *The CEO–CIO Partnership: Harnessing the Value of Information Technology in Healthcare,* edited by D. Smaltz, J. Glaser, R. Skinner, and T. Cunningham III, 99–110. Chicago: HIMSS Publications.

Southerton, L. 2007. "Mobile Device, Use, Reuse, and Disposal." *Journal of AHIMA* 78 (6): 68–70.

Squires, D. 2012. "Explaining High Health Care Spending in the United States: An International Comparison of Supply, Utilization, Prices, and Quality." Commonwealth Fund. Published May 2012. www.commonwealthfund.org/Publications/Issue-Briefs/2012/May/High-Health-Care-Spending.aspx.

Stacey, R., and R. Skinner. 2005. "Crystal Balls: The Elusive Art of Business and IT Strategic Alignment." In *The CEO–CIO Partnership: Harnessing the Value of Information Technology in Healthcare,* edited by D. Smaltz, J. Glaser, R. Skinner, and T. Cunningham III. Chicago: Healthcare Information and Management Systems Society.

Stahl, M. J. (ed.). 2003. *Encyclopedia of Health Care Management.* Thousand Oaks, CA: Sage Publications.

Standish Group. 2011. *CHAOS Manifesto*. Boston: Standish Group.

Sternberg, S. 2012. "Medical Errors Harm Huge Number of Patients." *US News Health*. Published August 28. http://health.usnews.com/health-news/articles/2012/08/28/medical-errors-harm-huge-number-of-patients?page=2.

Sundaresan, V. 2005. "Optimizing IT Service Delivery." *CIO Update*. Accessed January 29, 2007. www.cioupdate.com/insights/article.php/3502581.

Swayne, L. E., W. J. Duncan, and P. M. Ginter. 2005. *Strategic Management of Health Care Organizations,* 5th ed. Malden, MA: Blackwell Publishing.

Swayze, D. 2011. "9 Hot New Tech Trends You'll Want to Know About." Blog posting. Published January 7. www.trulia.com/blog/debraswayze/2011/01/9_hot_new_tech_trends_you_ll_want_to_know_about.

Taylor, A. 2004. "Success and Failure in IT Projects." *CIO Canada*. Accessed May 20, 2007. www.itworldcanada.com/publication/CIO.htm.

Taylor, R., A. Bower, F. Girosi, J. Bigelow, K. Fonkych, and R. Hillestad. 2005. "Promoting Health Information Technology: Is There a Case for More-Aggressive Government Action?" *Health Affairs (Millwood)* 24 (5): 1234–45.

Terry, K. 2012. "Natural Language Processing Could Eventually Change Medicine." *FierceHealthIT*. Published February 12. Accessed April 8. www.fiercehealthit.com/story/natural-language-processing-could-eventually-change-medicine/2012-02-05.

The Joint Commission. 2011. *Improving America's Hospitals: The Joint Commission's Annual Report on Quality and Safety 2011*. Oakbrook Terrace, IL: The Joint Commission.

———. 2003. "Using Aggregate Root Cause Analysis to Improve Patient Safety." *Joint Commission Journal on Quality and Safety* 29 (8): 434–39.

The Stationary Office (TSO). 2007. *The Official Introduction to the ITIL Service Lifecycle*. Norwich, UK: Office of Government Commerce.

Things People Said. 2011. "Yogi Berra Quotes." Accessed December 22. www.rinkworks.com/said/yogiberra.shtml.

Thompson, J. N. 2006. "The Future of Medical Licensure in the United States." *Academic Medicine* 91 (12): S36–S39.

Thorp, J. 2003. *The Information Paradox: Realizing the Business Benefits of Information Technology*. Toronto: McGraw-Hill Ryerson.

Thorpe, K. 2005. "The Rise in Healthcare Spending and What to Do About It." *Health Affairs* 24 (6): 1436–45.

TopTenReviews. n.d. "2012 Compare Best Voice Recognition Software." Accessed December 9, 2011. www.toptenreviews.com.

Trustee. 2011. "IT Spending: Providers Are Ramping Up IT to Qualify for Incentives." Dashboard. Accessed April 4, 2013. www.ahadataviewer.com/Global/knowledgecenter/data_dashboard_IT_spending_feb11.pdf.

Turisco, F. 2000. "How to Justify the Investment: Principles for Effective IT Value Management." *Health Management Technology* 21 (3): 12–13.

University of Texas Medical Branch (UTMB). 2007. "UTMB Electronic Health Network." Accessed February 17. www.digitalmedicalservices.com/EHN _Services.htm.

Upham, R., and A. Dorsey. 2007. "Living Day-to-Day with HIPAA Privacy: The Top 10 Most Inappropriate Responses Overheard in the Healthcare Workplace." HIPAAdvisory. Accessed January 4, 2008. www.hipaadvisory.com/action /privacy/daytoday.htm.

US Bureau of Labor Statistics (BLS). 2012. "Inflation and Prices." Databases, tables, and calculators by subject. Accessed June 21. www.bls.gov/data/#prices.

US Census Bureau. 2012. "Income, Poverty, and Health Insurance Coverage in the United States: 2011." Accessed June 1. www.commonwealthfund.org/Maps -and-Data/ChartCart/View-All.aspx?charttopic=Coverage.

US Department of Health & Human Services (HHS). n.d.(a). "Health Information Privacy." Accessed December 1, 2011. www.hhs.gov.

———. n.d.(b). "HITECH Act Enforcement Interim Final Rule." Accessed January 6, 2012. www.hhs.gov.

———. 2013. "New Rule Protects Patient Privacy, Secures Health Information." News Release. Published January 17. www.hhs.gov/news/press/2013pres /01/20130117b.html.

Vecchio, A. 2000. "Plan for the Worst Before Disaster Strikes." *Health Management Technology* 21 (6): 28–30.

Vest, J. R., and L. D. Gamm. 2010. "Health Information Exchange: Persistent Challenges and New Strategies." Viewpoint paper. *Journal of the American Medical Informatics Association* 17: 288–94. doi:10.1136/jamia.2010.003673.

Viscusi, W. 2004. "The Value of Life: Estimates with Risk by Industry and Occupation." *Economic Inquiry* 42 (1): 28–49.

Walker, J., E. Pan, D. Johnston, J. Adler-Milstein, D. Bates, and B. Middleton. 2005. "The Value of Health Care Information Exchange and Interoperability." *Health Affairs* Web Exclusive, January 19. Accessed February 2, 2008. http://content.healthaffairs.org/cgi/content/full/hlthaff.w5.10/DC1.

Waller, G., K. Rubenstrunk, and G. Hallenbeck. 2010. *The CIO Edge: Seven Leadership Skills You Need to Drive Results.* Boston: Harvard Business School Publishing.

Walshe, K., and T. G. Rundall. 2001. "Evidence-Based Management: From Theory to Practice in Healthcare." *Milbank Quarterly* 79 (3): 429–57.

Wanless, S., and T. Ludwig. 2011. *Business Intelligence and Analytics for Healthcare Organizations.* Peoria, IL: Ark Group.

Ward, J., and P. Griffiths. 1996. *Strategic Planning for Information Systems,* 2nd ed. New York: John Wiley and Sons.

Warner, K., and B. Luce. 1982. *Cost–Benefit and Cost-Effectiveness Analysis in Health Care: Principles, Practice, and Potential.* Chicago: Health Administration Press.

Washington Post. 2004. "Text of President Bush's 2004 State of the Union Address." Published January 20. www.washingtonpost.com/wp-srv/politics/tran scripts/bushtext_012004.html.

Watson, R., L. Pitt, and C. Kavan. 1998. "Measuring Information Service Quality: Lessons from Two Longitudinal Case Studies." *MIS Quarterly* 22 (1): 61–79.

Waymack, P. 2000. "Four Tips for Selecting Outsourcing Firms." *Health Management Technology* 22 (8): 19.

Weick, K. 1995. *Sensemaking in Organizations.* Thousand Oaks, CA: Sage Publications.

Weill, P., and J. Ross. 2004. *IT Governance: How Top Performers Manage IT Decision Rights for Superior Results.* Boston: Harvard Business School Press.

Weiner, N. 1954. *The Human Use of Human Beings: Cybernetics and Society.* Garden City, NY: Doubleday Anchor.

Weinstein, M., and W. Stason. 1977. "Foundations of Cost-Effectiveness Analysis for Health and Medical Practice." *New England Journal of Medicine* 298: 716–21.

Wennberg, J. E., and A. M. Gittelsohn. 1973. "Small Area Variations in Health Care Delivery." *Science* 183: 1102–8.

Whittleston, S. 2012. *ITIL Is ITIL.* Northhampton, UK: The Stationary Office (TSO), the Cabinet Office, Her Majesty's Government.

Wiig, K. 2000. "Knowledge Management: An Emerging Discipline Rooted in a Long History." In *Knowledge Horizons: The Present and the Promise of Knowledge Management,* edited by C. Depres and D. Chauvel. Woburn, MA: Butterworth-Heinemann.

Wilensky, G. R. 2006. "Consumer-Driven Health Plans: Early Evidence and Potential Impact on Hospitals." *Health Affairs* 25 (1): 174–85.

Wiley, V., and G. Daniel. 2006. *An Economic Evaluation of a Payer-based Electronic Health Record Within an Emergency Department.* Wilmington, DE: Health-Core, Inc.

Williams, C., F. Mostashari, K. Mertz, E. Hogin, and P. Atwal. 2012. "From the Office of the National Coordinator: The Strategy for Advancing the Exchange of Health Information." *Health Affairs* 31 (3): 527–36.

Wilson, T. D. 1989. "The Implementation of Information Systems Strategies in UK Companies: Aims and Barriers to Success." *International Journal of Information Management* 9 (4): 245–58.

Wilson, K. J., and C. E. McPherson. 2002. "It's 2002: How HIPAA-Ready Are You?" *Health Management Technology* 23 (1): 14–15, 20.

Wipke-Tevis, D. D., and M. A. Pickett. 2008. "Impact of the Health Insurance Portability and Accountability Act on Participant Recruitment and Retention." *Western Journal of Nursing Research* 30 (1): 39–53.

Wood, G. M. 2000. "The Changing Role of the Healthcare Chief Information Officer." *Managed Care Interface* 13 (9): 81–83.

Yasaitis, L., E. Fisher, J. Skinner, and A. Chandra. 2009. "Hospital Quality and Intensity of Spending: Is There an Association?" *Health Affairs* 28 (4): w566–72.

Young, I. B., L. Foster, A. Ailander, and B. J. Wakefield. 2011. "Home Telehealth: Patient Satisfaction, Program Functions, and Challenges for the Care Coordinator." *Journal of Gerontological Nursing* 37 (11): 38–46.

Young, C., and S. Mingay. 2003. *IS Process Improvement: Making Sense of Available Models.* No. DF-20–1898. Stamford, CT: Gartner, Inc.

Yu, F., N. Menachemi, E. Berner, J. Allison, N. Weissman, and T. Houston. 2009. "Full Implementation of Computerized Physician Order Entry and Medication-Related Quality Outcomes: A Study of 3364 Hospitals." *The American Journal of Medical Quality* 24: 278–86.

Zeltner, B. 2012. "Walmart to Send Employees to Cleveland Clinic for Heart Care." *The Plain Dealer,* September 12. Also available at www.cleveland.com/health fit/index.ssf/2012/10/wal-mart_to_send_employees_to.html.

OF SELECTED ABBREVIATIONS

A	Patient Protection and Affordable Care Act
HRQ	Agency for Healthcare Research and Quality
AI	artificial intelligence
ANSI	American National Standards Institute
ARRA	American Recovery and Reinvestment Act
ASP	application service provider
ASQ	American Society for Quality
ATM	asynchronous transfer mode
CDC	Centers for Disease Control and Prevention
CDDP	cellular digital data packet
CDS	clinical decision support
CDSS	clinical decision support system
CIO	chief information officer
CMIO	chief medical information officer
CMO	chief medical officer
CMS	Centers for Medicare & Medicaid Services
CPOE	computerized physician/provider order entry
CPU	central processing unit
CVO	credentials verification organization
DBMS	database management system
EDI	electronic data interchange
EBM	evidence-based medicine
EHR	electronic health record
EIS	executive information system
EMR	electronic medical record
ENIAC	Electronic Numerical Integrator and Calculator
ERP	enterprise resources planning (system)
FDDI	fiber-distributed data interchange
GAN	global area network
HIE	health information exchange
HIMSS	Healthcare Information and Management Systems Society
HIPAA	Health Insurance Portability and Accountability Act
HIT	Healthcare information technology

HITECH	Health Information Technology for Economic and Clinical Health Act
HITSP	Health Information Technology Standards Panel
HL7	Health Level Seven
HMO	health maintenance organization
ICD	International Classification of Diseases
IDS	integrated delivery system
IHI	Institute for Healthcare Improvement
IOM	Institute of Medicine
IP	Internet protocol
IRPQ	incidents, requests, problems, questions
ISDN	integrated services digital network
ISP	Internet service provider
ITIL	Information Technology Infrastructure Library
LAN	local area network
MPI	master patient/person index
NCQA	National Committee for Quality Assurance
NIC	network interface controller/card
OCG	Office of Government Commerce (United Kingdom)
OECD	Organisation for Economic Co-operation and Development
ONCHIT	Office of the National Coordinator for Health Information Technology
PACS	picture archiving and communication system
PDA	personal digital assistant
PHI	personal health information
PMO	portfolio management office
RAM	random access memory
RFI	request for information
RFID	radio-frequency identification
RFP	request for proposal
RJE	remote job entry
ROI	return on investment
ROM	read-only memory
SLA	service-level agreement
VDT	video display terminal
WAN	wide area network
WWW	World Wide Web

GLOSSARY

Administrative information system. An information system designed to assist in the performance of administrative support activities in a healthcare organization, such as payroll accounting, accounts receivable, accounts payable, facility management, intranets, and human resources management.

Algorithm. A step-by-step procedure for performing a task. Computer algorithms consist of logical and mathematical operations.

Analog signal. The representation of data by varying the amplitude, frequency, and/or phase of a waveform. See also *digital signal.*

Application service provider (ASP). An organization that contracts with a healthcare facility to provide access to online applications.

Applications program. A program that performs specific tasks for the computer user, such as payroll, order entry, and inventory control.

Arithmetic logic unit (ALU). A computer component that performs the computational and comparison functions. The ALU's speed is a primary consideration for applications involving image processing and other clinical applications.

Artificial intelligence (AI). A discipline that attempts to simulate human problem-solving techniques in a computer environment. See also *expert system.*

Asynchronous transfer mode (ATM). A networking technology that segments data into small fixed-length cells, directs the cells to the appropriate destination, and reassembles the data.

Bandwidth. A measure of the data-carrying capacity of a transmission medium. The higher the bandwidth, the larger the volume of data that can be moved across networks.

Bar code. A printed sequence of vertical bars and spaces that represent numbers and other symbols. The code can be read and translated automatically by specially designed computer input devices.

Bar-code scanner. An input device that allows a computer user to scan a bar code and transfer its contents to a computer.

Bit. A binary digit (0 or 1) that is part of a data byte. In most computer systems, eight bits make up one byte.

Bridge. An interface that connects two or more networks that use similar protocols.

Browser. A software application that enables users to view and interact with information on the World Wide Web.

Bus. (1) The physical network topology in which all workstations are connected to a line directly. (2) Within a computer, the signal path that links the central processing unit with primary memory and with input/output devices.

Byte. The smallest addressable piece of information in a computer's memory, typically consisting of eight bits, used to signify a letter, number, or symbol.

Cache memory. Primarily, short-term storage of data to facilitate high-speed processing. Although most cache data are deleted when the computer is powered down, some data-access tracking and application-specific information may be retained. Some cache memory must be deleted by command.

Client/server computing/architecture. A configuration in which users interact with their machines (called *clients*) and one or more other machines (called *servers*) that store data and do much of the computing.

Clinical data repository. A database that consists of information from various sources of care and from various departments and/or facilities. The database may represent a longitudinal description of an individual's care.

Clinical decision support system. An application that accesses structured databases of clinical information to aid a clinician provider in defining probable diagnoses or in selecting appropriate diagnostic tests or treatment options.

Clinical (or medical) information system. A system that provides for the organized storage, processing, and retrieval of information to support patient care activities.

Closed system. A completely self-contained system that is not influenced by external events. See also *cybernetic system, open system, system.*

Cloud computing. Remote access to data storage and processing functions via the Internet without use of or concern for the physical location in which the actual processing or storage systems are housed.

Computerized physician/provider order entry (CPOE). A process of electronically entering instructions or orders regarding the diagnosis and treatment of patients.

Configuration management database (CMDB). A knowledge store of solutions, answers, and temporary fixes; a knowledge store for system configuration settings that first-level technicians can use to potentially expedite the resolution of an end user's incident.

Cybernetic system. A self-regulating system that contains the following automatic control components: sensor, monitor, standards, and control unit. See also *closed system, open system, system.*

Data. Raw facts and figures collected by the organization from clinical encounters, empirical observations, or research. Data in and of themselves often have little value and take on meaning only after they are sorted, tabulated, and processed into a usable format (information).

Database. A series of records, containing data fields, stored together in such a way that the contents are easily accessed, managed, and updated.

Database management system (DBMS). Software that enables the creation and accessing of data stored in a database.

Data dictionary. A file that contains the name, definition, and structure of all the data fields and elements in a database.

Data field. One piece of information stored in a data record as part of a database. Patient date of birth is one example.

Data record. A group of individual fields, corresponding to a real-world entity, that are stored together in a database. Demographic and clinical information captured during a patient encounter is one example.

Data redundancy. A situation in which the same data item appears in several files of a healthcare organization's computer system.

Data warehouse. Collection and organization of data from disparate sources into an integrated subject-oriented repository to facilitate decision making.

Decision support system. A system designed to support the decision-making process of an individual or organization through the use of data retrieval, modeling, and reporting. See also *clinical decision support system.*

Deterministic system. A system in which the component parts function according to completely predictable or definable relationships with no randomness present.

Digital signal. The representation of data as a series of on/off pulses (1s and 0s). See also *analog signal.*

Distributed processing. A computer network topology in which the workload is spread out across a network of computers that can be located in different organizational units.

Documentation. Written information that provides a description and overview of a computer program or system and detailed instructions on its use.

Dumb terminal. A device that can provide input to and display output from a central computer but cannot perform any independent processing.

E-health application. Healthcare software delivered through the Internet and related technologies.

Electronic data interchange (EDI). The transfer of structured information between two computers.

Electronic health record (EHR). A system that consists of an individual's medical records from all locations and sources. Stored in digital format, an EHR facilitates the storage and retrieval of individual records with the aid of computers.

Encryption. The scrambling of an electronic transmission by using mathematical formulas or algorithms to protect the confidentiality and security of communications.

Enterprise resources planning (ERP) system. Bundled application that integrates operational information derived from financial, human resources, materials management, and other function-based areas into a robust database used to achieve business management objectives.

Ethernet. The trade name for a logical network topology used to control how devices on the network send and receive messages. The goal is to prevent "collisions" between two devices attempting to send messages simultaneously.

Evidence-based medicine (EBM). Also known as evidence-based management, EBM is a movement to explicitly use the most current, best scientific evidence available for managerial or medical decision making.

Executive information system (EIS). An organized data storage, retrieval, and reporting system that is designed to provide senior management with information for decision making.

Expert system. A decision support system that can approximate a human decision maker's reasoning processes. It can assist in reaching a decision, diagnosing a problem, or suggesting a course of action.

Extranet. A private computer network an organization shares with customers and strategic partners using Internet software and transmission standards (TCP/IP).

Fiber-distributed data interchange (FDDI). A network consisting of two identical fiber-optic rings connected to local area networks and other computers.

Fiber-optic medium. A communication-transmission medium that uses light pulses sent through a glass cable at high transmission rates with no electromagnetic interference.

File/server architecture. The physical and logical configuration of the data storage components of a networked system.

Firewall. Hardware and/or software that restricts traffic to and from a private network from the general public Internet network.

Front-end processor. The processor with which application users interact directly. In a client/server network, the front-end processor would correspond to the client.

Gateway. The interface between two networks that use dissimilar protocols to communicate.

Global area network (GAN). Use of wireless technology to extend a computing network beyond the geographic limits of a hard-wired network.

Graphical user interface (GUI). A particular interface between the human user and the computer to manage the functioning of the software and hardware that employs icons (graphical symbols on the monitor screen) to represent available operating system commands.

Grid computing. A distributed computing model whereby multiple Internet-connected computers emulate a supercomputer.

Groupware. Collaborative software that enables sharing of information via an interactive network.

Hardware. The physical components of a computer system.

Help desk. Also called *service desk*, a help desk provides in-person, telephone, or e-mail access to trained personnel who can assist IT users to resolve equipment malfunctions and incidents or to answer technology-related questions.

Healthcare information exchange. Smooth and safe coordination or transfer of patient data and information between two or more unrelated and disparate organizations.

Health Information Technology for Economic and Clinical Health (HITECH) Act. A component of the American Recovery and Reinvestment Act that specifically promotes widespread dissemination and adoption of EHRs through provider incentives.

Health Insurance Portability and Accountability Act (HIPAA). Federal legislation passed in 1996 to make health insurance more portable. The administrative simplification provisions of HIPAA establish standards for electronic transmission of administrative information related to health insurance claims. The privacy protection regulations are designed to limit the nonconsensual use and release of private health information.

Health Level Seven (HL7). A standard for data formatting that helps to facilitate the exchange of data among disparate systems within and across software vendors.

Host. A computer to which other, smaller computers in a network are connected and with which it can communicate.

Hub. A hardware device with multiple user ports to which computers and input/output devices can be attached.

Information. Data or facts that have been processed and analyzed in a formal, intelligent way so that the results are directly useful to clinicians and managers.

Information Technology Infrastructure Library. A framework of how HIT department processes should be interlinked to gain optimum proactive HIT service management.

Input. Data fed into a computer system, either manually (such as through a keyboard or bar-code device) or automatically (such as in a bedside patient-monitoring system).

Integrated system. A set of information systems or networks that can share common data files and can communicate with one another.

Internet protocol (IP). An addressing scheme that identifies each machine on the Internet and is made up of four sets of numbers separated by dots.

Interoperability. The ability of health information systems to effectively transmit and share medical information across organizations.

Intranet. A private computer network contained within an organization that uses Internet software and transmission standards (TCP/IP).

ISDN (integrated services digital network). A network that uses a telephone company branch exchange to allow separate microcomputer workstations, terminals, and other network nodes to communicate with a central computer and with each other.

Legacy system. A computer application designed to meet specific operational needs. Usually developed independent of a broad organizational information management/information technology plan and often is not compatible with newer integrated systems.

Lifecycle. The sequence of specification, design, implementation, and maintenance of computer programs. For models of computer hardware, the lifecycle is the sequence in market status—development, announcement, availability, and obsolescence.

Local area network (LAN). A computer network enabling communication among computers and peripherals within an organization or group of organizations over a limited area. The network consists of the computers, peripherals, communication links, and interfacing hardware.

Magnetic storage. Online or offline data storage in which each data character is stored as a 0 or 1 in magnetic form. Magnetic storage includes magnetic disks and tapes.

Mainframe. A large computer system that normally has very large main memories, specialized support for high-speed processing, many ports for online terminals and communication links, and extensive auxiliary memory storage.

Master patient (person) index (MPI). A relational database containing all of the identification numbers that have been assigned to a patient anywhere within a healthcare system. The MPI assigns a global identification number as an umbrella for all of a patient's numbers, thus permitting queries that can find all appropriate data for a particular patient regardless of where that person was treated within the system.

Meaningful use. Criterion used in incentive programs of the Centers for Medicare & Medicaid Services; payments are made to eligible healthcare providers who demonstrate meaningful use of EHR technology.

mHealth application. Health and healthcare–related information, tools, and other resources that can be accessed on mobile devices.

Microcomputer. A relatively small computer system in which the microprocessor, main memory, disk drives, CD-ROM, and interface cards and connectors are installed in a small case or box. See also *microprocessor.*

Microprocessor. A CPU contained on a single semiconductor chip.

Middleware. System architecture in which applications are connected to and distributed by networked systems.

Minicomputer. A computer with capabilities somewhere between those of a microcomputer and of a mainframe computer. See also *mainframe, microcomputer.*

Modem (modulator/demodulator). A data-communication device that modulates signals from output devices for transmission on a data link and demodulates signals destined for input devices coming from the transmission link.

Multiplexing. The process of combining two or more signals into a single signal, transmitting it, and then sorting out the original signals. The devices that combine or sort out signals are called *multiplexers.*

Multisourcing. Outsourcing information system functions and tasks to a number of different vendors. See also *outsourcing.*

Network. A collection of computer and peripheral devices interconnected by communication paths. See also *local area network, wide area network, global area network.*

Network computer. A low-cost personal computer that has minimal equipment and is designed to be managed and maintained by a central computing function.

Network configuration. The established connections between the components of a network; the physical and logical topologies.

Network controller. A mini- or microcomputer that directs the communication traffic between the host and the terminals and peripheral devices.

Network interface card (NIC). A plug-in board used in microcomputers and workstations to allow them to communicate with a host computer and other nodes in a local area network.

Open system. A system whose components are exposed to everyone and can thus be modified or improved.

Operating system. A set of integrated subroutines and programs that control the operation of a computer and manage its resources.

Optical disk. A disk in which data are written and read by a laser. Optical disk types include a number of variations of CDs and DVDs.

Output. Any data or information that a computer sends to a peripheral device or other network.

Outsourcing. Delegation of responsibility for specific organizational tasks or functions to an external entity on a contract basis. Examples include software development and accounts receivable collection.

Parallel processing. The use of multiple CPUs linked together generally for the purpose of more efficiently completing complex tasks.

Patient Protection and Affordable Care Act (ACA). This 2010 legislation extended the HIPAA rules by requiring a unique health plan identifier and by setting standards and rules for financial transactions.

Peer network. A decentralized computing environment in which each computer on the network has either data or some hardware resource that it can make available to the other users on the network.

Peripheral devices. A general term used to refer to input, output, and secondary storage devices on a computer.

Personal health information (PHI). Any health information, in any medium, that can be identified as related to an individual.

Picture archiving and communication system (PACS). A device that provides online storage and retrieval of medical images for transmission to user workstations.

Portfolio. A collection of programs and projects undertaken by an organization.

Portfolio management. The process of selecting and managing the organization's programs and projects, including valuing existing and proposed projects against strategic business and clinical objectives for investment decisions.

Portfolio management office (PMO). A central organization dedicated to improving the practice and outcomes of projects via holistic management of all projects. This includes the professional management and oversight of an organization's entire collection of projects. The terms *PMO*, *project management office*, and *program management office* are used interchangeably.

Primary storage. Internal memory where data to be processed are stored for access by the CPU.

Probabilistic algorithm. A decision support system that employs statistical probabilities rather than relies solely on knowledge collected from expert human beings.

Program. (1) An ordered set of instructions that a computer executes to obtain a desired result. (2) A group of related, often interdependent projects being conducted in an organization.

Programming language. A software system that has a specific format, or syntax, used for writing computer programs.

Radio-frequency identification (RFID). An automatic identification method that relies on storing and remotely retrieving data using devices called *transponders* or *RFID tags*. The RFID tag can be applied to a product, an animal, or a person for the purpose of identification using radiowaves.

Random access memory (RAM). Storage that permits direct access to the data stored at a particular address on a computer's hard drive. Data stored in RAM are deleted when the computer is powered off.

Read-only memory (ROM). Storage that contains permanent instructions or data that cannot be altered by ordinary programming.

Registers. High-speed CPU memory; employed during processing activity.

Real time. Describes a computer or process that captures data, performs an operation, or delivers results in a time frame that humans perceive as instantaneous.

Relational database. A type of database that stores data in individual files or tables, with data items arranged in rows and columns. Two or more tables can be linked for the purposes of ad hoc queries if at least one data item (the "key") is common in each of the tables.

Router. A device located at a gateway that manages the data flow between networks. See also *gateway.*

Secondary storage. Various devices and media designed to maintain small or large quantities of data.

Service continuity management. The process for restoring HIT services as quickly as possible after a service interruption.

Service-level agreement (SLA). Contract between an HIT department and specific customers that describes the services to be provided or the deliverable along with other details.

Software. The programs that control the operation of a computer, including applications, operating systems, programming languages, development tools, and language translators.

Synching station. A device wired to a computer that allows data to be exchanged between a personal digital assistant and a personal computer so that the same current data are available on both.

System. A network of components or elements joined together to accomplish a specific purpose or objective. Every system must include input, a conversion process, and output. See also *closed system, cybernetic system, open system.*

Systems analysis. The process of collecting, organizing, and evaluating facts about information system requirements and processes and the environment in which the system will operate.

Telecommunications. Transmission of information over distances through wired, optical, or radio media.

Telemedicine. Also referred to as *telehealth* and *e-health*, this is a rapidly developing application of clinical medicine that employs communications and information technologies to assist delivery of care (consulting, medical procedures, or examinations).

Terminal. A device consisting of a monitor and keyboard that allows a computer user to perform processing on a host computer directly. See also *dumb terminal.*

Terminal–host system. A centralized computer network configuration in which dumb terminals are connected to a large central host computer (typically a mainframe) and all the computing takes place on the host computer. See also *host, mainframe, terminal.*

Thin client. System architecture in which most processing is performed on a server remote from the end user or client.

Three-tier architecture. Configuration in which the user interface resides with the client, the relational databases reside on one server, and the application programs reside on a second server. Three-tier system offers faster information processing and distribution than does a two-tier system.

Throughput. The total time span from collection of the first data element to the preparation of the final report in a given system.

Total cost of ownership. A financial measure that incorporates both startup (one time) and recurring costs associated with technology purchases, such as training costs, costs associated with failure or outage and recovery from security breaches, and other hidden costs.

Transaction processing systems. Application programs that form the bulk of the day-to-day activities of an organization, such as financial, clinical, admissions, and business office systems.

Transmission control protocol/Internet protocol (TCP/IP). A collection of data communication protocols used to connect a computer to the Internet. TCP/IP is the standard for all Internet communication.

Two-tier client/server architecture. All back-end functions (database management, printing, communication, and applications program execution) are performed on a single server.

Web browser. Software that enables a user to view and interact with information stored on the Web.

Wide area network (WAN). A network in which long-distance lines allow computers and local area networks to communicate.

Workstation. (1) A microcomputer connected to a larger host computer in which some independent processing is performed. (2) A high-end microcomputer with a large amount of primary storage, a fast processor, a high-quality sound card, high-resolution graphics, a CD-RW drive, and in many cases a DVD drive. (3) Any computing device that allows users to input, process, or retrieve data or information necessary to perform their job duties.

INDEX

ABOUT THE AUTHORS

Gerald L. Glandon, **PhD**, is professor and chair of the Department of Health Services Administration at the University of Alabama at Birmingham (UAB). He is the interim program director for the Health Informatics Program and directs the Center for Health Services Continuing Education at UAB. Dr. Glandon has had a career in research, health administration education, and academic administration. His primary research interests have been technology evaluation (especially IT), the economics of aging, patient and physician satisfaction, and assessment of organizational performance. He has published in such journals as *JAMA, Journal of Gerontology: Social Sciences, Medical Care, Hospital & Health Services Administration,* and *Health Services Research* as well as written numerous books and book chapters.

Over the years, Dr. Glandon has kept his research and practice skills current by consulting with academic health centers, external agencies, and organizations. He has also worked in international health with engagements in Albania, Turkmenistan, Uzbekistan, Kazakhstan, Yemen, and Saudi Arabia. He has both developed and delivered management education in these countries and provided healthcare strategic analysis to ministries of health and to individual hospitals. Prior to coming to UAB, he was program director of the Department of Health Systems Management at Rush-Presbyterian–St. Luke's Medical Center in Chicago.

Detlev H. (Herb) Smaltz, **PhD**, **FACHE**, **FHIMSS**, is chairman, founder, and former CEO of Health Care DataWorks, Inc., an Ohio State University Technology Commercialization Company. Health Care DataWorks is a provider of enterprise data warehouse and business intelligence tools and strategic enterprise business intelligence consulting services.

Dr. Smaltz served as the chief information officer of the Ohio State University Medical Center (OSUMC), where he led an IT organization of 255 individuals with an annual operating budget of $42 million. He also served as an associate vice president for health sciences at OSUMC, leading collaborative initiatives between the three mission areas of the medical center: research, academics, and patient care. In addition, he was an adjunct professor at Capital College, Laurel, Maryland; an associate professor at University of Alabama at Birmingham; and a professor at Ohio State University, Columbus.

He has more than 25 years' experience in healthcare management, serving all but four of those years as CIO/CKO at various-sized organizations. He is a Fellow of the Healthcare Information & Management Systems Society (HIMSS) and served on the HIMSS Board of Directors (BOD) from 2002 to 2005 and as vice chair of the BOD from 2004 to 2005. In addition, he is a Fellow in the American College of Healthcare Executives (FACHE).

Dr. Smaltz holds certifications in knowledge management from the Knowledge Management Certification Board. He earned a BS in management information systems from the University of Tampa, an MBA from Ohio State University, and a PhD in information and management science from Florida State University. He has co-written a number of publications, including *Austin & Boxerman's Information Systems for Healthcare Management*, 7th Edition (Health Administration Press, 2008); *The Healthcare Information Technology Planning Fieldbook* (HIMSS Publications, 2008); *The Executive's Guide to Electronic Health Records* (Health Administration Press, 2007); and *The CEO–CIO Partnership: Harnessing the Value of Information Technology in Healthcare* (HIMSS Publications, 2005).

Donna J. Slovensky, PhD, RHIA, FAHIMA, is professor and associate dean for Student and Academic Affairs in the School of Health Professions at the University of Alabama at Birmingham (UAB). She holds secondary appointments in the Department of Management in the UAB School of Business and the UAB Graduate School. She is named as a scientist with the Center for Outcomes and Effectiveness Research and Education and as a scholar in the Lister Hill Center for Health Policy.

Dr. Slovensky has consulting experience in a variety of healthcare organizations, including inpatient and ambulatory facilities, home health programs, and physician practices, and academic programs. She has been on the UAB faculty for more than 35 years, teaching undergraduate and graduate courses in strategic management, quality management, information management, and clinical outcomes evaluation before her current administrative role.